S/REF

APR 2 8 2011

FOR REFERENCE

Do Not Take From This Room

D1506082

DALY CITY PUBLIC LIBRARY
DALY CITY, CALIFORNIA

DISEASES, DISORDERS, AND INJURIES

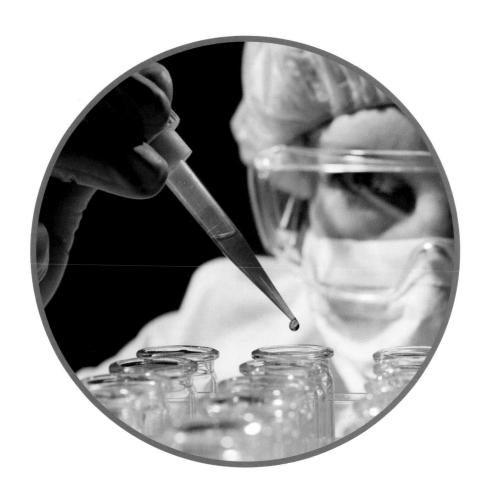

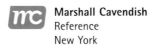 **Marshall Cavendish**
Reference
New York

S

R
616
DIS
2010

Marshall Cavendish

Copyright © 2011 Marshall Cavendish Corporation

Published by Marshall Cavendish Reference
An imprint of Marshall Cavendish Corporation

All rights reserved.

No part of this publication may be reproduced, stored in a retrieval system or transmitted, in any form or by any means, electronic, mechanical, photocopying, recording, or otherwise, without the prior permission of the copyright owner. Request for permission should be addressed to the Publisher, Marshall Cavendish Corporation, 99 White Plains Road, Tarrytown, NY 10591. Tel: (914) 332-8888, fax: (914) 332-1888.

Website: www.marshallcavendish.us

Library of Congress Cataloging-in-Publication Data

Diseases, disorders, and injuries.

   p. cm.

  Includes index.

  ISBN 978-0-7614-7935-2 (alk. paper)

  1. Medicine, Popular--Encyclopedias. 2. Diseases--Encyclopedias. 3. Wounds and injuries--Encyclopedias.

  RC81.A2D57 2011

  616.003--dc22

                   2010010057

Printed in Malaysia

14 13 12 11 10 1 2 3 4 5

MARSHALL CAVENDISH
Publisher: Paul Bernabeo
Project Editor: Brian Kinsey
Production Manager: Mike Esposito

THE BROWN REFERENCE GROUP PLC
Managing Editor: Tim Harris
Designer: Lynne Lennon
Picture Researcher: Laila Torsun
Indexer: Ann Barrett
Design Manager: David Poole
Editorial Director: Lindsey Lowe

This volume is not intended for use as a substitute for advice, consultation, or treatment by a licensed medical practitioner. The reader is advised that no action of a medical or therapeutic nature should be taken without consultation with a licensed medical practitioner, including action that may seem to be indicated by the contents of this work, since individual circumstances vary and medical standards, knowledge, and practices change with time. The publishers, authors, and medical consultants disclaim all liability and cannot be held responsible for any problems that may arise from use of this volume.

Other Marshall Cavendish Offices:

Marshall Cavendish International (Asia) Private Limited, 1 New Industrial Road, Singapore 536196 • Marshall Cavendish International (Thailand) Co Ltd. 253 Asoke, 12th Flr, Sukhumvit 21 Road, Klongtoey Nua, Wattana, Bangkok 10110, Thailand • Marshall Cavendish (Malaysia) Sdn Bhd, Times Subang, Lot 46, Subang Hi-Tech Industrial Park, Batu Tiga, 40000 Shah Alam, Selangor Darul Ehsan, Malaysia

Marshall Cavendish is a trademark of Times Publishing Limited

All websites were available and accurate when this book was sent to press.

PHOTOGRAPHIC CREDITS
Front Cover: Shutterstock: James Danel (br); Sebastian Kaulitzki (tr); Media 4D (bl); Tyler Olson (c); Vadim Ponomaenko (tl).
Back Cover: Shutterstock: Sebastian Kaulitzki. **Alamy:** 201; **Amplivox:** 99; **Phil Babb:** 116, 274b; **Tom Belshaw:** 206; **R. M. Bernstein:** 197l; **Steve Bicolschowsky:** 35; **Biofoto Associates:** 127, 174l, 174r, 207, 257, 290; **Paul Brevitt:** 242; **Camerique:** 253r; **COI Pictures:** 247r; **Corbis:** 14, 69, 289; Gideon Mendel 302; Stock Market 193, 217, 249; Wilson Wen/EPA 111; **Mike Courtney:** 33, 144; **Charles Day:** 304t; **Bernard Fallon:** 139l, 139r; **Frank Spooner Pictures:** 9t, 9b; **Getty Images:** 23, 209, 218; **Hammersmith Hospital:** 197r; **Hayward Art Group:** 24, 67t, 67b; **Hutchinson:** 239r; **Image Bank:** 175; **Institute of Dermatology:** 274t; Camilla Jessel: 169; **Frank Kennard:** 300; **Lifeline:** 59, 70; **London Scientific Films:** 261; **Frederick Mancini:** 220; **Medipics:** 65, 158; **Ken Moreman:** 12r; **Multiple Sclerosis Society:** 215; **Ron Murdoch:** 97; **Brian Nash:** 129; **PA Photos:** 132, 211; **Roger Payling:** 62, 63, 198; **PHIL:** 98, 107; **Photolibrary:** BSIP Index Stock Imagery/Thomas Craig 10; BSIP Medical 18b, 134; Scott Camazine 104; James Cavallini 84; Jaimie Duplas 260; Phototake Science 137; **Public Health Image Library:** CDC/Allen W. Mathies 284; N. Shah: 103b; **Shutterstock:** 262; Andresr 94, 282t; Galyana Andrushko 282b; Simone van den Berg 88; Carlos Caetano 281b; Stephen Coburn 130; Martin Garnham 281t; Vladimir Melnik 51; Photocreate 32b; Andrejs Pidjass 133; Alexander Raths 3; Mariusz Szachowski 231; Trialartinfo 124b; Triff 4; Maxim Tupikov 280; **Spectrum:** 103t; **SPL:** 30, 76, 131, 140, 153, 156, 162, 164, 166, 205, 230, 295; Simon Fraser 79, 238; P. Marazzi 42; Sovereign/ISM 254; **St. Mary's Hospital:** 180; **Still Pictures:** SIU 125; **Stock Boston:** 288; **Telegraph Colour Library:** 55, 244; **Topfoto:** Image Works 312; RIA Novosti 32t; **Venner Artists:** 38; **Vision International:** 191t, 191b, 297t; **John Watney:** 61, 305; **James Webb:** 189, 239l, 275t, 275tl, 275b, 286, 297b, 304b, 313; **Western Opthalmic Hospital:** 287; **Paul Windsor:** 27, 265; **Zefa:** 82, 83, 252.

Key to color coding of the articles

 BODY

 ILLNESS, INJURY, AND DISORDERS

Contents

Foreword 4

Abrasions and Cuts 5
Acne 6
AIDS and HIV 8
Allergies 11
Alzheimer's Disease 13
Anemia 14
Anorexia and Bulimia 16
Antibody and Antigen 19
Appendicitis 20
Artery 21
Artery Diseases and
 Disorders 22
Arthritis 25
Asthma 28
Athlete's Foot 30
Avian Influenza 31
Bacteria 33
Bacterial Diseases 34
Birth Defects 36
Blindness 38
Blood 40
Blood Diseases and
 Disorders 42
Body Systems 43
Bone 49
Bone Diseases and
 Disorders 50
Botulism 51
Brain 52
Brain Damage and
 Disorders 54
Bronchitis 57
Burns 58
Cancer 61
Carpal Tunnel Syndrome 64
Celiac Disease 65
Cells and Chromosomes 66
Cerebral Palsy 68
Chicken Pox 69
Cholera 70
Chronic Fatigue Syndrome 71
Circulatory System 72
Circulatory System
 Diseases and Disorders 73
Cold 76
Colon and Colon Diseases 77
Communicable Diseases 78
Creutzfeldt-Jakob Disease 79
Crohn's Disease 80
Cystic Fibrosis 81
Deafness 82
Dermatitis 84
Diabetes 85
Diarrhea 88
Digestive System 89
Digestive System Diseases
 and Disorders 92
Diphtheria 95

Down Syndrome 96
Dysentery 98
Ear and Hearing 99
Ear Diseases and
 Disorders 101
Eczema 104
Edema 105
Emphysema 106
Encephalitis 107
Endometriosis 108
Epidemic 110
Epilepsy 112
Eye and Sight 114
Eye Diseases and
 Disorders 116
Fibroids 120
Fibromyalgia 121
Fractures and
 Dislocations 122
Frostbite 125
Fungal Infections 126
Gallbladder and
 Gallstones 128
Gangrene 130
Gastroenteritis 131
Genes 133
Genetic Diseases and
 Disorders 134
Glands 135
Glaucoma 137
Gonorrhea 138
Gout 139
Guillain-Barré Syndrome 140
Gum Diseases 141
Hair and Scalp Disorders 142
Hamstring Injuries 144
Hansen's Disease 145
Heart 146
Heart Attack 148
Heart Diseases and
 Disorders 149
Heat Sickness 152
Hemochromatosis 153
Hemophilia 154
Hemorrhoids 155
Hepatitis 156
Hernia 157
Herpes 158
Hormones and
 Hormonal Disorders 159
HPV 161
Huntington's Disease 163
Hypertension 164
Hypoglycemia 165
Immune System 167
Immunodeficiency 169
Infectious Diseases 170
Infectious
 Mononucleosis 175
Influenza 176

Irritable Bowel
 Syndrome 178
Jaundice 180
Joint Disorders 181
Kidney 183
Kidney Diseases and
 Disorders 185
Legionnaires' Disease 188
Leukemia 189
Liver 190
Liver Diseases and
 Disorders 191
Lung 193
Lung Diseases and
 Disorders 194
Lupus Erythematosus 197
Lyme Disease 198
Lymphatic System 199
Lymphoma 201
Malaria 202
Malnutrition 203
Marfan Syndrome 205
Measles 206
Meningitis 207
Menstrual Disorders 208
Metabolic Disorders 209
Migraine 210
Motor Neuron Disease 211
Mouth 212
Mouth Diseases and
 Disorders 214
Multiple Sclerosis 215
Mumps 216
Munchausen Syndrome 217
Muscle 218
Muscle Diseases and
 Disorders 220
Muscular Dystrophy 222
Nervous System 223
Nervous System
 Disorders 225
Nonspecific Urethritis 227
Nosebleed 228
Nutritional Diseases 229
Obesity 230
Obsessive-Compulsive
 Disorder 231
Osteoarthritis 232
Osteoporosis 234
Paralysis 235
Parkinson's Disease 236
Pelvic Inflammatory
 Disease 237
Phenylketonuria 238
Plague 239
Pneumonia 240
Poison and Poisoning 241
Poliomyelitis 244
Premenstrual Syndrome 245
Rabies 246

Raynaud's Disease 248
Repetitive Strain Injury 249
Respiratory System 250
Respiratory System
 Diseases and Disorders 252
Retina and Retinal
 Disorders 254
Reye's Syndrome 255
Rheumatic Fever 256
Rickets 257
Rickettsial Diseases 258
Ringworm 259
Rubella 260
Salmonella 261
SARS 262
Sciatica 263
Scoliosis 264
Scurvy 265
Sexually Transmitted
 Diseases 266
Shingles 267
Sickle-Cell Anemia 268
Skeletal System 269
Skin 271
Skin Diseases and
 Disorders 273
Slipped Disk 276
Smallpox 277
Spina Bifida 278
Spinal Column 279
Sports Injuries 280
Sprains and Strains 283
Staphylococcal Infections 284
Streptococcal Infections 285
Stroke 286
Sty 287
Sunburn 288
Tennis Elbow 289
Tetanus 290
Thalassemia 291
Throat Diseases and
 Disorders 292
Tourette's Syndrome 294
Trichomoniasis 295
Tropical Diseases 296
Tuberculosis 299
Typhoid Fever 301
Typhus 302
Ulcers 303
Urinary System 305
Vein Disorders 307
Viruses 308
West Nile Virus 312
Whiplash Injury 313
Whooping Cough 314
Worms 315
Wounds 316
Yellow Fever 317

Index 318

Foreword

Most people at one time or another will have a disease, disorder, or injury. Having a health problem can be both frightening and daunting. Health problems range from mild to serious, acute to chronic, or barely noticeable to disabling. It is important to know when something is a temporary discomfort and when it may require professional attention. Some injuries can be treated with simple first aid techniques, while others require a visit to the doctor's office or hospital. At other times, the prevalence of public health dangers in the news, such as influenza outbreaks or the human papillomavirus (HPV), may prompt questions from people as yet unaffected.

Those kinds of questions and even more can be answered by *Diseases, Disorders, and Injuries*, which contains a selection of articles covering more than 200 topics. The articles are designed to give a basic understanding of the topics by providing important information about descriptions, causes, risk factors,

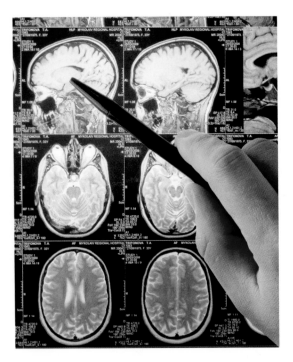

symptoms, diagnosis, treatments, pathogenesis, prevention, and epidemiology. Each topic has an easy-to-read layout with sidebar elements and detailed illustrations that provide vital information for quick reference. This layout gives the reader a snapshot of a particular medical problem without having to spend too long trying to explain complex technical details. The book addresses diseases such as cystic fibrosis, HIV/AIDS, and smallpox; disorders such as diabetes, Marfan syndrome, and obsessive-compulsive disorder; and injuries from repetitive strain injuries to nosebleeds.

Diseases, Disorders, and Injuries is not intended to replace medical textbooks or a physician but rather to help the readers understand a medical issue that may be affecting them or someone they know. The volume can help them understand what may have caused the ailment, some of the risk factors, what to expect when they see a physician, and some of the treatment options. It may offer comfort by empowering readers to learn how the disease, disorder, or injury formed in the first place and to prevent further risk to themselves or others.

Medicine has become a sophisticated, high-tech area with countless specialties and subspecialties. For most people, navigating through medical jargon and making decisions about treatment is intimidating. This volume can help readers to begin the journey of education in a particular area by offering simple language that makes medicine clear and understandable. In its simplicity, *Diseases, Disorders, and Injuries* offers the general reader a deeper insight and appreciation of the covered medical topics.

Dr. Rashmi Nemade
Rashmi Nemade is a biomedical writer and editor.

Additional related information is available in the 18-volume *Encyclopedia of Health*, fourth edition, and the corresponding online *Health Encyclopedia* database at www.marshallcavendishdigital.com.

Abrasions and Cuts

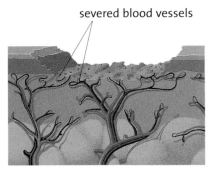

severed blood vessels

Abrasions are not usually as serious as they look, although they can be very painful and leave scars after they have healed. They must be cleansed thoroughly and checked for embedded objects.

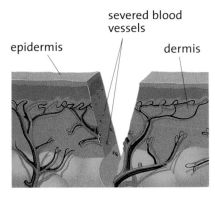

epidermis

severed blood vessels

dermis

Cuts sometimes bleed profusely and they must be kept closed to heal properly. They may need to be stitched, especially when they occur on the face.

Injuries that break through the surface of the skin are medically termed *wounds*. Some wounds are serious, but many are slight. Minor cuts and shallow abrasions (scrapes) are everyday happenings, but they still need proper treatment.

Abrasions and cuts need to be cleansed thoroughly because whenever the skin has been broken blood vessels may be torn, letting germs enter the body. Many cuts also need some sort of protective dressing. The wound bleeds at first. If the wound is minor, it may be best to leave it for a time so that the flow of blood can help wash away dirt and germs. However, any heavy bleeding should be stopped as soon as possible by using a clean pad and bandage and applying firm pressure to the wound for at least five minutes. If bleeding cannot be controlled, a doctor should be consulted, because stitches may be required.

Abrasions and cuts should be cleansed with soap and water, or with hydrogen peroxide (3 percent). First, any bits of dirt in the wound should be brushed away with small swabs of gauze or cotton soaked in solution. If a foreign object, such as a piece of glass, is deeply embedded in the wound, it should be removed only by a doctor. Once the wound is free from any loose particles of grit or dirt, it should be washed gently, from the center outward, with a fresh swab used for each stroke. If the wound is likely to get dirty again, it should be protected with antiseptic cream and a clean dressing.

Dry cuts and wounds are best left uncovered to heal, but all wet cuts and scrapes need to be covered to stop them from getting dirty and developing an infection. The edges of a small, clean cut can be held together with thin strips of adhesive butterfly tape. Nonstick sterile dressings, with a central pad of gauze surrounded by adhesive tape, are the best protection for small wounds because they can be easily removed and changed without harming the scab that forms as the wound heals. A larger wound should be covered with sterile gauze dressings. A pad of cotton should then be placed over the gauze to absorb any discharge and act as a buffer. This pad can be held in place with adhesive tape or with a bandage.

Most minor abrasions and cuts heal very quickly, but any signs of infection, such as redness, swelling and tenderness, pus, and fever, should be watched for. If any of these signs appear, a doctor should be consulted.

SEE ALSO

BACTERIA • SKIN • TETANUS • WOUNDS

Acne

Acne is a distressing skin condition that is extremely common in adolescence. It is a mixture of blackheads, whiteheads (pustules), and pink or reddish pimples present mainly on the face, the back of the neck, the upper back and chest, and sometimes even on the buttocks and in the armpits. Four out of five teenagers suffer from acne to some extent, and it can be particularly troublesome in boys. Most people outgrow it eventually, and if the blemishes are left to heal naturally, they should not cause permanent scars.

Causes

Acne starts in adolescence. The oil-producing sebaceous glands in the skin, which produce oil or sebum to keep the skin supple, become overactive. The extra sebum clogs the pores through which sebum is normally released onto the skin's surface. Sometimes, it forms a plug in the pore and has a raised top that turns black when it is exposed to the air. Blackheads are not caused by dirt or bacteria. Bacteria may multiply in the pore and cause a red pimple or a pus-filled whitehead.

Left undisturbed, pimples and blackheads usually clear up within about a week. They should not be picked at or squeezed. If the deeper skin tissues become bruised or damaged, a boil or abscess may form. This sort of secondary infection is one of the chief problems of acne, as it can lead to severe, permanent scars and pockmarks in the skin. A doctor will remove blackheads or can teach someone how to do it with a special instrument.

Treating acne

Although acne is not caused directly by dirt, keeping the skin as clean as possible plays an important part in controlling acne. Washing the skin with ordinary soap two or three times a day will help remove excess grease and encourage the top layer of the skin to peel away, taking some, if not all, of the plug of sebum with it. The skin should be kept dry, but not so dry that it becomes red and sore. If the skin has a tendency to become oily, excess oil can be removed between washes with alcohol or an astringent lotion applied with clean cotton balls. Acne wipettes are convenient for carrying around.

Q & A

I have bad acne, and the boys at school are teasing me and saying that it's because I don't wash properly. Is this true?

Definitely not. People who suffer from acne are likely to spend more time washing than anyone else, and excessive washing can actually make the condition worse. Neither does greasy hair cause acne or make it worse; acne is a condition caused by excessive oil production.

Does acne always leave scars on the skin?

No, but the chances of scarring are increased if you pick and squeeze the blemishes. If scars are severe, they can be partially removed by a minor surgical operation called dermabrasion, in which the top layers of skin are rubbed away, leaving the skin relatively smooth.

Is it true that eating chocolate causes acne?

It was once thought that eating fatty foods and sweets could make acne worse, but no evidence has been found to support this theory.

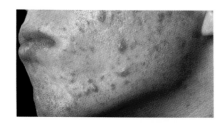

Although teenage acne is unattractive, it does not last forever. Difficult though it may be, the temptation to pick and squeeze blackheads must be resisted to avoid scarring the skin.

TEENAGE ACNE

Acne can make life miserable for many teenagers. They may be aware of their own pimples but fail to see those of their friends. They may feel unattractive and embarrassed and blame themselves for the condition. Feelings of unhappiness and stress can aggravate acne, so it should be remembered that acne is not anyone's fault.

Grease from the hair makes acne worse, so the hair should be washed often and kept away from the face. It is best not to use oil-based makeup products. There are many water-based, over-the-counter cosmetics available that not only conceal blemishes but also help dry the skin. Treatment creams and lotions containing substances such as calamine, sulfur, benzoyl peroxide, or resorcinol may also camouflage the pimples. People with severe acne should talk with their doctor, who may give them antibiotics, vitamin A cream, or some other form of treatment that is not generally available over the counter.

Preventing acne

Many people believe that acne is caused by eating too much junk food, or by not getting enough sleep, or by not washing enough. It is not. However, people can help keep their skin healthy by eating fresh fruits and vegetables, drinking water, and getting the right amount of sleep, all of which improve one's general health and help fight acne. Also, sunshine helps dry the skin, although sunburn should be avoided. Trying not to worry about the condition also helps, but nothing prevents acne; it is a normal adolescent condition that generally disappears in a person's early twenties.

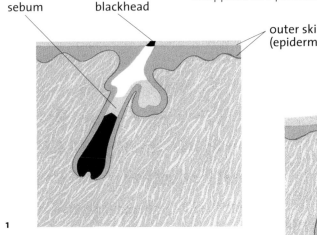

sebum   blackhead

1

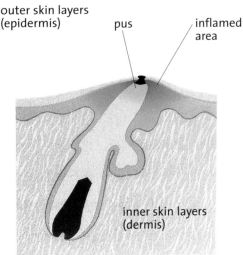

outer skin layers (epidermis)   pus   inflamed area

inner skin layers (dermis)

2

In acne, extra sebum clogs up the pores through which sebum is released to the skin surface. The sebum is trapped, forming a plug with a raised tip, which becomes a blackhead when exposed to air (1). The surrounding skin becomes inflamed and infected, resulting in pus-filled pimples (2).

SEE ALSO

BACTERIA • GLANDS • SKIN • SKIN DISEASES AND DISORDERS • SUNBURN

AIDS and HIV

Q & A

Can someone contract AIDS from being bitten by a mosquito?

A good deal of research has been conducted on this possible route of infection, mostly in Africa, where the mosquito is well-known for its ability to carry and transmit the organism that causes malaria. All the evidence indicates that people cannot be infected with the AIDS virus from the bite of any insect.

Can I tell if someone has been infected with the virus that causes AIDS?

A nonmedical person has no way of knowing if someone has been infected with HIV until AIDS develops, up to 10 years later. Three months after an infection, however, or often earlier, an antibody test can show whether the virus is present.

Where can I get more information and advice regarding AIDS?

The U.S. Public Health Service operates an AIDS hotline. The toll-free number is 1-800-342-AIDS. Your local Red Cross chapter can also give advice.

In 1981, the first cases of a new disease were reported in California and New York. In every case, it appeared that the body's immune system—its defense against infections—had broken down. The new disease was given the name AIDS, an abbreviation for acquired immunodeficiency syndrome. It is caused by the human immunodeficiency virus (HIV) and is most commonly transmitted from one person to another by sexual intercourse. HIV can also be passed from an infected mother to her newborn baby and spread by sharing intravenous needles used for heroin injection.

As yet, there is no known cure for AIDS. However, doctors and medical companies around the world are working to find treatments that will cure people who have the disease and safeguard others who are at risk.

Symptoms of AIDS

The body of a person with AIDS has little or no defense against infections that a healthy person could fight off without difficulty. Eventually, these infections are fatal. However, the average time between diagnosis of AIDS and death has increased markedly in recent years as a result of the use of combinations of anti-HIV drugs.

Symptoms of AIDS include a general feeling of tiredness and loss of energy; weight loss; enlarged lymph nodes; fever; night sweats; a persistent dry cough; bruising easily or unexplained bleeding; diarrhea; forgetfulness and loss of concentration; blurred vision; and skin cancer (Kaposi's sarcoma).

Tests show that many people who seem perfectly well have been infected with HIV. No one yet knows how long it will be before people who are HIV-positive develop AIDS, or if some of them will go on to live a normal lifetime without ever developing the disease. However, because they carry the AIDS virus, these people can infect others with it.

How AIDS is spread

The AIDS virus is present in the various body fluids, namely, blood, semen, vaginal and cervical secretions, saliva, and tears. The virus is passed from one person to another when infected body fluid gets into the bloodstream. The AIDS virus cannot survive long outside body fluids and is easily killed by disinfectant or even hot water.

The most usual way for infected body fluid to enter the bloodstream is during sexual intercourse with an infected person, through a tiny scratch or patch of broken skin. Infection can also happen if a drug addict uses someone else's unsterilized

Kaposi's sarcoma is a rare form of skin cancer that affects many people who have AIDS. It is other causes, rather than the AIDS virus itself, that lead to death in many HIV-positive patients.

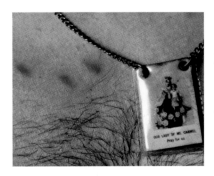

needle after it has been used. A woman can pass AIDS to her unborn baby through blood exchanged in the placenta. Infected blood or blood products that carry the AIDS virus can pass on HIV if they are used for transfusions or the treatment of hemophiliacs. Health workers who might accidentally puncture their own skin with needles used on an AIDS patient are also at risk.

Sexually promiscuous people, drug users, and partners of these people make up the largest group of AIDS patients and known carriers. Taking drugs makes people careless, and heavy users often share needles without sterilizing them.

Anyone who belongs to one of the high-risk groups—highly promiscuous people, homosexuals or bisexuals, drug users, prostitutes, people with a number of short-term sexual relationships—or anyone who has been the partner of someone in one of these groups over the past few years may be infected.

Outlook

Although there is no cure for HIV, advances in drug treatments have allowed patients in the developed world to lead near-normal lives, with the virus virtually suppressed. However, in the last few years there have been worrying cases of new drug-resistant strains of the virus. In developing countries, where there is little money for drug treatments, the outlook is poor, with most infected people dying within 10 years of becoming infected with HIV.

Until a cure can be found, the widespread implementation of educational programs on the prevention of HIV is crucial to check the spread of the virus. People worldwide must be made aware

Since it was discovered that AIDS could be transmitted through blood transfusions, great efforts have been made to identify and discourage high-risk donors.

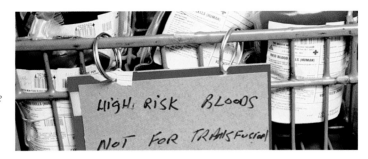

This man is able to lead a near-normal life, even though he is HIV-positive. A range of drugs helps prevent the virus from spreading and slows down the progression of the disease.

A VACCINE FOR AIDS

Scientists have been exploring ways of controlling AIDS by developing a vaccine that would provide immunity to the disease. So far, such projects have been unsuccessful. Vaccines introduce weakened forms of disease-causing organisms into the body. These organisms put the immune system on guard and stimulate the body's defenses to destroy a particular organism. The problem with the AIDS virus is that it frequently changes, or mutates, into a different strain. It has not yet proved possible to find a vaccine that would work against all the different forms of the virus.

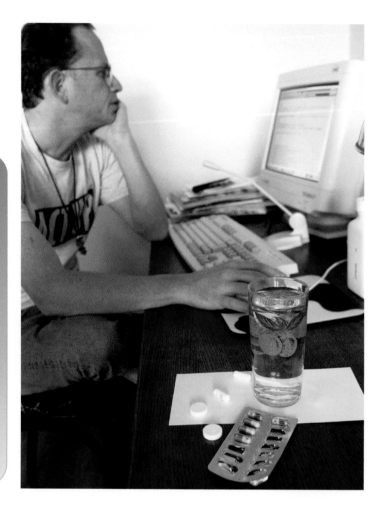

of the importance of using condoms during sex and of using clean needles for injecting drugs. Understanding HIV can also help reduce prejudice toward infected people.

It is perfectly safe for AIDS patients to live a completely normal life in the community. During the time between diagnosis of the disease and death, which can be a period of several years, AIDS patients become less and less able to fight off infections. However, for much, if not all, of this time, they can live at home with the loving help and support of family and friends.

SEE ALSO
BLOOD • IMMUNE SYSTEM • IMMUNODEFICIENCY • INFECTIOUS DISEASES • SEXUALLY TRANSMITTED DISEASES • VIRUSES

Allergies

If a person has an allergy, he or she has a bad reaction to, or is unusually sensitive to, a substance that does not normally cause people any harm. Allergies can affect any part of the body and can be caused by an enormous range of substances. Common symptoms include rashes, sneezes, and headaches.

Although allergies can be very painful and sometimes even dangerous, they are seldom life-threatening. The process is now fully understood and is extremely complex. However, it can be explained to some extent in the following terms. When the body comes into contact with an allergen (a substance to which it is allergic), the immune system reacts as if the allergen were a dangerous infectious organism. The body makes a special antibody to fight the invader. In the process, some of its cells release a substance called histamine, which makes tiny blood vessels widen, causing redness, itching, and swelling. Histamine also makes some tissues, such as the membranes lining the nose and eyes, produce extra fluid.

Common complaints caused by allergies

Among the common complaints caused partly or entirely by allergies are hay fever, asthma, dermatitis, hives, and migraine headaches. Among the most common allergens are foods, such as eggs, milk, and shellfish; pollens and spores; insect bites (especially bee and wasp stings); mites and animal dander; cosmetics; metals; and some drugs and chemicals. Food allergens are absorbed into the blood, so they produce a wide variety of symptoms, including upset stomach, skin rash, headache, and difficulty breathing.

Some people are allergic to drugs such as penicillin. Such people should always carry a medical tag or card that states this fact, in case of an emergency. The most severe of the allergic reactions is called anaphylaxis. This is a sometimes life-threatening reaction in which, among other effects, the lining of the voice box may swell to block the air intake. People who have reacted in this way should carry a hypodermic syringe containing adrenaline for emergency use.

Peanut allergy

Genuine food allergy is rare, affecting only about one person in 100,000 per year. However, when food allergy occurs, some of its forms can be

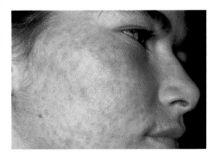

Q & A

My younger brother is allergic to cats, and touching one makes him break out in a rash. Will he grow out of this problem?

Possibly. Children who suffer from allergic rashes often do grow out of the problem. However, they may suffer from other forms of allergy—asthma, for example—when they are older, because they have a basic tendency to be allergic.

Can you be allergic to people, places, or animals?

You cannot be allergic to a person, but allergy to body fluids or material on the skin is possible. Some people who are acutely allergic to fish can get swollen lips from kissing someone who has just been eating fish. Allergy to animals is common and is caused by the fine pieces of hair or feathers from the animal. You can be allergic to a place only if you are allergic to something found there, such as pollen.

Some people are allergic to penicillin, often developing a rash when they take it. If this reaction occurs, the prescribing doctor should be told immediately.

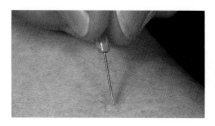

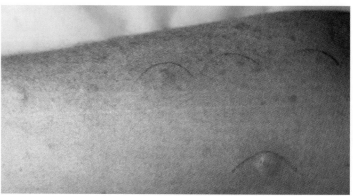

Skin tests (above) are often carried out to help determine the cause of an allergy. The skin of the arm is pricked several times with a needle, and a small amount of solution containing an allergen is dropped on to test for a reaction. This allergy sufferer (right) has been tested with a number of solutions. The large welt on her arm has been caused by a dust mite solution.

serious. One of the most dangerous is peanut allergy or, more accurately, allergy to peanut protein. About one in three people with this allergy will suffer anaphylaxis. Peanut allergy is no more common than many other food allergies, but it is likely to be more severe than most. It is especially dangerous in asthmatic children. Unfortunately, peanut proteins are widely used by food manufacturers and occur in foodstuffs in which they might not normally be expected to be present.

Treating allergies

The first step in treatment is to find out what is causing the allergy. Sometimes, it is obvious—if, say, eating strawberries always causes a rash. More often, skin tests carried out by a doctor are needed. Food additives, such as sulfur dioxide, preservatives, and dyes may cause allergic reactions. Special diets help identify foods that may be causing trouble. Once people know what they are allergic to, a doctor may be able to desensitize them, but the treatment does not last long and is not always effective.

Drugs cannot cure allergies but they sometimes relieve symptoms. Antihistamines prevent the inflammation caused by the release of histamines, but they often make people drowsy.

It may be necessary to take steroid drugs in life-threatening cases of acute allergic reactions. However, long-term use of these drugs in less serious cases can have harmful side effects. People with an allergy can best help themselves by avoiding the allergens as much as possible.

SEE ALSO

ANTIBODY AND ANTIGEN • ASTHMA • DERMATITIS • MIGRAINE • SKIN

Alzheimer's Disease

Alzheimer's disease is a deterioration of the brain, or dementia, that usually affects people over 60. The disease is caused by a chemical deficiency in the brain cells, which prevents them from passing messages to one another. There is no known cure, but there are drugs that may slow the progress of the disease.

Symptoms of Alzheimer's disease

The first signs of Alzheimer's disease are forgetfulness and loss of memory for recent events. Victims may be able to remember quite clearly things that happened long ago but are unable to recall what they had for breakfast or where they left their purse only a few minutes before. As the disease progresses, the patient may have difficulty in speaking and in understanding things, be less able to reason, and lose interest in familiar pastimes and activities, sometimes even in news of relatives and friends.

Victims can become emotionally unbalanced, tending to swing between apathy and aggressive behavior. They no longer keep themselves clean. Eventually, they may be so confused that they wander around in a daze and cannot safely be left alone. They may eventually need full-time care in a residential institution.

The underlying cause of Alzheimer's disease is still unknown, but genetic forms of the disease are known and other possible causes are being intensively investigated.

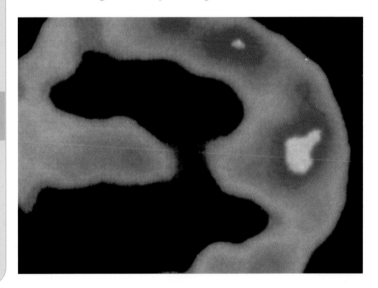

SEE ALSO
BRAIN • BRAIN DAMAGE AND DISORDERS • GENES • GENETIC DISEASES AND DISORDERS

Q & A

How common is Alzheimer's disease among people under age 60? Is there any lower age limit for who can get it?

Alzheimer's disease is uncommon below the age of 60 and virtually unknown below the age of 45.

My mother is 47, and she keeps forgetting where she puts things. Could she have Alzheimer's disease?

It is very unlikely. Everyone gets absentminded at times, especially when rushed or under stress. If your mother stays calm and takes things slowly, she will be less likely to lose things.

Is there any way of preventing Alzheimer's disease?

Despite a huge amount of research that has improved knowledge about the brain degeneration underlying Alzheimer's disease, no method of preventing it has been found. However, there are several drugs that may slow its progress.

This scan of the brain shows the enlarged dark area that indicates the presence of Alzheimer's disease.

Anemia

Anemia is a disorder that is caused by an abnormally low level of hemoglobin in the blood. It occurs when the number of red blood cells that contain hemoglobin is low or when the cells contain low levels of hemoglobin.

Hemoglobin picks up oxygen in the lungs and carries it to the body tissues, where it provides energy. If the hemoglobin in the blood falls below normal levels, too little oxygen reaches the tissues. That produces the classic symptoms of anemia: skin pallor, breathlessness, and lack of energy. These symptoms may be accompanied by palpitations (rapid and noticeable heartbeats), fainting, dizziness, and sweating.

Types of anemias

A common cause of anemia is a lack of iron, which is an essential component of hemoglobin. Women are particularly likely to experience this deficiency, because of the amount of blood they lose each month in menstruation, especially if they have very heavy periods. Other causes include ulcers that produce slow but steady internal bleeding, cancer of the stomach or intestine, hemorrhoids, and parasites such as hookworms and tapeworms that feed on the blood. Thirst is a symptom of iron-deficiency anemia; anemic children may be irritable and have a tendency to hold their breath.

Without vitamin B_{12} and folic acid, fewer red blood cells can be made, and those that are produced are enlarged. In the United States, people's diets usually contain plenty of B_{12}, but in some people, the stomach lining fails to produce a substance known as intrinsic factor. Without this factor, B_{12} cannot be absorbed, and red blood cell production falls. This condition is known as pernicious anemia. It can cause tingling sensations in the hands and feet, nosebleeds, and, in severe cases, heart failure and nerve damage, as well as the usual symptoms of anemia.

Folic acid deficiency

Folic acid is usually supplied by green vegetables in the diet. A deficiency of folic acid generally occurs in elderly people who are not eating properly, in pregnant women who use extra folic acid to nourish the developing baby, and in people who drink excess amounts of alcohol. These anemias can be treated by increasing supplies of the deficient substance. Iron tablets or shots rectify deficiency anemia in a few weeks. Folic acid deficiency can be treated with tablets and an adequate diet.

Q & A

My mother is pregnant and is getting paler and paler. Could she be anemic?

During pregnancy, the body's demand for essential nutrients, such as iron and folic acid, is increased. The developing fetus depletes the mother's store of nutrients via the placenta, and the mother may then become deficient in one or more of them, causing anemia, unless extra iron and folate are given. Your mother should check with her doctor, who will give her a prescription for supplements if they are necessary.

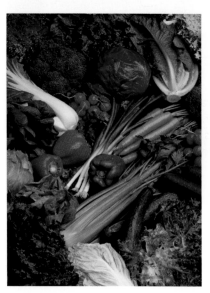

Green leafy vegetables such as salad leaves and spinach are an important source of folic acid and iron, a lack of which can cause anemia.

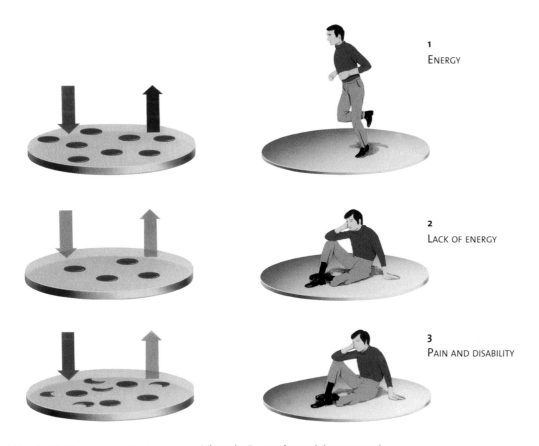

1
ENERGY

2
LACK OF ENERGY

3
PAIN AND DISABILITY

Red blood cells play an important part in anemia. (1) When there are enough chemicals to produce the required number of blood cells, the cells carry adequate oxygen supplies around the body to give energy. (2) When there are not enough chemicals to produce the number of red blood cells required, less oxygen reaches the tissues, resulting in tiredness. (3) Sometimes there are enough chemicals, but a number of red blood cells are malformed. They may block small arteries and cause severe pain and disability.

Vitamin B$_{12}$ and pernicious anemia
If the stomach lining has ceased to produce intrinsic factor, it will never be able to absorb vitamin B$_{12}$. Regular shots of vitamin B$_{12}$ for the rest of the patient's life will keep pernicious anemia under control, although it will recur if shots are missed.

Hereditary anemias
Sometimes, red blood cells are destroyed more quickly than they can be replaced, causing hemolytic anemia. Two serious types of hemolytic anemias are hereditary. Sickle-cell anemia is present largely in black communities. Thalassemia is present in Mediterranean, Middle Eastern, and Southeast Asian communities. Both types of hereditary anemia are serious and incurable, but they can be helped with blood transfusions.

SEE ALSO

BLOOD • BLOOD DISEASES AND DISORDERS • SICKLE-CELL ANEMIA • THALASSEMIA

Anorexia and Bulimia

Q & A

My friend has been told she is anorexic but doesn't believe it. Why can't she realize how emaciated she looks?

She is suffering from an abnormal mental state. When she looks in a mirror she sees a distorted body image that initiates, and prolongs, the disease. Your friend should get help from a counselor or doctor.

Sometimes I eat a bag of cookies. Then I'm sorry, so I make myself vomit afterward. Am I suffering from bulimia?

Not unless these binges have become uncontrollable and frequent. Many dieters go on an eating binge after they have been on a strict diet for some time. A binge is not good for the body, but it does no lasting harm. Only when it becomes a way of life should you seek treatment. You seem to feel guilty about overeating, but try to be less emotional about it and attempt to lose weight in a more sensible way.

Anorexia, or anorexia nervosa, is a compulsive desire to lose weight, which goes far beyond any ordinary wish to become thin. Left untreated, it can be fatal. It usually affects young people between the ages of 11 and 30 and occurs more often in girls than in boys. Anorexia nervosa used to be rare, but it is becoming increasingly common, particularly in people from middle-class homes. This is a serious disorder of perception in which the sufferer—a girl, for example—is convinced she is too fat when, in fact, she may be desperately thin. The affected girl may also be frightened of her developing sexuality and feel that if she can keep her childish figure, then she will not have to face up to the problems of adult sexuality. The danger of anorexia must never be underestimated; skilled management by experts is required. Up to 20 percent of cases end fatally.

Some emotionally insecure girls and boys diet drastically to increase their sexual confidence. The idea that being thin is a desirable state is reinforced constantly by television and magazine advertizing that promotes thinness by glamorizing unnaturally thin supermodels.

Addicted to dieting

Normal people who diet drastically can usually stop whenever they choose, perhaps when they have reached their target weight. Their problem is usually to keep to a diet when there is food around them, since hunger is such an unpleasant sensation. Anorexics, once started, cannot go into reverse. They are as addicted to dieting as if they were taking drugs. They may even experience some of the same light-headedness.

Anorexics go to great lengths to hide what they are doing. They may be unusually energetic and insist that they are well. They cook large meals for other people, while eating nothing themselves. They tell lies, saying that they have eaten elsewhere, and become very skilled at hiding food while pretending to eat normally. Some make themselves vomit to get rid of food they have been coaxed to eat, or they use laxatives, diuretics, and even enemas to prevent their bodies from absorbing nourishment. Some anorexics develop a binge-and-vomit pattern called bulimia. They eat large quantities and then make themselves vomit so that they can eat without putting on weight.

Symptoms of anorexia nervosa

The first, obvious symptom of anorexia nervosa is continued loss of weight. It may not be easy for the anorexic's family to recognize the symptom until it has become severe. An unmistakable symptom in a girl is that once her weight has fallen more than around 26 pounds (12 kg) below normal, she stops menstruating. Girls or boys who diet excessively and seem to have a false image of being overweight should be seen by a physician as soon as possible. They may simply need advice and information on the weight they should try to achieve and on a proper diet. However, if they have anorexia nervosa, it is important to begin treatment as soon as possible. The longer the condition goes untreated, the more difficult it is to cure.

Perhaps one in five anorexics eventually dies of starvation or from infections caused by undernourishment. Some become so depressed that they commit suicide. Cures seldom take place without treatment, because victims take pride in their condition. The more distorted their self-image, the more difficult the cure.

Treating anorexia nervosa

The first step is to increase body weight, at least above the danger level. Research indicates that when a patient is below a certain weight, psychotherapy cannot break through the strange mental isolation caused by voluntary starvation. Until a more normal weight is reached, no real communication can take place.

It is usually better to treat anorexics at a hospital. Their food intake must be checked carefully because they tend to hide or throw away food to avoid eating. There is also the possibility that they will fake their weight gain by putting weights in their pockets before they step on scales. This behavior can be monitored more easily in a hospital. Sometimes, patients are made to rest in bed, very often in a room alone, and their food intake is strictly monitored by the nursing staff. In the early phases of treatment, patients may also be given a form of tranquilizer and be fed intravenously. Sometimes, a system of rewards and withdrawal of privileges is used to coax the patient to eat normal food and gain a certain amount of weight.

Once the patient has gained enough weight to be out of danger, psychotherapy can begin. This approach may be required for months or years after the patient is at normal weight. Often, the whole family is given counseling, so that the parents can understand the nature of their child's illness and what causes it.

Bulimia

Bulimia is another eating disorder. It may appear on its own, but it often goes with anorexia nervosa. Its severe form is called bulimia nervosa. This condition is most often present in girls and young women who become convinced that they are overweight, although in most cases, their weight fluctuates between a little above and a little below normal.

EMACIATION AS A SENSE OF ACHIEVEMENT

The longer the illness lasts and the more weight the anorexic loses, the greater is her sense of achievement. She believes that being thin makes her significant and outstanding as an individual. Her behavior focuses attention on herself and sometimes gives her a satisfying form of rebellion against the authority of her parents.

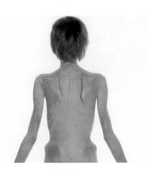

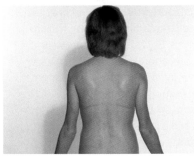

Before and after: This 19-year-old anorexic girl needed hospital treatment. After two months she had a normal body weight.

Many teenagers with anorexia nervosa enjoy cooking for other people, but they are reluctant to eat the food themselves, even if they are hungry.

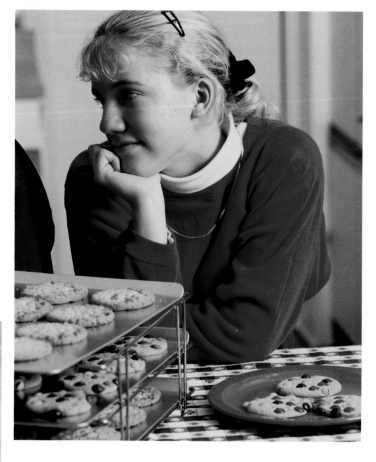

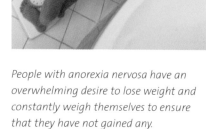

People with anorexia nervosa have an overwhelming desire to lose weight and constantly weigh themselves to ensure that they have not gained any.

People with bulimia eat very large meals, or binge. The fear of becoming overweight then prompts self-induced vomiting. They tend to eat in secret and are unable to control themselves. During binges, they may eat up to 12,000 calories in just a few hours. These binges are often triggered by stress and may take place several times a week or several times a day. The patient may not eat at all between binges. Bulimics do not usually become seriously underweight, as anorexics do, but they can cause themselves physical harm by overloading their systems with food and through the subsequent taking of laxatives. They suffer from weakness and cramps, as well as dehydration, and their teeth may become damaged by gastric acid. Treating their underlying psychological problems often helps the condition.

SEE ALSO

MALNUTRITION • NUTRITIONAL DISEASES

Antibody and Antigen

Antibodies are proteins produced in the body to fight harmful foreign substances such as disease-causing microorganisms. These microorganisms carry chemical groups called antigens. The antibodies lock on to the antigens and immobilize the germs so that they can be killed by cells of the immune system.

The first time that the body recognizes a foreign substance, the immune system makes specific antibodies to fight it. The manufacturing process may take a little time, during which the germs multiply. The symptoms of the illness are caused by poisons produced by germs and by the interaction between antigenic substances and the immune system. After the disease is cured, some antibodies remain in the body's system. The next time the same types of organisms invade the body, the antibodies recognize them. Reinfection leads to the formation of large numbers of these antibodies. As a result, therefore, the illness is prevented or cured.

When someone is vaccinated against an illness, dead or harmless antigens are introduced into the body. These antigens may have minor side effects but they will not make a person ill. They stimulate the body to produce antibodies, which remain in the blood to fight the same germs another time, thus giving the person immunity to the disease.

Q & A

I've heard that antibodies are all the same. Is that true?

No. Substances that are foreign to the body, such as bacteria, viruses, dust, and pollen all contain protein markers called antigens. The human immune system makes antibodies specific to the antigen of each foreign substance.

FIGHTING THE COMMON COLD

Viruses are infectious agents. Those that cause the common cold are continually changing. Antibodies to a virus causing one cold do not recognize the antigens of the next and cannot fight it. So, people never become immune to colds.

Infecting microorganisms, such as bacteria, have specific parts called antigens. Y-shaped protein molecules called antibodies bind to specific antigens and neutralize the invaders. Antibodies are produced by the immune system.

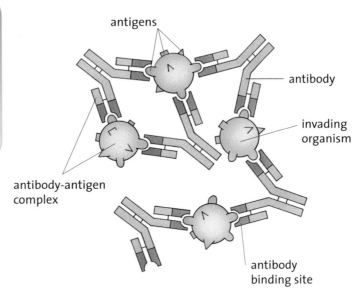

antigens

antibody

invading organism

antibody-antigen complex

antibody binding site

SEE ALSO

ALLERGIES • BACTERIA • IMMUNODEFICIENCY • VIRUSES

Appendicitis

Appendicitis is inflammation of the appendix, a narrow, tubelike piece of intestine that resembles a tail. One end of the appendix joins the large intestine on the lower right side of the abdomen; the other end is closed. This small organ has no obvious function and can be removed with no ill effect.

Appendicitis can occur at any age, but it is most common between the ages of 10 and 30. It may be due to the lack of fiber in the modern western diet. Fiber eases the passage of food through the intestine. Food residues or intestinal worms obstructing the appendix cause it to inflame and fill with pus.

Symptoms of appendicitis

The first sign of appendicitis is a colicky, on-and-off pain around the navel. After six to 12 hours, as inflammation builds up around the appendix, the lining of the abdomen becomes irritated, and the pain increases. The pain usually moves down to the lower right abdomen, although it can move to the upper abdomen or down to the pelvis. The patient feels nauseated and feverish and may be constipated (or, more rarely, have diarrhea). The inflamed appendix often affects the right leg muscle where it joins the back. That makes the leg stiff, and the patient will bend the leg up for relief. Stretching the leg down produces pain, and the muscles in the front wall of the abdomen may also go into spasm to protect the appendix from any painful movements. The whole abdomen feels as hard as a board.

Surgical removal

The appendix must be removed before it ruptures (bursts), because pus spreading into the abdominal cavity can result in a serious inflammation called peritonitis. Peritonitis is dangerous and can happen within hours. A small incision is made in the patient's abdomen, and the appendix is tied off securely and cut away. A plastic drain is inserted to allow any infected material to drain away. The patient leaves the hospital after a few days and will be back to normal in two or three weeks, although active sports should be avoided for a time. Twinges of pain may occur during the healing stage but they disappear within a month or so.

Q & A

My father, who is 45 and has never had appendicitis, claims that he will probably never have it. Is this true?

Yes. The appendix shrivels as you get older, so it should be completely shriveled (and unlikely to become irritated and inflamed) by the time you are 45.

An inflamed appendix can be removed in a simple operation under general anesthesia. The patient is usually able to leave the hospital a few days later but should avoid strenuous activity for several weeks afterward.

inflamed appendix

small intestine

rectum

SEE ALSO

BACTERIA • DIARRHEA

Artery

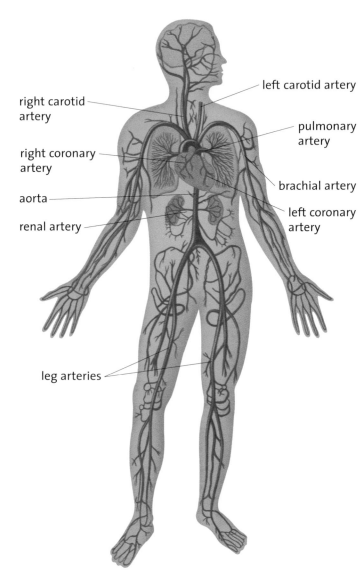

right carotid artery

right coronary artery

aorta

renal artery

leg arteries

left carotid artery

pulmonary artery

brachial artery

left coronary artery

The arterial system carries blood containing nutrients and oxygen to every part of the body. Arterial diseases can therefore be very dangerous, so preventive measures are essential and early treatment is vital.

Arteries are thick-walled blood vessels that carry blood containing nutrients and oxygen to all parts of the body. The heart pumps out oxygen-rich blood from the lungs through the large main artery called the aorta. Smaller arteries called coronary arteries branch off the aorta and carry blood to the muscles of the heart; other arteries carry blood to the rest of the body.

The arteries branch many times, getting smaller and narrower each time. The smallest arteries connect with a network of tiny blood vessels called capillaries, from which oxygen and nourishment enter the body tissues. The blood picks up carbon dioxide and other waste products from the body and carries the waste products through the veins and back to the heart. This oxygen-poor blood is then pumped via the pulmonary arteries to the lungs, where it collects more oxygen and releases carbon dioxide, which is breathed out via the lungs. Oxygen-rich blood then travels back to the heart before being pumped around the body again via the aorta.

Structure of the arteries
Arteries have strong walls that can stand up to the pressure of the blood pumped through them. The outer wall of an artery is a loose, fibrous tissue sheath. Inside this sheath is a thick, tough elastic sheath that gives the artery its strength. This elastic tissue contains rings of muscle fiber that encircle the artery. The inner layer of the artery is called the endothelium. It is made of a smooth layer of cells that allows the blood to flow freely through the arteries. The thick elastic walls of the arteries continue to push the blood forward in the pause between two heartbeats.

SEE ALSO

BLOOD • BODY SYSTEMS • CIRCULATORY SYSTEM • HEART

Artery Diseases and Disorders

The arteries play such an important part in taking oxygen and nourishment around the body that any disease affecting them is extremely serious. If an artery becomes blocked or narrowed over time, the part of the body that is supplied by it can die from oxygen starvation. Arterial disease is the most common serious illness in the developed world.

Blockages are the result of atherosclerosis, in which deposits of a porridgelike substance called atheroma collect in the inner lining of the arteries. Blockages begin when cholesterol from the blood leaks into the inner surface of the artery and forms a plaque (fatty streak) in the arterial wall. Rupture of the plaque causes the blood to clot, and a plug of fibrous tissue forms. This mixture of fatty and fibrous tissue is called an atheromatous plaque. As the plaque grows, it blocks the central space, or lumen, of the artery, which reduces the flow of blood past the plaque. That, in turn, may activate the clotting system at the site of narrowing. The resulting clot may then produce a total obstruction, known as a thrombosis. An embolism is the blockage of an artery by an embolus, a fragment of material—usually a blood clot—that has been carried in the bloodstream.

Heart attacks and strokes

Atheroma are most likely to form in the body in places where an artery branches and is under stress. The coronary arteries that supply blood to the heart are under more stress than practically any other artery in the body because they are constantly

Q & A

Three of my male relatives, including my father, have died of heart attacks. Are men more prone to atherosclerosis than women?

Yes, this seems to be true for several reasons. First, female hormones seem to protect women from atheroma, the buildup of fatty deposits that cause blockages in the arteries. After menopause, when hormone levels fall, atheromas increase. Second, in the past men smoked more than women. As that pattern changes, however, the number of women suffering from atherosclerosis is rising.

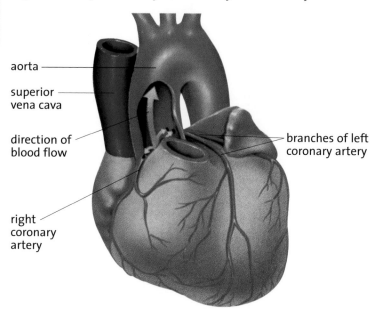

aorta

superior vena cava

direction of blood flow

branches of left coronary artery

right coronary artery

The coronary arteries supply the heart muscle with the oxygen and nutrients it needs. There are really three coronary arteries—the two branches of the left coronary artery, and the right coronary artery. These arteries are particularly prone to blockages and obstructions, which cause heart attacks.

stretched and relaxed as the heart beats. When a coronary artery becomes completely blocked, the blockage causes a heart attack, or coronary thrombosis. If the artery is partly blocked by atheroma, the supply of blood to the heart muscle may be adequate to keep it going only when the body is resting. However, exercise uses more oxygen than the reduced blood supply can provide, and that situation brings on chest pain, which is called angina.

When atherosclerosis reduces the supply of blood to the brain, it can cause a gradual loss of memory and some types of dementia. It may also cause a stroke, which occurs when an artery becomes completely blocked by a blood clot on a plaque or by an embolism. Alternatively, the artery wall becomes weakened until eventually blood leaks into the brain. Some strokes are minor (if the blocked artery is extremely small), and the patient can make a complete or partial recovery over time. However, a severe stroke can cause death. The most devastating and fatal strokes are caused by hemorrhage from a small artery in the brain.

The risk of artery disease increases with age and often runs in families. People at risk should have regular health checkups, stick to a low-fat diet, avoid smoking,

Atheroma in the arteries of the leg can limit blood supply to the leg, and exercise can cause pain. If the blockage is extremely bad, the tissues of the leg may die and the limb may have to be amputated. Kidney failure may also be caused by atherosclerosis.

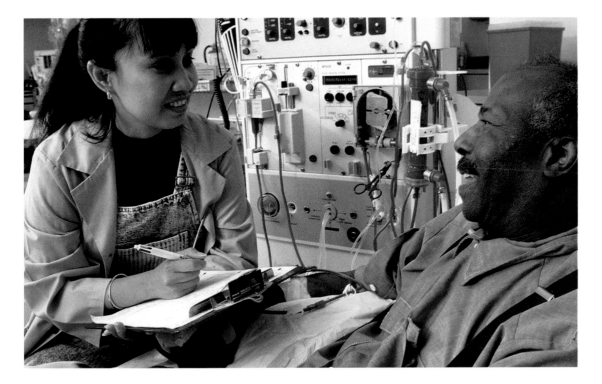

Sometimes a weakness in the wall of an artery, usually caused by inflammation or atherosclerosis, makes the artery bulge out in an aneurysm, or saclike swelling. The swelling may burst, causing internal bleeding and loss of blood supply to part of the body, or it may press against surrounding tissues and damage them. A burst aneurysm in the aorta or arteries of the brain can sometimes be fatal.

What can be done?

The main cause of atherosclerosis is age, and people can do nothing about that. However, there is a great deal that can be done to reduce the risk of atherosclerosis. The condition is caused above all by a diet that includes too much animal fat and cholesterol. In recent years, many people have become more aware of this danger and have changed their eating habits, cutting down on foods such as meat, dairy products, and eggs. As a result, the rate of deaths from arterial disease has decreased and in some places the number of deaths has even fallen. People who have high blood pressure, are overweight, are under stress, or smoke are also at risk. Men are more likely to suffer than women, and the condition seems to run in families.

The best way of preventing arterial diseases is to eat a healthy and balanced diet, cut down on animal fats, watch one's weight, give up smoking, and exercise regularly. Three 20-minute sessions of exercise a week, sufficient to cause mild breathlessness and raise a sweat, are recommended to increase cardiovascular efficiency. Regular gentle exercise, such as walking, is also recommended to raise fitness levels and to help keep the arteries working properly.

This thermograph, or heat-sensitive picture, shows the effects of smoking on the circulation. The pale areas indicate the decreased blood flow, particularly to the patient's fingertips.

SEE ALSO

ARTERY • CIRCULATORY SYSTEM • CIRCULATORY SYSTEM DISEASES AND DISORDERS • HEART ATTACK • OBESITY • STROKE

Arthritis

Arthritis is inflammation of the joints. It ranges from brief discomfort to severe, long-lasting pain and serious disablement. Arthritis occurs in people of all ages and can affect one joint or several. In many cases, no one knows for sure what causes arthritis. There are two main kinds of arthritis: osteoarthritis and rheumatoid arthritis.

Osteoarthritis

Osteoarthritis happens as part of the aging process, and almost every adult has some signs of it. It is caused by degeneration of the cartilage, which is the strong, elastic tissue that protects the surface of the joints. The cartilage becomes rough and cracked, compressing the underlying bone and inflaming the tissue lining above it. Osteoarthritis mainly affects the hands and the weight-bearing joints of the hips, knees, and spine. The first symptoms are pain and loss of use of the affected area, followed by stiffness and swelling. In time, the affected joints become distorted. Osteoarthritis gets gradually worse and can be disabling if it occurs in a weight-bearing joint and is severe.

Rheumatoid arthritis

Rheumatoid arthritis is an autoimmune illness in which the body's immune (defense) system works incorrectly, producing antibodies that react against the tissue lining of the joints, causing inflammation, tenderness, pain with movement, and stiffness. This form of arthritis may be triggered by an illness, emotional stress, or shock, which causes a chain of biochemical reactions in the body. Rheumatoid arthritis usually affects adults between the ages of 20 and 55. Rheumatoid arthritis may appear suddenly, starting with a fever or rash, or develop over several weeks. A common symptom is inflammation of the knuckles and toe joints, and the patient may lose weight, become lethargic, and feel generally unwell. The knees, hips, shoulders, wrists, elbows, ankles, and bones of the neck may also be affected. The patient may have great difficulty in moving around and may have to stay in bed. It may be several months before the inflammation dies down, and further attacks can occur. The joints may become deformed and the bones around them weakened.

Still's disease

When rheumatoid arthritis occurs in children, it is known as Still's disease. This condition is fortunately rare. It mainly affects children between the ages of one and three, or between 10 and 15, and the child may have several attacks over the years, ending with the onset of puberty. Each attack may last for several weeks.

Q & A

Is it safe for my father to take a lot of aspirin to ease the pain caused by arthritis?

Yes and no. Because aspirin reduces inflammation and temperature and eases pain, it is often used as a first-line treatment for arthritis. However, when aspirin is taken for a long time, there are two possible side effects: tiny gastric ulcers can bleed or an existing ulcer can flare up.

My grandmother always wears a bandage wound tightly around her arthritic knee. Is this really helpful?

It can be of some help. Bandaging or supporting an acutely inflamed joint can stop jarring movement and, therefore, ease some of the pain. When a joint is swollen, the tissues feel stretched. A support under these circumstances gives a sensation of stability. However, she should always be careful not to make the bandage too tight, because a very tight bandage can reduce the circulation of blood to the lower part of the leg.

The child may have a rash and a temperature that rises from normal in the morning to about 103°F (39.4°C) in the evening; other symptoms can include swollen glands in the neck and armpits, and painful, red eyes. Eye inflammation in Still's disease is serious because it can permanently damage the vision; it requires skilled ophthalmic care.

Other forms of arthritis

Arthritis can be caused by infections, including tuberculosis, rheumatic fever, gonorrhea, and psoriasis. Once the infection is cured, the arthritis disappears. However, it can be triggered at a later date by an injury, such as a blow to a joint. Bacteria in the joint fluid can cause a damaging and dangerous septic form of arthritis. Another type of arthritis that affects the spine and pelvic joints is ankylosing spondylitis.

Many cases of arthritis are treated with drugs such as aspirin and ibuprofen, which help combat inflammation and ease the pain. Steroid drugs such as cortisone can also help the condition but they may have unpleasant side effects. Regular, sensible exercise helps prevent stiffness and loss of movement in the joints and helps muscles keep their strength. Heat treatment can ease painful joints, and swimming in a warm pool is also good exercise for people with arthritis.

A normal knee (below left) compared with an osteoarthritic knee. The smooth cartilage that cushions the joint has degenerated and worn away, leaving the bones to grind against each other. As the bone seeks to heal itself, its surface becomes rough and painful.

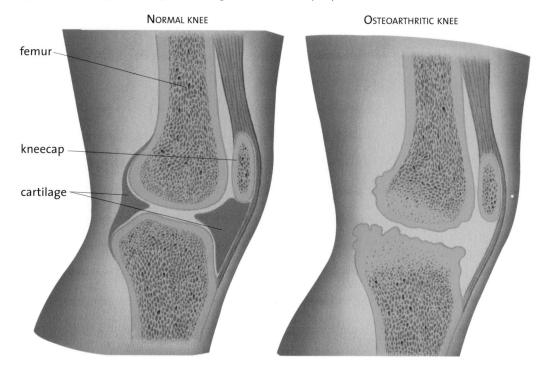

NORMAL KNEE

OSTEOARTHRITIC KNEE

femur

kneecap

cartilage

Relieving the strain of arthritis

Claims are made that special diets ease arthritis, but there is as yet no real proof of this. Too much weight puts unnecessary strain on the joints, so heavy people with arthritis should reduce their weight by eating sensibly and exercising. Operations to replace the hip, the knee, and other joints damaged by arthritis are now common. The damaged joint is replaced by an artificial one made of metal or metal and plastic. This operation is usually successful and gives the patient increased movement and relief from pain. Surgery can also relieve pressure around a joint, can free ligaments that have become stuck together, or can remove inflamed tissue lining a joint if it is greatly affected.

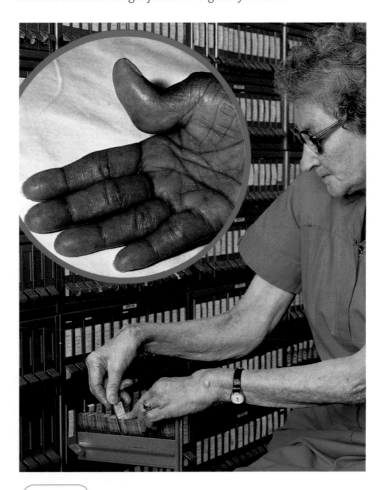

Fine movements with the hands are often difficult and painful for someone suffering from arthritis. People with rheumatoid arthritis need to keep their hands as mobile as possible, but movements may be painful and difficult to make. Sometimes, a joint (inset) becomes so deformed that it cannot be used.

SEE ALSO

IMMUNE SYSTEM • JOINT DISORDERS • OSTEOARTHRITIS

Asthma

Asthma is a common condition that involves considerable difficulty in breathing. During an attack, asthmatics tend to breathe in with short gasps and force their breath out again with a long wheeze. Asthma is caused by a narrowing of the bronchial tubes when the muscles that line them contract. These tubes lead from the windpipe (trachea) to the lungs.

Asthma attacks are quite common in children, but most people outgrow them in adolescence. Some attacks are mild but others can be extremely bad. Asthma is brought on by a number of different causes, from breathing polluted air to emotional stress. All the different causes of asthma result in the release of one of two chemicals in the body. These chemicals are histamine and acetylcholine, both of which cause the bronchial muscles to contract.

Histamine release is the most common cause of asthma. It is triggered by an allergic reaction to all sorts of substances, including the following: pollen; house dust; certain foods, such as shellfish, eggs, chocolate, and milk; and some preservatives. Sudden strenuous exercise and emotional upsets also cause attacks or make them worse, and the more anxious the patient becomes, the worse the attack gets.

Most asthmatics are prescribed a bronchodilator, which they can use if they have an attack. The bronchodilator contains a substance that opens the bronchial tubes. People with asthma should always carry their inhaler with them, in case they have an attack when they are away from home.

Q & A

What can I do if I forget my inhaler and then suffer an asthma attack?

If you suffer a severe attack, you must go to a doctor or to a hospital emergency room immediately. Otherwise, try to sit still and save your breath.

My father had asthma, and my sister and I now have it. Can asthma run in families?

Asthma does tend to be inherited, especially those types of asthma that are a strong response to an allergy. However, the inherited link is not yet fully understood.

My young brother is asthmatic. Should he play sports?

Yes, all asthmatic children should be encouraged to exercise. Some sports are more likely to cause asthma than others; swimming is the least likely to bring on an attack. Your brother should use his inhaler before taking part.

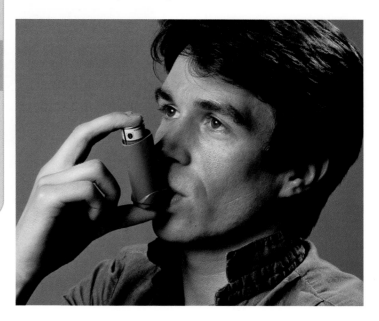

Easy to use and convenient to carry in a pocket, this type of aerosol inhaler relaxes and widens the airways in all but the worst asthma attacks.

PREVENTING ASTHMA ATTACKS

Cause	How to prevent
Infections such as common cold and other viruses, sinusitis, bronchitis	Avoid people with colds, eat a balanced diet, get enough sleep and exercise.
Allergic reaction to pollen, house dust, fungal spores, animal hair	Keep home as dust-free as possible. Do not sit on carpets or rugs. Use foam pillows. Avoid animals. Use air cleaners.
Irritants breathed in, such as gasoline fumes, cigarette smoke, fresh paint, bad odors, cold air	Avoid fumes and smoky atmospheres. Avoid going out in cold air.
Exercise or unusual physical exertion	Avoid strenuous exercise. Use gentle relaxation techniques.
Sudden changes of temperature or air pressure	Avoid sudden temperature changes.
Emotional upset and stress	Identify cause of problem or stress and seek help for it.
Food allergies to milk, eggs, strawberries, fish, tomatoes	Consult allergist to identify allergen and avoid it.
Drug allergies to aspirin, penicillin, vaccines, and anesthetics	Avoid the drugs. A doctor can provide alternatives.

FIRST AID FOR ASTHMA

When a person with asthma has a bad attack, give any drug that the doctor has prescribed and make a note of the exact time. Sit the patient up, leaning slightly forward (resting on the elbows can help). Make sure that he or she can get plenty of fresh air. Give more medication after 30 minutes if the doctor has said that this will be all right. If the attack does not seem to be getting better, telephone the doctor and get ready to take the patient to a hospital if necessary.

This is a photograph of a house dust mite, viewed from below and magnified many times. These mites are about 0.12 inch (3 mm) long and can be seen only with a magnifying glass. They are found in dust and bedding in even the cleanest home and can trigger an asthma attack.

Treatment of asthma

People with asthma should regularly monitor the state of their bronchial tubes with a peak flow meter, which is prescribed by doctors and is available in large drug stores. This simple device measures the ease with which air can enter and leave the lungs and gives warning of the probability of a dangerous asthma attack. Asthmatics can take inhaled steroids to prevent attacks or help cope with minor ones. These steroids now play an important part in the control of asthma and can reduce the likelihood of permanent lung damage. More severe attacks need prompt treatment from a doctor or sometimes hospitalization. If a severe attack is not treated quickly, the patient may even die. A doctor can inject a drug such as aminophylline, which relaxes

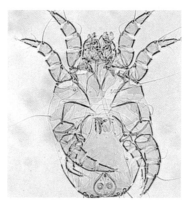

the bronchial muscles and takes effect immediately. Hydrocortisone injections also relieve an attack very quickly. Asthmatics should have tests to find the cause of their attacks. Regular, steady exercise, particularly swimming, helps sufferers, but they must be careful not to overdo it. There is no cure for asthma, but current research may lead to one.

SEE ALSO

ALLERGIES • BRONCHITIS • LUNG • RESPIRATORY SYSTEM

Athlete's Foot

Athlete's foot is probably the most common foot complaint. It is a fungal infection, like ringworm, that can affect almost everyone, although small children seem immune to it.

The fungus settles in the moist, sweaty areas between the toes, where it lives on dead skin, which the body sheds every day. Athlete's foot may cause inflammation and damage to the living skin. The first signs are irritation and itching between the toes, and then the skin begins to peel. The condition may smell unpleasant. In more severe cases of athlete's foot, painful red cracks appear between the toes and even the toenails can become infected. The nails become either softer or more brittle as the fungus invades the nail substance. In extreme cases, the whole foot swells and blisters.

The fungus that causes athlete's foot can be present on floors and in clothing. People with sweaty feet are particularly likely to develop it. Wearing plastic shoes, which prevent air from circulating around the feet, makes the problem worse. Locker rooms and showers are breeding grounds for the fungus.

Treatment for athlete's foot is simple and soon successful. Antifungal creams should be applied daily while the condition lasts, and for two or three weeks after the symptoms have disappeared, to prevent it from coming back. If the condition does not clear up, the person should see his or her doctor, who may prescribe a drug to take by mouth. To prevent athlete's foot from recurring, the feet, shoes, and socks should be dusted regularly with antifungal powder and the feet should always be washed and dried carefully. Clean cotton or wool socks (not nylon socks) should be worn every day.

Q & A

I have a severe form of athlete's foot that keeps recurring. Will my feet be permanently scarred?

No, because the fungus causing athlete's foot lives only on the superficial layers of the skin, eating dead skin cells.

Can athlete's foot spread to other parts of the body?

The athlete's foot fungus can live on various parts of the body but is not contagious and is unlikely to spread. However, there is a condition similar to athlete's foot that can affect the hands. That should be diagnosed and treated by a doctor.

My sister has athlete's foot. Can she infect the rest of the family?

Not if all family members wash and dry their feet carefully using separate towels and use antifungal powder.

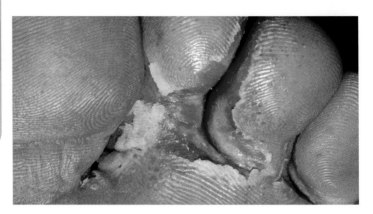

In severe cases of athlete's foot, the skin between the toes becomes painful, red, and cracked. The fungus responsible for the infection grows readily in these warm, moist areas, feeding on dead skin cells.

SEE ALSO

FUNGAL INFECTIONS • INFECTIOUS DISEASES • RINGWORM

Avian Influenza

Avian influenza, or bird flu, is an infection caused by type A influenza viruses that are common among birds. Wild birds carry the viruses but they do not usually get sick from them. However, these viruses are extremely contagious among domesticated birds, such as chickens, ducks, and turkeys, and can make them very sick and even kill them.

There are many different subtypes of type A influenza viruses. All known subtypes of influenza A viruses can be found in birds. In medicine and research, one of the most contagious subtypes is known as the H5N1 virus. The disease was first identified in Italy more than 100 years ago and occurs worldwide.

Although the avian influenza virus infects mostly birds, infections with these viruses can occur in humans. The risk from avian influenza is low for most people, but confirmed cases of human infection have been reported since 1997. In these cases, humans have had contact with infected poultry. For example, a farmer who has chicken, ducks, and turkeys on his or her farm probably has a great deal of contact with poultry and can become infected. However, the spread of avian influenza viruses from one ill person to another has been reported very rarely.

Symptoms of avian influenza in humans have ranged from typical human influenza-like symptoms, such as fever, cough, sore throat, and muscle aches, to eye infections, pneumonia, severe respiratory diseases (difficulty in breathing), and other severe and life-threatening complications. Studies done in laboratories suggest that some of the prescription medicines approved in the United States for human influenza viruses should work in treating avian influenza infection in humans. However, influenza viruses can become resistant to these drugs, so these medications may not always work. The best approach is to prevent infection in the first place by finding a vaccine.

Developing a vaccine

A vaccine has been difficult to develop because all type A influenza viruses, including those that regularly cause seasonal epidemics of influenza in humans, are genetically labile. That means their genes are constantly changing. To find a vaccine, the virus must be stable long enough to study it, create the vaccine, and vaccinate a large population before the virus changes again. However, the H5N1 virus changes too quickly for all of these steps to be completed.

Although there has been some human-to-human spread of H5N1, it has been limited and inefficient. Nonetheless, because all influenza viruses have the ability to change, scientists are concerned that one day the H5N1 virus might be able to infect

Q & A

I got flu last winter but wasn't that sick. What's the big deal about bird flu?

Avian influenza (or bird flu) is not the same as other flu infections. Bird flu is extremely contagious among birds and can be deadly to them. So far, bird flu has spread mainly from one bird to another and from bird to person—rarely from person to person. However, it is possible that the virus could mutate (change) and become more easy to pass from person to person. At present there is no vaccine available to protect people from catching bird flu.

I've heard people talk about bird flu becoming a pandemic. What is that?

An influenza pandemic is a worldwide outbreak of disease that occurs when a new influenza A virus appears, causes serious illness, and spreads easily from person to person worldwide. Past influenza pandemics have led to high levels of illness, death, social disruption, and economic loss.

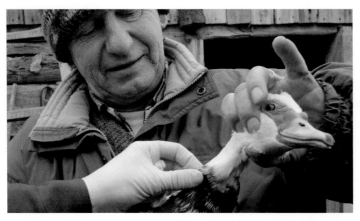

A farmer holds a goose while a veterinarian examines it for signs of avian influenza. If the disease is identified, close contact with poultry should be avoided as far as possible.

humans and spread easily from one person to another. If that happened, an influenza pandemic (worldwide outbreak of disease) could begin. In human history, influenza pandemics have occurred regularly—on average, three to four times each century, when new virus subtypes emerge and are readily transmitted from person to person. However, the occurrence of influenza pandemics is unpredictable. In the twentieth century, the influenza pandemic of 1918–1919, which caused an estimated 40 million to 50 million deaths worldwide, was followed by pandemics in 1957–1958 and 1968–1969. Experts agree that another influenza pandemic is inevitable.

When cases of avian influenza occur in humans, information on how many birds and humans have been infected is urgently needed to help protect the rest of the population. A thorough investigation of each case also helps give clues about what kind of virus subtype might be circulating in the population. The World Health Organization (WHO) and members of its global influenza network with other agencies, such as the Centers for Disease Control and Prevention (CDC) in the United States, work together to collect and keep this information available.

Although a pandemic is likely to take place at some time in the future, on April 17, 2007, the U.S. Food and Drug Administration (FDA) announced its approval of the first vaccine to prevent human infection with one strain of the avian influenza H5N1 virus. If and when it is needed, the vaccine will be distributed by public health officials. Meanwhile, scientists worldwide are developing other H5N1 vaccines against different H5N1 strains.

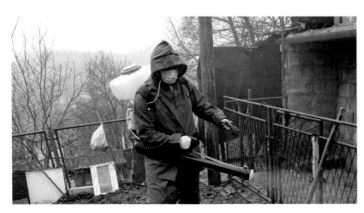

Wearing full protective clothing, a health worker disinfects a poultry farm. Avian influenza is controlled by culling (killing) infected and exposed birds and by quarantining and disinfecting farms.

SEE ALSO

COLD • EPIDEMIC • INFECTIOUS DISEASES • INFLUENZA • PNEUMONIA • VIRUSES

Bacteria

Bacteria are minute living organisms far too small to be seen with the naked eye. They live everywhere—in the air, water, soil, and oceans. Countless millions of them of many different species (types) live on and inside every person. Bacteria can even live in hot springs, boiling mud, frozen soil, and ice. There are more bacteria on Earth than any other type of organism. Scientists have already found more than 10,000 species of bacteria, and probably many thousands more have yet to be discovered.

Each bacterium consists of a single life unit, or cell, bound by a tough wall. The largest bacterium measures less than one-thousandth of an inch. Bacteria are among the most successful living organisms. They reproduce simply by splitting in two and can multiply at great speed. At body temperature and in places rich in material for them to feed on, they divide in this way once every 30 minutes. In less than 10 hours, one bacterium will have multiplied to form more than half a million replicas of itself.

Some bacteria help plants feed and others have a vital role as recyclers, breaking down dead organic material and releasing the chemicals into the soil. That process makes the soil rich in nutrients and provides plants with food. Bacteria also help make certain vitamins in the human intestine, assist in the production of food such as yogurt and cheese, and make drugs. Some bacteria live in the digestive system of animals, such as cattle and plant-eating insects, where they help digest tough plant fibers. However, bacteria also cause serious diseases, such as anthrax and typhoid. Some bacteria live in people's mouths and develop a coating called plaque that eats away at teeth and gums.

Q & A

How many bacteria can a person tolerate and still stay healthy?

The answer varies from person to person and from time to time. It also depends on the type of bacteria. Everybody harbors bacteria on the skin and within the digestive tract. Some bacteria do no damage, because they are either tolerated or destroyed by the body's white blood cells and antibodies. If, however, the body becomes run down, resistance to bacteria is lowered and harmful bacteria may multiply. They then have the power to penetrate the body's defenses.

I had an infection recently, which did not clear up. My doctor said I had a "resistant strain." What does that mean?

Antibiotics were once almost always effective in combating infections. Now, some bacteria have become resistant to antibiotics and are known as resistant strains.

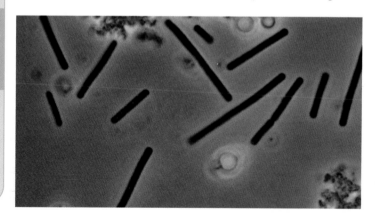

Not all bacteria are harmful to humans. The rod-shaped ones, shown here greatly magnified, ferment milk to make yogurt.

SEE ALSO

BACTERIAL DISEASES • INFECTIOUS DISEASES • TYPHOID FEVER

Bacterial Diseases

Q & A

I've heard that many bacteria are harmful but that there are good bacteria as well. Is that true?

Yes. Some bacteria cause infections, but other bacteria are helpful to humans and the environment. Bacteria that normally live in humans can prevent infections. Bacteria living in the stomachs of cows and sheep enable them to digest grass. Bacteria are also essential to the production of yogurt, cheese, and pickles.

Why doesn't the doctor give me an antibiotic to cure me when I am sick?

There are usually two types of infections that can make you sick: viral infections and bacterial infections. Although bacterial infections, such as strep throat (streptococcal infection of the throat), respond to antibiotics, viral infections, such as the common cold, do not. If you do have a bacterial infection, your doctor will have to decide if an antibiotic is necessary. This decision can depend on how bad the infection is.

Billions of bacteria live around, on, and in the human body. Some, called pathogenic bacteria, can cause harm. They enter the body in contaminated food or water, through wounds in the skin, or by being breathed in, especially in the minute droplets of water that infected people cough, sneeze, or breathe out of their lungs. Some bacteria are also transmitted by direct contact. These bacteria enter the bloodstream through a cut or scratch or push their way into the tissues of the digestive, respiratory, urinary, or genital system. Then, they go through a growth or incubation period, which ranges from a few hours to more than a year.

Toxins and types of bacteria

Pathogenic bacteria produce tiny quantities of extremely powerful poisons (toxins), which are capable of killing almost any type of body cell. These toxins either act remotely (exotoxins) or damage only the tissues with which they are in direct contact (endotoxins). They are among the most powerful toxins known.

Disease-carrying bacteria exist in three main forms, based on their shape. Spherical cocci include staphylococci, which are responsible for infections such as boils and abscesses; streptococci, which cause strep throat and scarlet fever; and gonococci, which cause the disease gonorrhea. Rod-shaped bacilli cause typhoid fever, cystitis, and tuberculosis. Spirochetes are tiny, elongated spirals and cause syphilis, relapsing fever, trench mouth, and other diseases. The cocci are immobile, but many bacteria can move by waving whiplike projections called flagella or, in the case of spirochetes, by making twisting movements.

Combating bacteria

When bacteria invade, the body mobilizes its defense systems. The area becomes inflamed as its blood supply increases to bring extra white cells to attack and engulf the invaders. The body also starts making antibodies that attack the invaders, but this reaction can take several days. However, antibiotics and sulfonamides are extremely effective against bacteria; diseases that were once killers can now be cured with little difficulty.

Bacterial infections can be prevented by destroying breeding grounds, by killing bacteria, and by immunization. Favorite breeding grounds for bacteria include water and feces, both of which can be cleared by improving standards of hygiene and by better housing. Most bacteria can be killed by boiling, by the ultraviolet radiation in sunlight, and by disinfectants and antiseptics. Immunization is available against some bacterial infections and has helped make these diseases far less common and less dangerous than they used to be.

BACTERIAL DISEASES

Type	How transmitted	Bacterium
Abscess	Through skin contact with contaminated object	Staphylococcus
Acute tonsillitis	Droplets in air	Streptococcus
Anthrax	Contact with infected animal	*Bacillus anthracis*
Bacillary dysentery	Contaminated food or water	*Shigella*
Bartonellosis	Through sand fly bite	*Bartonella*
Boils	Through skin contact with contaminated object	Staphylococcus
Botulism	Contaminated food and water	*Clostridium botulinum*
Brucellosis	Contact with infected cattle or their products	*Brucella*
Cholera	Contaminated food and water	*Vibrio cholerae*
Diphtheria	Droplets in air	*Corynebacterium diphtheriae*
Food poisoning	Contaminated food and water	*Salmonella, staphylococcus,* and others
Gastroenteritis	Contaminated food and water	*Salmonella* and others
Gonorrhea	Sexually transmitted	*Neisseria gonorrhoeae*
Hansen's disease (leprosy)	Droplets in air	*Mycobacterium leprae*
Infectious arthritis	Through wound or injury or from other infected site	Numerous organisms
Leptospirosis	Contact with infected animals or their products	*Leptospira*
Meningitis, bacterial	Droplets in air	*Hemophilus* and *Neisseria*
Middle ear infection	Droplets in air	Staphylococcus and others
Osteomyelitis	Through wound or injury or from other infected site	Staphylococcus and others
Pharyngitis	Droplets in air	Streptococcus
Plague	Contact with infected animals and droplets in air	*Yersinia pestis*
Pneumonia	Droplets in air	Pneumococcus
Relapsing fever	Lice or tick bite	*Borellia* and others
Scarlet fever	Droplets in air	Streptococcus
Syphilis	Sexually transmitted	*Treponema pallidum*
Tetanus	Contaminated soil entering wound	*Clostridium tetani*
Toxic shock syndrome	Mostly infected tampons	Staphylococcus
Tuberculosis	Droplets in air or (rarely) contaminated food	*Mycobacterium tuberculosis*
Tularemia	Contact with infected animal	*Francisella tularemia*
Typhoid	Contaminated food and water	*Salmonella*

DORMANT BACTERIA

Some bacteria become dormant when conditions are unfavorable. They change into spores, with a tough outer wall that is extremely difficult to destroy. The bacteria can be destroyed only at very high temperatures produced under conditions of high pressure. Therefore, spores are extremely dangerous. The spores of the tetanus bacteria are common in the soil, but people can easily be immunized against them. Some people have disease-causing bacteria living in their body, but they show no signs of illness. However, they can still pass on such bacteria to other people, who then become ill. People who harbor such infections are called carriers; the most dangerous are carriers of the diseases typhoid and diphtheria.

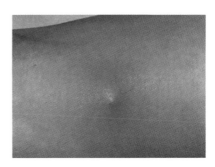

Staphylococcal bacteria are known to cause a variety of infections and diseases, such as this painful boil.

SEE ALSO

ANTIBODY AND ANTIGEN •
BACTERIA • IMMUNE SYSTEM

Birth Defects

Birth defects are imperfections or abnormalities in the structure or functioning of the body that are present, although not necessarily apparent, at birth. Birth defects are also called congenital defects. Many defects are slight and cause few problems. Some birth defects affect the structure of the baby's body and are immediately obvious. The child may have a cleft palate and lip, or extra fingers or toes, or spina bifida. Some babies look normal but have defects that affect the working of the body. A baby is given a blood test in its second week of life to see if it has phenylketonuria (PKU), a disorder that, unless detected early and treated, can cause mental retardation.

Q & A

How does Down syndrome occur?

Down syndrome is caused by a chromosomal abnormality in the genes of the father or mother. People usually have 23 pairs of chromosomes. Down syndrome occurs when one chromosome makes three copies of itself instead of two. This syndrome affects one in 800 babies. Older mothers have a greater chance of giving birth to a baby with Down syndrome.

Genetic defects and environmental disorders

Some birth defects are inherited, or genetic; they are passed down to the baby by one or both of its parents. A woman may carry the gene for a blood disease called hemophilia, for example. She is perfectly healthy, as are any of her daughters, because it is extremely rare for women to have this disease. However, some of her sons may have the disease, and some of her daughters may be carriers of the gene.

Other defects are caused when something damages the fetus as it develops in its mother's uterus. Such defects are known as environmental disorders. Some of them are beyond the mother's control—she may be exposed to radiation, for example, which can cause malformations. Other birth defects are caused by the mother's behavior; drugs, smoking, alcohol, and poor diet can all cause birth defects. Illness in pregnancy, particularly rubella, is also dangerous. Often, heredity and environment act together. The chance of having a baby with Down syndrome increases once the mother is over the age of 40.

Treatment of birth defects

Many birth defects can be treated, often extremely successfully, with surgery, medicines, a special diet, and physical training. As experts learn more about their causes, people can do more to prevent birth defects. People who know that there are hereditary problems in their family can go to a genetic counselor, who will carefully study the family's medical history.

The counselor may also test them to see if they carry the genes for a disease. Then, the counselor will figure out the chances of their child's having a birth defect. The prospective parents must decide whether the risk is worth taking. Tests such as amniocentesis or chorionic villus sampling provide fetal DNA samples from which any of a wide range of genetic defects can be detected early in pregnancy.

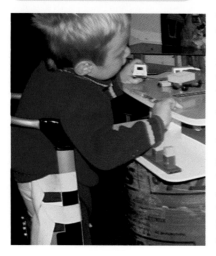

This child is severely affected by spina bifida, but he is able to stand with the aid of a supportive frame. Spina bifida is a birth defect in which one or more of the vertebrae fail to develop completely in a fetus, leaving the spinal cord exposed.

SOME BIRTH DEFECTS

Defect	Type	Result	Treatment
AIDS syndrome	Environmental	Defective immune system	Anti-HIV medication
Cleft lip and/or palate	Hereditary and/or environmental	Feeding and later speech problems	Surgery
Clubfoot	Hereditary and/or environmental	Misshapen foot	Physical therapy and/or surgery
Congenital heart malformations	Hereditary and/or environmental	Structural defects	Surgery and medication
Congenital rubella syndrome	Environmental	Defects of heart, eye, and brain	Surgery, physical training, and therapy
Congenital syphilis	Environmental	Various physical and mental defects	Medication
Cystic fibrosis	Hereditary	Disorders of respiratory and digestive system	Physical therapy, special diet, respiratory therapy
Down syndrome	Chromosomal abnormality	Mental retardation and physical defects	Special education, sometimes surgery
Galactosemia	Hereditary	Inability to digest milk and sugars; mental retardation	Special diet
Hemophilia	Hereditary	Blood does not clot	Medication and blood transfusions
Huntington's disease	Hereditary	Neurological illness in adulthood	None
Low birthweight	Hereditary and/or environmental	Risk of brain damage and physical defects	Intensive care and special diet
Muscular dystrophy	Hereditary	Weakness and wasting of muscle	Physical therapy
Phenylketonuria (PKU)	Hereditary	Inability to digest certain proteins	Special diet
Polydactyly	Hereditary	Extra fingers or toes	Surgery
Sickle-cell anemia	Hereditary	Malformed red blood cells	Medication and blood transfusions
Spina bifida	Hereditary and environmental	Spinal cord not covered	Surgery and physical therapy
Tay-Sachs disease	Hereditary	Progressive mental retardation and death	None
Thalassemia	Hereditary	Blood disease	Blood transfusions

SEE ALSO

AIDS AND HIV • BLOOD DISEASES AND DISORDERS • BODY SYSTEMS • CYSTIC FIBROSIS • DOWN SYNDROME • GENES • GENETIC DISEASES AND DISORDERS • HEART DISEASES AND DISORDERS • HEMOPHILIA • HUNTINGTON'S DISEASE • MUSCULAR DYSTROPHY • PHENYLKETONURIA • RUBELLA • SICKLE-CELL ANEMIA • SPINA BIFIDA • THALASSEMIA

Blindness

Blindness is the loss of sight. Some people have no sight at all; others may be able to see only light or shade. Still others may have part of the normal area of vision missing. There are many causes of blindness. Some people are born blind because their eyes have not developed properly or because of some illness that affected their mother during pregnancy. All sorts of eye disorders and infections can cause blindness. Another cause is damage to the optic nerves that carry information from the eyes to the brain. These nerves can be inflamed by a virus infection or by poisons such as methanol, quinine, lead, and arsenic. Pressure on the nerve from a tumor, hemorrhage, or swollen blood vessel can also cause loss of vision. So can damage to the part of the brain that is concerned with sight. Some cases of blindness have no physical cause but are the symptom of a psychological problem.

Sometimes, blindness can be cured by surgery; cataracts (the clouding of the eye lens) can be removed in a simple operation under local anesthesia, for example, and an artificial lens can be inserted. Sudden blindness caused by a clot in the vein leading from the retina often gradually gets better. However, many people face being unable to see ever again.

Blindness in children

Children who are born blind usually have congenital cataracts or a serious visual defect. Cataracts can be surgically removed, but a condition called nystagmus, which is a fine involuntary tremor of the eye, often occurs and makes focusing difficult. Infections that cause blindness are rare in developed countries, but the most common cause of blindness, trachoma (a virus disease of the eyelids), is still widespread in underdeveloped tropical regions. If a pregnant woman contracts rubella, her child may be

Q & A

I keep getting spots in front of my eyes, and I worry that they mean that I am going blind. Might this be true?

This is a common experience that doctors call muscae volitantes; the little black spots are quite normal and tend to be seen when a person is young and a little anxious. They are not connected with failing vision or blindness in any way at all.

My 17-year-old brother was recently blinded in an accident. What should I do to help him adjust to this life change?

Helping him to adjust will need all the understanding and love you and your family can give. You can get lots of practical help from your local institution for the blind. Because of the many modern aids for the blind, your brother still has a great deal of choices left open to him.

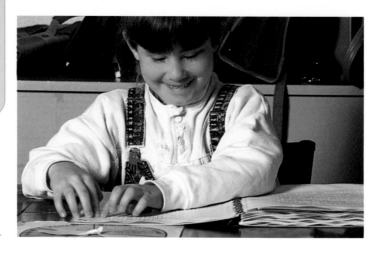

This little girl is learning to read braille with her fingers. Later, she will learn to use a braillewriter, a machine like a typewriter that punches dots on paper. Computer programs that can read saved or typed text are also now commonplace.

born with cataracts. If she becomes infested with a parasite called *Toxoplasma gondi*, the child may be born blind. Young children who are contaminated with dog excreta run a risk of contracting a worm parasite, *Toxocara canis*, that can affect the eye and cause chronic inflammation of the retina.

Effects of aging

People who are over 70 may suffer macular degeneration of the retina, for which there is no cure. The cells of the retina age and die, particularly those in the area called the macula, which is responsible for fine vision.

Magnifying glasses help some people. Sometimes, closed-circuit television can be used to magnify print and project it onto a screen for easier and closer viewing.

Detached retina and glaucoma

Retinal detachment is most common in people with a high degree of short sight (myopia). Detachment occurs when eyeball enlargement leads to stretching and degeneration of the retina so that a small tear or hole occurs. Then, fluid from the eye passes through the tear and gathers behind the retina, pushing it off the underlying coat of the eye. Laser treatment is widely used to seal detected holes and small tears before detachment occurs. Younger people may suffer a detached retina after a severe blow to the eye.

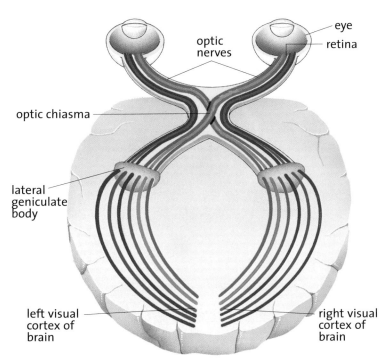

The optic nerves carry information from the retinas to the brain. At the optic chiasma, information from each eye is transferred to the opposite side of the brain. Depth is analyzed in the part of the brain called the lateral geniculate body. The remaining image is processed in the visual cortexes.

Older people are also prone to glaucoma, when the pressure of the fluid within the eye is raised. The delicate nerves transmitting sight become compressed and damaged and the eye becomes red. If the condition is left untreated, vision will be lost completely and permanently. In chronic glaucoma, the rise in pressure is slow and progressive, so the condition is symptomless. The outer boundaries of vision are gradually lost until only tunnel vision remains.

> **SEE ALSO**
>
> **EYE AND SIGHT • EYE DISEASES AND DISORDERS • GLAUCOMA**

Blood

Blood is the vital fluid that maintains life. Blood picks up oxygen from the lungs, and the heart pumps the blood around the body, delivering oxygen, digested food, and other essential substances to the tissues. In return, blood extracts carbon dioxide and other waste products that might poison the system.

Blood consists of a colorless liquid called plasma, in which float millions of red cells (also called erythrocytes), white cells (called leukocytes), and extremely small cell fragments called platelets. Plasma is mostly water, but it carries vital chemicals around the body, including glucose and other sugars, vitamins, minerals, fats, and proteins. The red blood cells act as transporters, carrying oxygen from the lungs and returning with carbon dioxide and waste water. The red cells contain hemoglobin, the substance that gives blood its color.

Plasma

Plasma is the liquid part of the blood, in which the red and white blood cells are transported around the body. It is a clear, slightly yellowish fluid that consists mainly of water, but it also contains salts, proteins, antibodies, and blood-clotting factors. Plasma makes up about 55 percent of the blood.

Since plasma is liquid, it can diffuse through the walls of the small blood vessels called capillaries and can combine with the fluid bathing the surface of the body's cells. This mixing allows

Q & A

My sister asked me if kings and queens really have blue blood. What is the origin of this saying?

Veins, which contain blood, appear blue where they show through the surface of the skin. The saying "blue-blooded" came about because aristocrats, in the past, were not exposed to the sun, so their veins showed up more clearly than those of laborers with weathered skin.

I've been told that I need a blood test. What exactly does this involve?

A doctor or other medical worker will draw out the blood using a needle with a syringe and then send the sample to a laboratory. The number and condition of the cells will be checked, and chemical tests will be performed to check the amounts of certain substances such as sugar. Tests will also be run to check for the presence of antibodies that form against attacking viruses or bacteria. If an illness is discovered after getting the results, your doctor will be able to treat it properly.

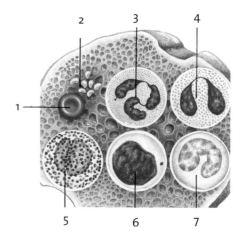

Specialized blood cells. Red blood cells (1) carry oxygen; platelets (2) are concerned with clotting; and there are many kinds of white cells: neutrophils (3), eosinophils (4), basophils (5), lymphocytes (6), and monocytes (7). They fight bacteria, prevent allergies, prevent clotting of circulating blood, and remove the debris resulting from bacterial attack.

plasma to carry many substances from cells in one part of the body to cells in another part. Nutrients from the digestive tract, iron to make hemoglobin, hormones to regulate functions, and waste products are all carried through the body by plasma.

The body cannot function without sufficient plasma in circulation, because the heart cannot beat effectively. Someone who loses a lot of blood will need a transfusion. The new liquid may be whole blood, or it may be just plasma, or even a simple solution of salt in water (saline).

White blood cells

White blood cells protect the body against invasion by bacteria. They are larger than red blood cells and are of several different kinds. White blood cells move with a creeping motion, whereas red cells only float. There are three basic kinds of white cells: polymorphs, lymphocytes, and monocytes. Polymorphs engulf bacteria and kill them. One group of polymorphs, known as basophils, make heparin, a substance that prevents blood from clotting inside the veins and arteries.

Lymphocytes produce substances called antibodies to counteract the damaging effect of invading bacteria. The two main types are B lymphocytes (B cells) and T lymphocytes (T cells). Monocytes remove the debris of cell remains resulting from bacterial attack.

Platelets and red blood cells

The small blood-cell fragments called platelets have sticky surfaces. If the capillaries, which are the smallest blood vessels, are damaged, chemicals are released that make the platelets stick to the broken ends and plug them to stop the bleeding.

Red blood cells are made in bone marrow. They have a life of around 120 days. Other cells made in the bone marrow remove worn-out red blood cells and break them down into their chemical parts. Polymorphs, which have a maximum life of only about 12 hours, are also made in the bone marrow, as are monocytes and platelets. Lymphocytes live for about 200 days. They are made in the spleen, lymph nodes, and other glands. If blood is lost, the body steps up the production of new blood cells to replace the lost volume.

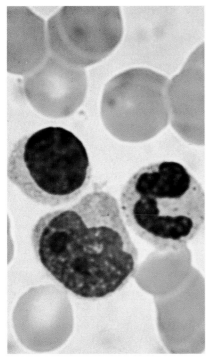

The sample of blood on this slide shows a mixture of red cells (erythrocytes) and white cells (leukocytes).

SEE ALSO

ANTIBODY AND ANTIGEN • BLOOD DISEASES AND DISORDERS • BONE • CELLS AND CHROMOSOMES • CIRCULATORY SYSTEM

Blood Diseases and Disorders

The blood is the supply line to and from every part of the body. Disorders and diseases often cause changes in the blood, so blood tests are important for finding out what is wrong with a person. The blood itself has a range of disorders, which can be serious unless they are treated.

Red blood cells

Red blood cells, or erythrocytes, carry oxygen around the body. A disorder that reduces the number of red blood cells and stops them from carrying oxygen efficiently is called anemia. Anemia may be the result of an insufficient diet, or the body may not be using vitamins or minerals efficiently. Sometimes, the bone marrow may produce abnormal red blood cells or it may not produce enough red cells. Red cells may be dying off faster than they can be replaced or may be lost through bleeding. In the condition called polycythemia, too many red blood cells are produced, making the blood thick and sluggish.

Diseases that affect blood clotting

Normally, the blood clots to stop bleeding. Two blood disorders, hemophilia and purpura, stop this process. Hemophilia is an inherited disease in which the body does not make a blood-clotting factor. In purpura, tiny bruises and bleeding spots appear on the body as the blood, containing too few platelets, bleeds into the skin and joints. Platelets are cell fragments that help the blood-clotting process. Purpura can be caused by viruses, bone marrow diseases, and drug treatments; by platelets that are not working normally because of allergies or scurvy; or by fragile capillaries.

White blood cells

The most serious blood disorder is leukemia, in which the bone marrow or lymphatic system produces large numbers of abnormal white cells. Infections such as infectious mononucleosis cause an overproduction of white cells, a condition known as leukocytosis. Allergies can also result in the overproduction of white cells. Tuberculosis, typhoid, and some virus infections can lead to too few white cells; that can also be a side effect of drugs and radiation treatment.

Q & A

Can stress and strain cause anemia? I'm in high school and have an after-school job, and I seem to be tired all the time.

Anemia cannot be caused by emotional problems alone; there is always an organic basis. Chronic depression, for example, may be accompanied by a poor diet. That may lead to anemia through vitamin and iron deficiency. It is best to discuss your tiredness with your doctor. You may just need a break from your normal routine.

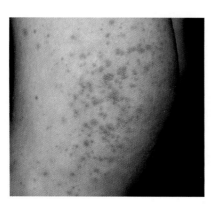

These red-purple spots on the skin are a sign of a condition called purpura. The blood contains too few platelets and therefore bleeds into the surrounding skin and joints.

SEE ALSO

ANEMIA • BLOOD • CIRCULATORY SYSTEM • HEMOPHILIA • IMMUNE SYSTEM • LEUKEMIA • LYMPHATIC SYSTEM

Body Systems

The organs of the body are major units such as the heart, lungs, stomach, liver, kidneys, skeleton, and brain. Each organ is made of tissues, which in turn are made of cells. The cells are complex collections of cell organs (organelles) bathed in a chemical-rich fluid. Each cell contains deoxyribonucleic acid (DNA), which incorporates the genes that determine the characteristics, such as skin and eye color, that children inherit from their parents.

There are several main types of tissues, and each organ contains at least one kind of tissue. Epithelial tissues, for example, are sheets of tissues that cover or line the organs of the body. Epithelial tissues include the skin, which covers the outside of the body.

Connective tissues are those that connect or fill out the structures of the body. They include ligaments and tendons.

Skeletal tissues include all the bones of the skeleton and the soft gristle known as cartilage. Muscle tissues enable the body and its component parts to move and work.

Nervous tissue is the communication network of the body, linking all the parts and carrying messages to and from the brain.

Q & A

Can people's state of mind really affect their immune system and make them prone to illness?

Yes. Current medical thinking holds that the interaction of the mind and all body systems is so intimate and interdependent that hardly anything can happen in one area without affecting another. This certainly holds true for the emotions and the immune system. There is a discipline called psychoneuroimmunology that studies this relationship.

What is it about the "funny bone" that causes such a strange and painful sensation if I hit it?

This sensation concerns the ulnar nerve, which passes behind the elbow and into the forearm. A slight knock here can cause a volley of signals in the nerve's sensory fibers, which can be excruciatingly painful.

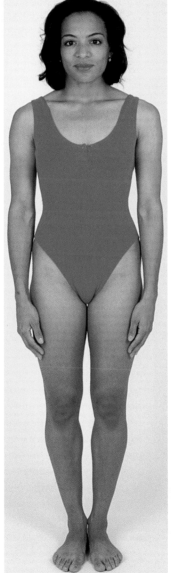

Right: The human body consists of a number of systems, each with its own job to do, yet all working together as a unit.

Far right: Muscle tissue consists of fibers that contract. Epithelial tissue lines and covers the surface of internal organs.

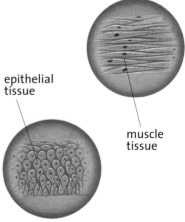

epithelial tissue

muscle tissue

The skeletal system

The skeleton, or skeletal system, is the framework that supports the body. The bones that form the skeleton are linked by flexible joints so that the body can bend and move. The bones are held in place at the joints by bands of tissue called ligaments.

The skeleton is made mostly of bone. While a baby is in the uterus (womb), however, its skeleton is made of a softer, more flexible substance called cartilage. As a child grows, the cartilage is gradually replaced by hard bone. Adults still have cartilage in the lower part of the nose and ears, at the ends of long bones, and between the front ends of the ribs and the breastbone.

The muscles that enable a person to move make up most of the body's flesh. Many muscles, known as skeletal or voluntary muscles, are attached to the bones by cordlike tissues called tendons. These muscles are stimulated by messages from the brain that are carried along the nerves. As a result, muscle movement can be controlled. Other muscles, known as smooth or involuntary muscles, work automatically. They include the muscles of the digestive system and the heart. Heart muscles have the power to contract spontaneously and rhythmically.

The circulatory system

The heart is a pump that drives the blood around the body. Together, the heart and blood make the circulatory system. Blood is used to carry food and oxygen to all the cells of the body and to take away their waste products. The blood flows through a complicated network of tubes, known as the blood vessels, which forms the body's plumbing system. This pipeline system of vessels is extremely long; in a full-grown man, it can total more than 60,000 miles (97,000 km). The system carries about 10 pints (4.7 l) of blood. The blood picks up oxygen from the lungs and is then pumped through the biggest blood vessels, known as the arteries, to all parts of the body. The arteries divide into smaller blood vessels, called arterioles. From there, the blood flows through fine tubes called capillaries to all the body's tissues. The capillaries distribute oxygen and other nutrients to the tissues and collect waste products. The blood then flows back to the heart through a series of medium-size tubes, known as the veins. Blood is returned to the lungs, where it gets rid of carbon dioxide and picks up fresh oxygen.

The immune system

All around are bacteria and viruses that can make people ill. The body's immune system helps protect people against disease. The first barrier in the immune system is provided by the skin.

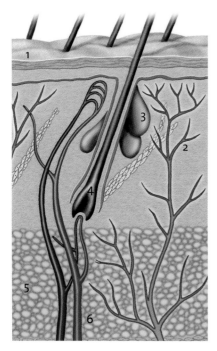

Skin is a kind of epithelial tissue that covers the surface of the body. The surface that can be seen is made of dead cells (1). Below is living tissue containing nerve cells (2), sweat glands (3), hair follicles (4), fat cells (5), and blood vessels (6).

Below left: The skeleton is made of hard, living bone tissue. The bones are hinged at joints. The knee joint allows up-and-down, but not sideways, movement. The ball-and-socket hip joint allows the thigh bone to rotate. The joints between the bones of the toes are highly flexible.

Below middle: The power to move the bones is provided by muscles. A single muscle acts not alone, but with one or more other muscles. When a muscle contracts, it pulls on a bone; its opposing muscle relaxes to let the bone move.

Below right: Blood supply is vital to bones, muscles, and all the other tissues. Blood flows through blood vessels, carrying food and oxygen to the cells and waste materials away from them.

However, germs can enter through wounds or be injected by insects such as mosquitoes. Germs can also enter the lungs through breathing if they are not trapped and expelled in the mucous lining of the respiratory system. Once inside the body, germs encounter white cells in the blood, which attack and kill them with the aid of antibodies. If germs are swallowed, acids in the digestive system help destroy them. If the immune system breaks down, the consequences are serious.

The respiratory system

The organs of the respiratory system consist of the mouth and nose, trachea (windpipe), and lungs. Just as the heart is a pump for the blood, the muscles between the ribs and the diaphragm act as pumps for air, contracting to increase the volume of the chest so that air is drawn into the lungs. Like the heart, this mechanism works automatically, pulling in fresh air, rich in oxygen, and expelling waste air that contains carbon dioxide. Unlike the heart, the lungs are not completely automatic.

Oxygen absorbed from the air is used by the body to convert food into energy. The converted food is carried to the cells by the

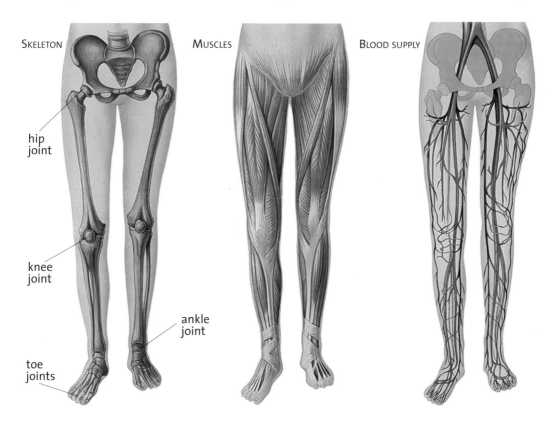

SKELETON   MUSCLES   BLOOD SUPPLY

hip joint

knee joint

ankle joint

toe joints

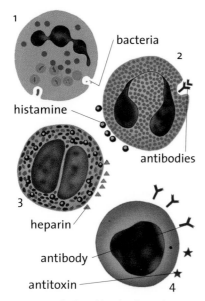

A variety of white blood cells performing their various jobs: swallowing bacteria (1); reacting to antibodies and histamine (2); releasing heparin to stop blood from clotting (3); and releasing antitoxin to neutralize antibodies (4).

blood. In the cells, waste carbon dioxide gas is picked up by the blood and returned to the heart. It is then pumped to the lungs and expelled from the body. This process is called respiration.

Breathing is known as external respiration. Air is drawn in through the nose and filtered to get rid of harmful substances such as dust and bacteria. As air goes down through the trachea to the lungs, it is warmed and moistened.

The trachea divides into two smaller pipes called bronchi, located inside the lungs. In turn, the bronchi split into a network of smaller tubes called bronchioles. The bronchioles branch into tiny sacs, called alveoli, where oxygen is delivered to the blood and carbon dioxide is returned.

The digestive system
Food and drink are the body's fuels and the raw materials from which the body can replace or repair worn-out and damaged cells. Before the blood can take these supplies to the cells, they must be broken down into a form in which they can be used. This process is called digestion. Digestion begins in the mouth when the food is chewed to break it into small pieces before swallowing. The saliva in the mouth is the first of many powerful substances that act on the food. From the mouth, the food passes down a long tube, called the esophagus, to the stomach. Muscles in the stomach wall knead the food to soften it further, and chemicals called gastric juices act by breaking down proteins.

The respiratory system consists of the nose (1), mouth (2), trachea, or windpipe (3), and lungs (4). During breathing, most of the work is done by the diaphragm (5), a large sheet of muscle that lies below the lungs. The lungs are protected by the rib cage (6).

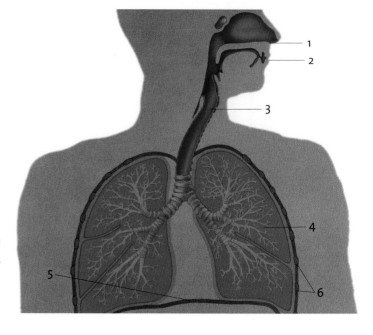

From the stomach, the partly digested, semiliquid food passes into the intestines. First, it enters the small intestine, a coiled tube around 20 feet (6 m) long, where the food is finally broken down into the form of fats, amino acids, and glucose. In this state, the food is absorbed into the bloodstream through tiny projections, called villi, on the walls of the small intestine.

From the small intestine, what remains of the food passes into the large intestine. Most of the useful substances have by now been absorbed into the blood. The remainder is waste, including roughage, such as vegetable fibers and seeds, living and dead bacteria, dead cells from the walls of the upper part of the digestive system, waste gastric juices, and water. As this waste material passes through the large intestine, most of the water is removed, and the solid waste is eventually expelled from the body through the rectum and anus in the form of feces.

The urinary system

Waste substances that have been broken down in the body are carried by the blood to the kidneys. They remove waste materials and surplus water from the blood, producing a liquid known as urine. Urine then passes, via the ureters, into the bladder, where it is stored. Once there is a sufficient buildup of urine in the bladder, the body is stimulated to excrete it via the urethra.

The glandular system

The glands are the body's factories, making substances that the body needs and processing waste products. There are two kinds of glands: exocrine and endocrine. Exocrine glands secrete their products into ducts, or channels, that carry them inside or outside the body. Exocrine glands include the liver, tear ducts, salivary and digestive glands, and mammary glands (which produce milk). Endocrine glands are ductless; they secrete hormones straight into the blood. They include the pituitary gland, thyroid gland, and adrenal glands. These hormones control growth, reproduction, the rate at which food is burned, the level of blood sugar, and the body's emergency response to fear and stress. Hormones can also be released by other organs, such as the brain, the kidneys, and the placenta, or fetal life-support system, in a pregnant woman.

The nervous system and senses

The nervous system is the control mechanism for the body. Its central switchboard is the central nervous system (CNS), which comprises the brain and the spinal cord. The central nervous system receives and interprets messages from the rest of the body and sends instructions through nerves to the muscles,

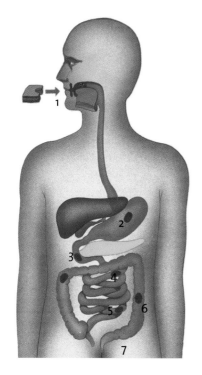

This diagram shows the digestion of a cheese sandwich. Proteins, fats, and carbohydrates are broken down into small molecules and absorbed into the blood to be used by the cells. Digestive juices in the mouth (1) act on the food, which passes into the stomach (2) and on to the duodenum, the first part of the small intestine (3), and the jejunum (4) and ileim (5). The broken-down food passes through the intestine walls. Waste matter enters the large intestine (6), where water passes into the blood. Finally, waste passes through the rectum (7), which is the end of the intestine, and out of the body.

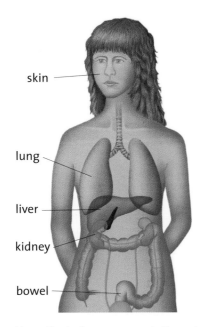

skin

lung

liver

kidney

bowel

Above: The body removes waste through the skin (water and salt), lungs (carbon dioxide), liver and gallbladder (bile), kidneys (urea), and bowel (feces).

Right: Glands regulate metabolism, aid digestion, produce sweat, and control growth and reproduction.

Far right: The central nervous system consists of the brain and spinal cord, from which pairs of nerves radiate all over the body to form the peripheral nervous system.

Below: The female reproductive system consists of the ovaries, fallopian tubes, uterus (womb), and vagina.

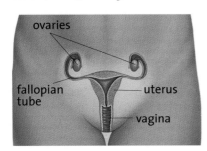

ovaries

fallopian tube

uterus

vagina

organs, and glands. The nerves are like telegraph wires, along which the electrical messages travel to and from the body's senses. The senses link the brain with the world outside the body.

Humans are sensitive to sights, sounds, tastes, smells, touch, heat, cold, hunger, thirst, tiredness, and pain. The eyes are the organs of sight. The ears hear sounds and help people maintain their balance. Taste and smell are linked to the digestive system. Aromas trigger the saliva needed for digestion. People's senses tell them when the body needs to have food or rest, when it needs to avoid danger, or when there is a malfunction or pain.

The reproductive systems

A man's and woman's reproductive organs enable a male sperm to fertilize a female egg to produce a baby. Women have ovaries, which produce ova (egg cells). Once a month, one or more ova pass down the fallopian tubes to the uterus, where the egg can be fertilized. Men have testes, glands that produce sperm cells.

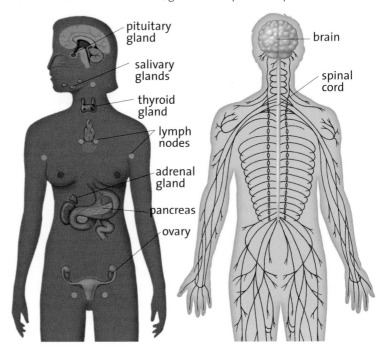

pituitary gland

salivary glands

thyroid gland

lymph nodes

adrenal gland

pancreas

ovary

brain

spinal cord

SEE ALSO

CIRCULATORY SYSTEM • DIGESTIVE SYSTEM • GLANDS • IMMUNE SYSTEM • LYMPHATIC SYSTEM • NERVOUS SYSTEM • RESPIRATORY SYSTEM • SKELETAL SYSTEM • URINARY SYSTEM

Bone

Bones make up the skeleton, or skeletal system, the rigid frame that supports the body. There are 206 bones in all, which not only hold up the body, but allow it to move. The bones are connected at joints and are moved by pairs of muscles attached to them by ligaments. Most bones do not form until after birth. The skeleton of the fetus consists largely of soft, pliable cartilage. As the child grows, the cartilage gradually hardens into bone.

Bone is made of two types of tissues, called compact and cancellous. Compact tissue is the hard outer part of the bone; cancellous tissue is the spongy part on the inside. Most of the bony tissue's weight consists of the minerals calcium and phosphorus and a fibrous material called collagen. The insides of most bones are hollow, filled with a soft substance called bone marrow, where blood cells are made.

There are several different kinds of bones, with varying functions. Long bones (forming the limbs in the arms and legs) and short bones (present for example at the wrist and ankle) are basically cylinders of hard bone with marrow inside. Flat bones consist of a sandwich of hard bone with a spongy layer in the middle. Some bones, such as the skull and the rib cage, provide protection for the internal organs. Other bones, such as the shoulder blades, provide a large surface area to which muscles are attached. Irregular bones include the vertebrae (spine bones) and facial bones.

Q & A

Why do people suffer so much from backache?

When humans began walking on two legs, they used the same skeleton that had evolved for four-legged animals. So while humans are well adapted horizontally, vertical postures create strain in the lower back.

rings of mineral salts and collagen fibers

bone cell

blood vessel

strong, hard bone

marrow

light, spongy bone

CROSS SECTION OF LONG BONE IN ARM

flat bone (skull)

vertebra (spine bone)

humerus (arm)

short bones (foot)

There are several different kinds of bones: flat bones such as the skull bones, irregular bones such as vertebrae (spine bones), short bones as in the hands and feet, and long bones as in the arms and legs. A long bone is a cylinder of hard bone. Inside is spongy bone, and inside that is bone marrow. New blood cells are made in the marrow.

SEE ALSO

BONE DISEASES AND DISORDERS •
SKELETAL SYSTEM

Bone Diseases and Disorders

The most common problem with bones is breakage, or fractures. However, bones are good at healing themselves, and if a bone is set in the right position, a fracture may repair itself so well that there are no obvious signs that the break ever happened. Most broken bones can be diagnosed only by X-ray, unless the fracture is open with the bone protruding through the skin.

Osteomyelitis and bone cancer

Infections of the bone are called osteomyelitis (*osteo* means "bone"). Osteomyelitis is far more common in children than in adults. The infection may be carried to the bone by the blood from an infection elsewhere in the body; sometimes, bacteria enter an injured bone. The infected area becomes inflamed, and pus forms. The bone around the infection becomes painful and tender, and the patient has a fever. Within a day or so, the area is swollen. However, antibiotics can quickly cure the infection.

Tumors in the bone are usually formed when the blood carries malignant (cancerous) cells there from tumors in other places, such as the breast, prostate, and lung. These secondary tumors usually cannot be cured, but they can be controlled by hormones, drugs, and radiation treatment. Tumors that begin in the bone—primary tumors—are less common, but when they do occur, they tend to affect young people rather than adults.

Rickets, osteomalacia, and osteoporosis

Until recent times, many children did not get enough vitamin D in their diet. That lack caused rickets, a disease in which the bones soften and bend; in particular, the leg bones buckle under the body's weight. The skull may also be misshapen. Vitamin D deficiency can also result from lack of sunlight.

Sometimes adults lack vitamin D, or their body cannot use it properly. That condition results in osteomalacia, a softening of the bone. The long bones bend, and the skeleton becomes deformed. Massive doses of vitamin D help cure this problem.

As people get older, their bones become more porous and spongy from loss of collagen and minerals. This condition is called osteoporosis and is most likely to occur in elderly women. Their bones become thin and weak and break easily. People with osteoporosis may become round-shouldered and have back pain. Exercise, calcium, and vitamin D will help prevent osteoporosis.

This deformed leg belongs to a person with Paget's disease, which causes irregular bone growth. In this condition, new bone is formed unusually quickly but is thin and weak. Paget's disease particularly affects the skull, pelvis, and leg bones, which can become badly deformed and may ache all the time.

> **SEE ALSO**
>
> BONE • CANCER • FRACTURES AND DISLOCATIONS • NUTRITIONAL DISEASES • OSTEOPOROSIS • RICKETS

Botulism

Botulism is a rare but deadly food poisoning. It is caused by the bacterium *Clostridium botulinum*. This microorganism grows and produces its toxin (poison) in places where there is no oxygen, such as in canned food and foods sealed in airtight packs. Foods that may be contaminated include home-canned goods, sausages, meat products, seafood, and canned vegetables. The bacteria are harmless on fresh food, but their spores germinate and produce their toxin on food left around at room temperature. Spores are the bacteria's reproductive bodies that can develop into new individual organisms. These spores can survive boiling and can be killed only by cooking food in a pressure cooker at 250°F (120°C) for at least 15 minutes.

Q & A

My mother insists on using a pressure cooker for canning vegetables. Is that necessary?

Commercial canners plan their sterilization programs to kill botulism spores, so if you can vegetables at home, pressure cooking is advisable.

Can you get botulism from dented cans of food?

No, but dented cans present problems with other types of bacterial poisoning, so it is wise to choose undented food cans.

Home-canned food should be prepared properly to avoid the risk of poisoning with Clostridium botulinum.

Processing foods

Home-canned foods should be sterilized by pressure cooking after the canning process, and unless the canning process was inadequate, the food is then safe. As a precaution, home-canned food should be boiled briskly for 15 to 20 minutes to destroy any toxins that may be present.

Commercial food processors are well aware of the risk of botulism, and they design their food preservation procedures to prevent it. Outbreaks of botulism have almost always been associated with home-preserved foods such as canned vegetables rather than with commercial foods.

Symptoms and treatment of botulism

Symptoms of botulism develop 18 hours or more after the affected food is eaten. They include dizziness, double vision, headache, nausea, vomiting, diarrhea, and increasing paralysis. Once the paralysis affects the lungs and the ability to breathe is lost, the person dies. Victims can be treated with antitoxins, but around 30 percent still die. However, patients who survive the initial paralysis will make a full recovery. Even the tiniest amounts of the toxin can cause severe damage. The toxin is so potent that just 0.5 pound (225 g) could kill everyone in the world. However, cases of botulism are extremely rare, and commonsense cooking prevents the spread of the disease.

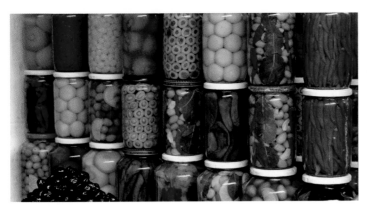

SEE ALSO

BACTERIA • SALMONELLA

Brain

The human brain is more sophisticated than the largest computer, yet it fits neatly in the skull. It contains around 10 billion nerve cells, or neurons, and directs and monitors all the body's activities, even when a person is asleep or unconscious. The brain is the center of a network of nerves that runs through the body.

Together with the spinal cord, the brain makes up the central nervous system. The central nervous system controls the whole body by means of messages that are continually passing up and down its nerve pathways. The messages are transmitted by minute electrical impulses. The brain receives information about the world outside the body through the sense organs: the eyes, ears, nose, tongue, and sense receptors in the skin. Once the brain has decided what action to take, it sends instructions down the nerves to the relevant parts of the body.

Parts of the brain

Brain cells form a mass of soft, jellylike tissue, called gray and white matter. White matter surrounds gray matter in the spinal cord and brain stem; gray matter surrounds white matter in the upper part of the brain. Gray matter consists of neurons, the white area of nerve fibers, which connect to other parts of the brain. The brain cells are surrounded by three layers of protective membranes, called meninges.

The brain is divided into the hindbrain, midbrain, and forebrain. Each region contains sections that have specific functions. The hindbrain contains the cerebellum, which controls balance and coordination. Part of it, the brain stem, connects the brain with the spinal cord. All the functions of the left side of the body are controlled by the right side of the brain, and vice versa.

Q & A

Why do old memories flood back when I smell certain aromas?

The connections in the brain for the sense of smell are closely linked with the circuits of the limbic system, which deals with emotions. Smells can thus take on emotional significance, whether pleasant or unpleasant. Events associated with strong emotions are often firmly stored in memory, so the smell itself can bring them back.

My memory is poor. Is there anything I can do to improve it?

It is not your memory that needs improving; it is the way you try to remember things. To make sure that something is firmly stored, it must be presented in a way that arouses the most links with other knowledge already in the brain. For example, written directions are more difficult to recall than a map. A humorous map is even easier to recall, because emotions are involved.

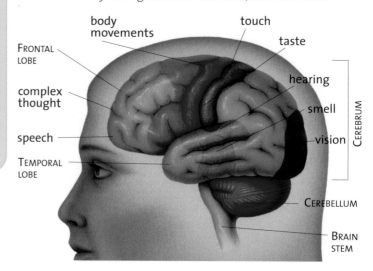

The brain consists of the brain stem, cerebellum, and cerebrum. Specific body activities are controlled by certain areas within the brain.

body movements

touch

taste

FRONTAL LOBE

hearing

complex thought

smell

speech

vision

TEMPORAL LOBE

CEREBRUM

CEREBELLUM

BRAIN STEM

A cross section of the brain, showing the cerebral cortex (gray matter) and cerebrum (white matter). The two hemispheres of the brain are joined at the bottom by a thick bundle of nerve fibers called the corpus callosum. The brain stem links the brain to the spinal cord and contains structures that control heart rate, breathing, blood pressure, and other vital bodily activities that the body does not control consciously. The thalamus is surrounded by the limbic system, which is concerned chiefly with memory, learning, and emotions. The cerebellum is in charge of balance and coordination.

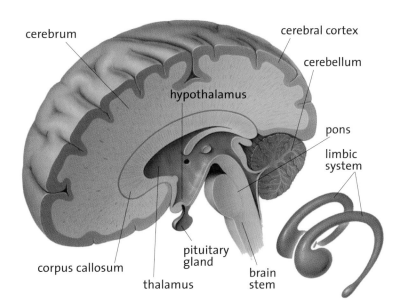

The brain stem also controls other activities such as heart rate, blood pressure, swallowing, coughing, breathing, and consciousness. Eye movements are controlled in the midbrain. The forebrain is divided into four lobes, each with different functions. It contains the thalamus, a sort of relay station for incoming information; the hypothalamus, which controls bodily functions such as hunger, thirst, and sleep, as well as regulating body temperature; and the limbic system, where emotions such as rage, excitement, and fear are controlled.

Memory and learning

No particular area of the brain stores all memories. Memory is not a bank of information but a process. When an electrical message passes through a brain cell, the cell changes physically. As a person learns something, new electrical pathways are set up that enable the new fact to be remembered for a few minutes. To remember something for a longer period of time, closer attention has to be paid to it and it has to be gone over repeatedly. As a result, a permanent physical change takes place in the brain cells, which makes the memory a part of the person. Sometimes a special trigger is needed to recall a memory, and some memories seem to be buried so deep that they are lost.

> **SEE ALSO**
> BODY SYSTEMS • BRAIN DAMAGE AND DISORDERS • EYE AND SIGHT • NERVOUS SYSTEM • SPINAL COLUMN

Brain Damage and Disorders

Q & A

I've heard that brain damage is less serious in children than in adults. How can this be?

Any substantial brain damage is tragic, but a child's brain is less rigid than an adult's, so other parts of the brain can take over the function of a damaged section more easily. For example, speech loss (or aphasia) after brain injury is usually not permanent in extremely young children.

I enjoy watching boxing fights with my father, but what does he mean when he says that a boxer is punch-drunk?

Some of the repeated blows to the head that boxers suffer cause tiny hemorrhages, or bleeding, in various parts of the brain. Over the years, the brain damage mounts up. That causes the boxers to slur their speech and makes them unsteady on their feet. In addition, a boxer's mind may become a little less sharp, with some confusion and loss of memory. All these symptoms make the boxers appear drunk.

The brain is a delicate structure. It is well protected by the skull, but even so, it can be damaged. For example, brain damage may occur as a baby develops in the mother's uterus (womb) or during birth. It can also be caused by an illness or infection. It may be the result of an accident. Anything that interrupts the normal blood supply to the brain, and so starves it of oxygen, can damage it, sometimes permanently.

The results of brain damage depend on the area of the brain that is unable to work properly. The functions normally controlled by that part of the brain will be partly or completely lost. That may mean loss of movement in part of the body or loss of speech, sight, or understanding. However, other areas of the brain may be able to take over at least some of the work of the damaged cells. A key factor is how badly the brain stem has been damaged. All the body's messages to the brain pass through the brain stem, and it contains areas that help control breathing and blood circulation. If the brain stem has been too badly damaged, the patient will die.

Some children with brain damage suffer from cerebral palsy, in which one or more of their limbs may be paralyzed or out of control. Depending on how much of the brain has been damaged, the child may or may not have a mental handicap, although many people with cerebral palsy are of average intelligence. A baby's brain may also be damaged by hydrocephalus, the presence of excess fluid on the brain.

Injuries to the brain

A common cause of injury to the brain is a blow to the head. A hard blow can shake the brain violently, causing dizziness and possibly loss of consciousness. Although patients may lose their memory and have headaches for a time after the blow, the brain generally heals with no aftereffects. If the brain has been bruised, some of the cells and fibers will be damaged.

People such as boxers who have had a number of concussions may eventually develop slurred speech, unsteady movements, and a confused mind as the result of so many small injuries.

Some blows are so hard that the bones of the skull are fractured (broken). In itself, that fracturing is not serious, and the bones heal well. However, if the broken part of the skull bone presses down onto the brain, it can damage the area underneath. An operation to lift away the bone fragments must then be done. Injuries from sharp objects that pierce the skull are especially dangerous, because they expose the brain to infection. Death commonly results from uncontrolled bleeding within the skull that compresses the brain or forces it downward.

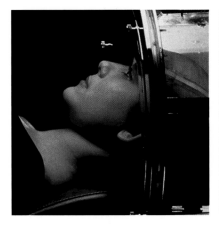

Radioisotope scanners (left) are used to diagnose brain damage or disease. A radioactive substance is injected into the brain before a computed tomography (CT) scan is carried out. That helps make any abnormalities visible. The scanner is linked to a computer that shows the brain in horizontal layers. This scan (right) reveals a serious tumor, shown in the concentrated area of red. A technique called magnetic resonance imaging (MRI) is also used to detect tumors and damaged tissue.

Strokes and tumors

The cells in the brain soon die if they do not receive a sufficient supply of oxygen. That happens during a stroke, when the blood supply to part of the brain is cut off completely. Signs of resultant brain damage include total loss of movement in part of the body, usually on one side only, and a loss of speech. However, many people recover almost completely from a stroke.

Leaking blood in the skull and abnormal growths called tumors cause pressure on the brain tissues. Symptoms include severe headaches, nausea, drowsiness, and confusion. Some tumors, both malignant (cancerous) and benign (noncancerous), can be removed, and others can be shrunk by radiation or drug treatment. Recovery depends on where the tumor is and if it has damaged the surrounding brain tissue.

Brain diseases

Infections of the brain cause encephalitis (inflammation of the brain), and infections of the membranes that surround the brain cause meningitis. The brain may also be affected by an illness called multiple sclerosis, in which the insulating material around the nerves of the brain and spinal cord is damaged. In another condition, epilepsy, unusual electrical signals in the brain cells may cause loss of consciousness.

As a person grows old, the cells in the brain begin to die. Sometimes that happens unusually early and quickly, causing various diseases. For example, Parkinson's disease results in trembling fingers, slowness of movement, stiff muscles, and an expressionless face; Huntington's disease causes uncontrollable, jerking movements of the limbs, head, and tongue. Among other symptoms, Alzheimer's disease usually leads to increasing confusion, loss of memory, loss of intellect, and eventual

MAIN BRAIN DISEASES

Symptoms	Cause	Comments
Dementia Loss of recent memory, patient is easily confused, gradual loss of intellectual function; at the end, speech impairment and incontinence	Alzheimer's disease, degeneration of cells of cerebral cortex, tumors, alcoholism, vitamin deficiency, and chronic infection	Mostly in older people; some causes treatable, so must be investigated
Encephalitis Fever, drowsiness, and speech impairment	Virus infection of brain itself	Needs early treatment; may permanently damage the brain
Epilepsy Convulsive seizures, which may be major, causing unconsciousness and jerking of the limbs; or minor, with odd sensations and lapses of unconsciousness; or confined to jerking of the limbs	Electrical storm in brain due to abnormal excitability of some neurons; may come on later in life and be caused by tumors or brain injury or have no known cause	Treatment will control seizures; may need special tests to establish cause
Meningitis Headache, fever, general illness, stiff neck, rash, intolerance of light	Infection of brain's surrounding membranes, or meninges, by bacteria or viruses	If bacterial, requires urgent hospital treatment with large doses of antibiotics; viral meningitis requires no treatment
Multiple sclerosis Sudden blurring of vision, unsteadiness, or loss of use of a limb; patient tends to recover and then relapse; gradual increase in disability over the years	Patchy degeneration of insulating material around nerves in brain and spinal cord; basic cause remains unknown	Usually affects younger people; wide variation in disability; some will lead nearly normal lives for many years; others will gradually deteriorate
Parkinson's disease Stiff muscles, difficulty starting movements, expressionless face, trembling fingers	Degeneration of cells deep in the base of the brain	Treatment with the drug levodopa (L-dopa) helps control the symptoms
Stroke Sudden weakness or loss of use and numbness of one side of body and/or loss of speech or other brain function	Blood vessel blockage, known as cerebral thrombosis, or rupture of blood vessels (with cerebral hemorrhage), referred to as a cerebrovascular accident (CVA)	Usually affects older people; disability always worse at onset, gradually improving to some degree

speech impairment and incontinence. Some of the symptoms of Alzheimer's disease can be caused by alcoholism and vitamin deficiency, because the brain can be affected by substances carried in the bloodstream.

SEE ALSO

ALZHEIMER'S DISEASE • BRAIN • CANCER • CEREBRAL PALSY • ENCEPHALITIS • EPILEPSY • HUNTINGTON'S DISEASE • MENINGITIS • MULTIPLE SCLEROSIS • NERVOUS SYSTEM • NERVOUS SYSTEM DISORDERS • PARKINSON'S DISEASE • STROKE

Bronchitis

Bronchitis is an inflammation of the mucous membrane that lines the bronchi (singular, bronchus), which are the main airways of the lungs. Bronchitis may be caused by a bacterium or a virus, which is often spread to the bronchi from a cold or throat infection. These infections usually clear up fairly rapidly and are known as acute bronchitis. Many people have acute bronchitis from time to time. People who smoke heavily or breathe in harmful fumes, dust, or other particles may have chronic, or long-lasting, bronchitis.

Q & A

My uncle has difficulty in walking very far. He blames this on his bronchitis. Is he right?

Yes. The worse the bronchitis, the less exercise the person can tolerate. Doctors divide bronchitis into four stages: one, a slight cough; two, breathlessness on exertion; three, breathlessness so severe that the patient is unable to leave the house; and four, breathlessness so severe that the patient cannot converse normally.

Symptoms and treatments

The first symptoms of acute bronchitis are a head cold, a runny nose, fever and chills, aching muscles, and sometimes back pain. These symptoms are followed by a persistent cough, which is dry at first but later produces phlegm. The patient may feel wheezy and breathless. A spasmodic cough with phlegm is the main symptom of chronic bronchitis. Some people who suffer from chronic bronchitis are overweight and have a bluish tinge to the lips. The blueness is caused by a lack of oxygen in the blood. Exercise makes these people short of breath. If the infection damages the smaller airways (bronchioles) and air sacs (alveoli) in the lungs, they will have emphysema. They will be short of breath all the time and tend to be underweight. That condition can eventually lead to respiratory failure and heart failure.

The best treatment for acute bronchitis is to rest in bed in a warm room. Aspirin brings down a high temperature, and medicines can relieve the cough. The doctor may give antibiotics if the infection has been caused by bacteria. Acute bronchitis usually clears up in a week. Chronic bronchitis is more difficult; bronchodilator drugs widen the airways, and breathing exercises may help the condition. Anyone with bronchitis should stop smoking, avoid polluted air, and if possible live in a warm, dry place.

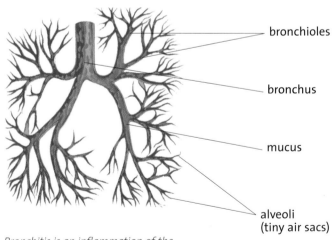

bronchioles

bronchus

mucus

alveoli
(tiny air sacs)

Bronchitis is an inflammation of the bronchi (main air tubes in the lungs), which causes irritation and persistent coughing. These result in an increased production of mucus, which blocks the alveoli and causes shortness of breath.

SEE ALSO

LUNG • LUNG DISEASES AND DISORDERS • RESPIRATORY SYSTEM • RESPIRATORY SYSTEM DISEASES AND DISORDERS

Burns

Burns are among the most common and most serious accidents, injuring or even killing countless people every day. The most obvious cause of burns is fire, but they can also be caused by touching any hot object (such as an electric iron) or by scalding. Scalding is a form of injury or damage to tissue resulting from being in close contact with a hot liquid (usually boiling water or a hot cup of coffee) or vapor (such as steam). Contact with a corrosive chemical, harsh friction, and electric shock can also cause burns. Excessive exposure to sun can cause serious burns. Young children and old people are particularly at risk of burns.

Depth of burns

Burns may be superficial or deep and are divided into four types. In a first-degree burn, only the outer layer of the skin and perhaps a little of the tissue beneath are damaged. This type of burn is not serious, because the basic structure of the skin, including the hair follicles and sweat glands, is not damaged. The skin becomes red and painful but does not blister. These burns include mild sunburn and accidental burns from, say, hot pans. The deeper layers of the skin tissue are not damaged, so first-degree burns heal quickly with no scars.

In second-degree burns, the damage goes through to the thicker layers of the skin and causes the formation of blisters. All but the deepest cells, hair follicles, and glands are destroyed. Healing takes several months, and the new skin that forms is likely to be rougher and less elastic than before.

In a third-degree burn, the whole thickness of the skin, including hair follicles and sweat glands, is destroyed. If the burn is deep, muscles and bone may be exposed. There is nothing from which new skin can grow, except at the very edges of the burn. Therefore, healing is extremely slow and uncertain.

In a fourth-degree burn, all the tissue beneath the skin is burned and destroyed, including the muscles, tendons, ligaments, and bones. Skin grafting is usually needed to close the burned areas. Fourth-degree burns often result in the loss of hands and feet and are sometimes fatal.

After a severe burn, plasma (the colorless liquid part of blood) oozes out from the damaged blood vessels in the surrounding area. When people lose plasma, they develop a condition known as shock. The coating of plasma on the burned area also makes it more likely to be infected by bacteria. The larger the area of the burn, the more serious these problems are. Any second-degree burn covering an area greater than 3 inches (7.5 cm) square and all third- and fourth-degree burns need medical treatment as soon as possible.

Q & A

Should I see a doctor if I get sunburned on vacation?

Yes, if the sunburn is severe or is combined with sunstroke. You should take care to get used to the sun gradually if you are fair-skinned or unused to strong sunlight. You can even get sunburned on ice and snow on a mountaintop, owing to the reflected ultraviolet radiation from the sun. Also, if you are on a beach, the sun is much more intense near the sea and sand than elsewhere.

FIRST AID FOR BURNS

Minor burns can be treated at home. For 10 minutes or until the pain stops, the area should be cooled by holding it under cold running water, immersing it in cold water, or covering it with a frequently changed cloth soaked in cold water. Cream or lotion should never be applied to a burn. Any blisters that form over a burn should not be burst but covered with a sterile, nonfluffy dressing. If the blisters then burst, the area should be kept scrupulously clean.

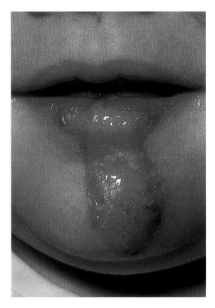

A blistered and infected second-degree burn is the result of this child's having a drink that was far too hot.

Treatment for burns

When fire victims breathe in smoke and fumes, their windpipe and lungs may be damaged or obstructed. If the lungs are swollen and inflamed, the victim may need an emergency operation to insert an artificial tube or may need to be put on a respirator. The other main concern is to combat shock. If patients have burned more than 15 percent of their total body area (10 percent in a child), they need a transfusion of blood or plasma. Antibiotics are given to prevent infection; painkilling drugs are also given.

Skin grafts

A large third- or fourth-degree burn cannot heal on its own, because there is no skin tissue left to regrow. Beneath the damaged tissue is a raw area, and skin grafts are needed to cover it. Skin grafts are pieces of skin (complete with hair follicles and sweat glands) from an undamaged part of the patient's body. The area from which the skin has been taken will heal itself. Skin grafts allow the donor area to regrow, while providing cover for the burned areas. Grafts are pressed onto the burned area and gradually grow and spread to form a new skin surface. This process takes a long time, during which the patient needs skillful nursing to ensure that the burn does not become infected and that the graft grows properly. At the same time, the hospital staff will check that the patient's other organs have not suffered harm

Burns are classified according to the extent of the body they cover and the depth of tissue that is injured. First-degree burns affect only the surface layers. Second-degree burns leave enough skin intact to heal. In third-degree burns, all the skin tissue may be destroyed. In fourth-degree burns, all the tissue beneath the skin is burned and destroyed, including the muscles, tendons, ligaments, and bones.

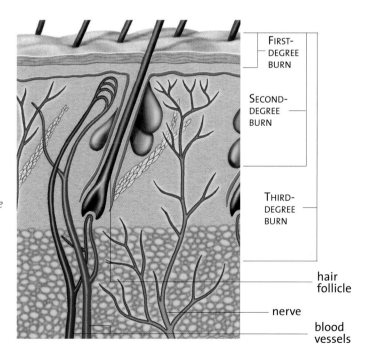

STOP, DROP, AND ROLL

If your clothing catches fire, you must extinguish the fire instantly. The best way to do this is STOP where you are, DROP to the ground, and ROLL out the fire. If someone else's clothes catch fire, you may have to push him or her to the floor. If there is a blanket or rug available, use it to help smother the flames. When the fire is out, COOL the area that is burned with cold water and cover it with a clean, dry cloth. If the burn is severe, get medical help as fast as possible.

The kitchen is the most hazardous room in the house—full of electrical appliances, hot objects, and liquids. Loose mats and clutter on the floor could cause people to fall onto a hot stove. Loose cloths on tables can cause hot food or drinks to spill over people. Electrical cords can be accidentally caught, and frayed ones can cause electric shocks or fires. Gas, cooking oil, and food can all catch fire easily. Find out, before it is too late, the correct way to cope with different types of fires if they do break out.

during the time that the patient was in shock—when the blood supply to various organs would have been reduced. Some hospitals have special burn units with the most advanced equipment and a specially trained staff to take care of burn victims. Recovery depends partly on the area of the body affected and the depth of the burn.

Helping a burn victim

If someone is seriously burned and on fire, any flames should be put out with water (if it is not an electrical fire), the clothing should be doused with water, or the flames should be smothered with a rug or large piece of material. An ambulance should be called immediately. During the wait for medical assistance, the burn should be covered with a cloth soaked in cold water. This cloth should be cooled repeatedly with more cold water. Any clothing that is stuck to the wound should not be removed, but exposed burn areas should be covered with a clean, dry cloth. The victim should lie down and be kept warm.

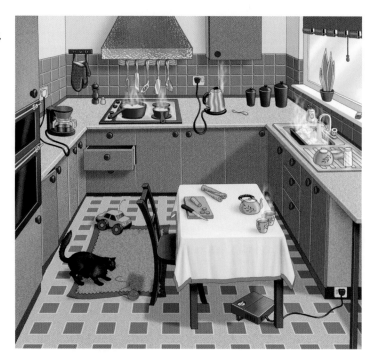

SEE ALSO

ABRASIONS AND CUTS • SKIN • SUNBURN • WOUNDS

Cancer

The body is made up of many different types of cells, such as muscle cells, tissue-forming cells, and blood cells. Each cell grows into its own particular shape. A tissue-forming cell and a muscle cell look completely different, for example. In all parts of the body, cells die off through ordinary wear and tear and are replaced with new ones through cell division. The rate at which new cells are made is controlled by the body so that exactly the right number of new cells is produced to replace those lost.

Cancer is a serious condition in which some of the cells in the body behave abnormally. These malignant (harmful) cells grow and reproduce too quickly. They spread into surrounding tissues and damage them before spreading to other parts of the body. Unless cancer is treated, it can kill, and it is one of the most feared of all diseases. However, treatment for many types of cancers is now so effective that patients have a good chance of being cured, particularly if the cancer is discovered and treated at an early stage.

The spreading of abnormal cells

In cancer, abnormal cells appear that are modified versions of the cells in the tissues around them. These cells grow without the normal controls, reproducing at their own speed and forming a mass of tissue known as a tumor. The abnormal cells invade the surrounding tissues and damage them. What makes cancer so serious is that the cells can spread through the body. Cells break off from the original, or primary, cancer and float in the tissue fluid. These cancerous cells are usually trapped in glands called lymph nodes, which filter out dead cells and infections, and most of the cancer cells will die. Sooner or later, however, one will live

Q & A

My brother has needed a lot of X-rays recently. Can the X-rays give him cancer?

The risk of developing cancer from X-rays is so small as to be virtually insignificant. Doctors are aware of what risk there is and will advise a patient to have an X-ray only if it is absolutely necessary.

My grandfather has cancer. I enjoy being around him, but I'm worried that the cancer might be contagious. Is it possible?

No. There is no risk of catching cancer from a relative or a friend with the disease.

Can cancer ever be hereditary?

Not usually. There are a few cancers that run in families, but they are rare. Only if cancer is particularly common in your family is there any increased risk. If so, take better care of yourself, and report any persistent symptoms to your doctor.

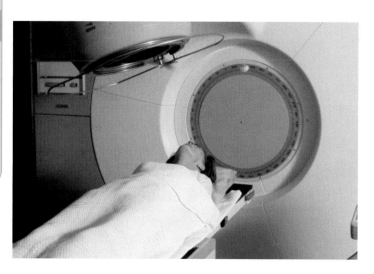

Tumors can be treated with radiotherapy, using a linear accelerator. Only the malignant cells are targeted and killed.

and start to grow in the node, forming what is called a secondary growth. Later, cancer cells are carried through the lymph nodes into the bloodstream. The blood takes the cancer cells to various organs of the body, such as the lungs, liver, bone, and brain, and they may form secondary growths in these organs.

Kinds and causes of cancers

There are more than 100 different kinds of cancers. Those cancers that start in membranes, such as the skin and intestines, are called carcinomas. Those that start in other tissues, such as bone and muscle, are called sarcomas. Carcinomas are far more common than sarcomas. Leukemia is a cancer of the blood. The most common cancers are lung and intestinal cancers. Breast cancer in women and prostate cancer in men are also common.

Doctors do not know what causes cancer cells to form, although many research workers are studying cancer and developing various theories. Experts do know, however, that some substances called carcinogens can trigger cancer. Smoking causes lung cancer, and some workers in the petroleum industry develop skin cancer from the substances they handle. Long exposure to bright sun can also lead to skin cancer. Diet may play a part in cancer of the intestine. Too much radiation can cause cancer. Certain cancers result from viral infection; others result from a fault in the body's immune system, which allows an abnormal cell that should have been destroyed to live and develop into cancer. Certain cancers are linked with hereditary factors. However, no single cause of any cancer has been established, and it seems likely that cancer has many different causes, some of which are unknown.

Oncogenes

An oncogene is one of a number of genes that contribute to cancerous changes in cells. Oncogenes are mutations of normal cell genes and must work together to cause cancer. Similar or identical genes are present in viruses known to cause cancer. If one of the three virus genes known as "gag," "pol," or "env" is replaced by an oncogene, such as "ras," the virus becomes capable of causing cancer.

Treatment for cancer

Cancer treatments aim to kill or remove every cancer cell in the body, so that the cancer cannot spread. Treatment is now often successful, and thousands of people are cured who would have died without modern techniques. A small amount of cancer is

---

PREVENTIVE MEASURES

- Cancer is most common in late middle age. Healthy habits should be developed early in life.
- A balanced diet should be eaten. Smoking and too much alcohol should be avoided.
- Sunburn should be avoided, especially by fair-skinned people.
- Women should check for breast lumps at least once a month. If a lump is found, a doctor should be consulted at once. Mammogram screening is essential.
- Men should check their testicles regularly for lumps.
- Women should have a yearly test for cervical cancer, the second most common cancer in women.
- Any lump, persistent pain, or bleeding should be investigated.

This boy has lymphoma, or cancer of the lymph nodes. The sites of these nodes are marked on his chest. If radiotherapy is not successful, chemotherapy may be needed.

easier to cure than a large amount, so it is important to tell a doctor about any symptoms as soon as possible. If there is a possibility of cancer, special tests are carried out. These tests include examining suspect cells under a microscope, as well as X-ray and scanning tests. If cancer is detected, further tests are carried out to see if the disease has spread to other parts of the body. Cancer is treated by surgery and radiation and with drugs called chemotherapy. Surgery for cancer removes all the cancer cells that can be seen, together with some normal tissue from around the growth to try to ensure that every cancer cell has been removed. Lymph nodes that are close to the cancerous growth are also removed in case cancer cells have lodged in the nodes, and neighboring organs are checked.

Treatment with radiation and with drugs kills cancer cells more readily than healthy body cells, but it can also have unwelcome side effects. Sometimes a combination of treatments is used. Once treatment has been finished, doctors will keep a careful check on the patient just in case the cancer should come back. If cancer is treated early enough, there is a very good chance that the patient will recover completely.

Surgery, radiotherapy, and chemotherapy often result in unpleasant side effects and complications, for which treatment is also necessary. In addition, psychiatric help may be given, especially for patients whose cancer is known to be terminal. Often, people are led into unnecessary suffering by unethical people who promise miracle cures. They should be avoided at all costs. Anyone needing help or advice should contact the American Cancer Society or the National Cancer Institute.

MANAGING BREAST CANCER

A new concept in the treatment of breast cancer and some other types of cancer involves examining the sentinel nodes—a type of lymph node. The sentinel nodes are thought to be the first nodes to be affected by breast cancer or other cancers. Sentinel node biopsy is the identification and removal for examination of the sentinel node. Experts claim that examination of this single lymph node can accurately predict in 97.5 percent of cases whether or not a breast cancer has spread to the lymph nodes and caused a secondary cancer. In the case of breast cancers, sentinel nodes in the armpit can be examined prior to surgery.

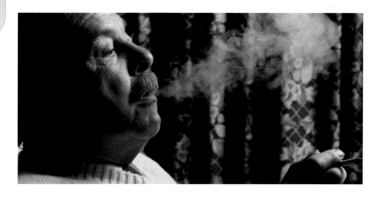

Cigarette smoking accounts for more than 90 percent of lung cancer cases in men and about 70 percent in women. Air pollution and some industrial substances have also contributed to the rise in cancers over the last 40 years. A smoker's lungs become unhealthy and black, but soon return to a healthy pink color if their owner quits the habit. It is never too late to stop smoking.

SEE ALSO

BODY SYSTEMS • CELLS AND CHROMOSOMES • IMMUNE SYSTEM • LYMPHATIC SYSTEM • LYMPHOMA

Carpal Tunnel Syndrome

Q & A

Does carpal tunnel syndrome affect only the hands?

Similar conditions can occur if the nerves at the ankle or elbow become trapped, although both of these conditions are far less common than carpal tunnel syndrome.

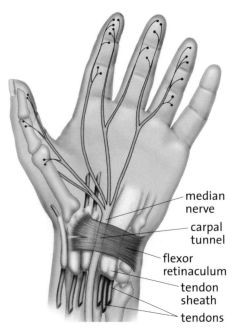

median nerve

carpal tunnel

flexor retinaculum

tendon sheath

tendons

The carpal tunnel is tightly packed with tendons, arteries, and nerves. If the median nerve is compressed, this can cause pain and tingling in the fingers and forearm.

Most of the movements of the fingers are brought about by muscles in the forearm. The muscles that pull the fingers into a fist are called the flexor muscles. They have long, thin tendons that pass over the front of the wrist. These flexor tendons are kept in place by a narrow but strong band of fibrous tissue called the flexor retinaculum that bridges across the wrist from side to side. The narrow space between the flexor retinaculum and the wrist bones is a short tunnel under which the tendons and other structures pass into the hand. The wrist bones are called the carpal bones, so this tunnel is known as the carpal tunnel.

Without the flexor retinaculum, any attempt to bend the wrist would cause the flexor tendons to spring away from the bones. In addition to the flexor tendons, four other important structures pass under the flexor retinaculum. These are the two arteries to the hand (the radial and the ulnar arteries) and two nerves (the large median nerve centrally and the smaller ulnar nerve lying on the little finger side). The carpal tunnel is therefore tightly filled with five tendons, two arteries, and two nerves, and there is very little room to spare. That is the cause of all the trouble.

Carpal tunnel syndrome is a condition in which a minor degree of swelling of the tissues under the retinaculum causes compression of the tiny blood vessels that keep the median nerve healthy and functional. All nerves require a good blood supply, and if that is reduced, the nerves cease to work properly. The cause of the swelling in the tunnel remains unknown, but the condition is eight times as common in women as in men.

Symptoms and treatment

The ulnar nerve provides sensation to the little finger and the outer half of the ring finger on each hand. Sensation in the rest of the hand is provided by the median nerve, and it is in this area that the symptoms of carpal tunnel syndrome are felt: a burning pain, tingling, and numbness, which is usually worst at night.

The median nerve is concerned with movement as well as sensation, and in severe cases there may also be wasting of the bulky muscle at the base of the thumb.

Carpal tunnel syndrome can be cured by cutting the flexor retinaculum where it lies over the median nerve. That allows more room for expansion without interfering with the normal operation of the tendons.

SEE ALSO

MUSCLE DISEASES AND DISORDERS • NERVOUS SYSTEM

Celiac Disease

Celiac disease is a particular condition in which food, especially fats, cannot be properly absorbed. Celiac disease is a genetic disorder in which there is a sensitivity to gluten, the insoluble protein present in wheat and other grains, which causes the stickiness in dough. Gluten is a mixture of two proteins: gliadin (which causes the problem) and glutenin. In people with this genetic mutation, the immune system is sensitive to gliadin, treating it as a foreign substance and developing antibodies to it, which attack the intestinal lining.

For digested food to be absorbed, a large surface area is needed. Although the small intestine is about 20 feet (6 m) long, its internal surface would not provide nearly enough area if it were plain and smooth. To aid absorption, the surface area is increased by millions of tiny, fingerlike protrusions called villi. Molecules of digested food pass through these villi to get into the bloodstream, before being carried to other parts of the body.

In celiac disease, the antibodies that attack the intestine have their most obvious effect on the villi, which become stunted and almost flat. The diagnosis can be positively confirmed by performing a biopsy. The patient swallows a small, spring-loaded device (Crosby capsule), which is attached to a tube. When it is triggered, a sample of intestinal lining is retrieved through the tube. Microscopic examination reveals the defects in the villi.

Symptoms and treatment

Celiac disease causes weight loss, diarrhea, abdominal pain, anemia, bloating, distension, and bulky and fatty stools. There may also be bone softening from mineral and vitamin deficiency. These symptoms are due to food retention in the intestine and nutritional losses from failure of absorption. Treatment involves excluding gluten from the diet. That is difficult, because gluten is used widely in foods such as bread, cakes, soups, sauces, hot dogs, and even ice cream. Expert advice is necessary. Extra vitamins and minerals may be required.

Q & A

My brother has celiac disease. Am I likely to develop it as well?

Celiac disease does run in families, though just how it is passed on is not clear, and not everybody with celiac disease has relatives who suffer from it. There is a controversial theory that celiac disease can be brought on by feeding infants foods containing gluten at too early an age, before their immune system can cope with foreign proteins. So it may be due to a combination of hereditary and dietary factors.

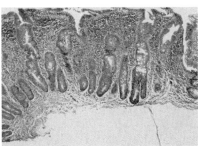
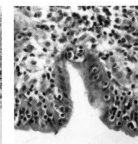

The above biopsy shows normal villi, the projections that line the small intestine and absorb nutrients. The stunted villi on the right show celiac disease.

SEE ALSO

ANEMIA • DIGESTIVE SYSTEM DISEASES AND DISORDERS

Cells and Chromosomes

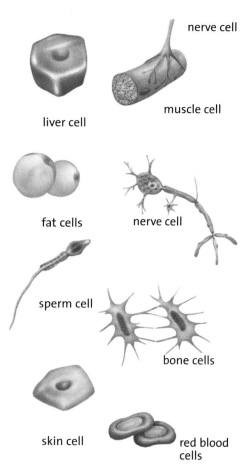

nerve cell

muscle cell

liver cell

fat cells

nerve cell

sperm cell

bone cells

skin cell

red blood cells

There are many types of cells in the human body, some of which are shown here. All cells produce energy and use it, but different cells do different jobs. In a process called differentiation, one cell gives rise to other kinds of cells. As they divide and multiply, the cells become specialized. Some become bone cells, some brain cells, some liver cells, and so on, until the whole body is created.

Cells are the basic units of life. In humans, they are the minute building blocks of the body. Every part of the body consists of living cells. Each cell contains chromosomes: microscopic threads that carry genes, which determine the characteristics of each human. Life begins as a single, fertilized egg cell that divides many times to produce a new human. By adulthood, the human body contains about 100 trillion cells. An average cell is so tiny it can be seen only when magnified using a microscope.

Cell structure and function

Cell shape varies. Nerve cells are long and thin, red blood cells are concave disks, and still other cells are spherical. However, all cells have the same basic structure. Each cell contains a watery gel called cytoplasm, surrounded by a thin membrane that protects the cell. Nutrients pass through the membrane into the cell, and waste material passes out through the membrane. The cytoplasm contains a number of structures, of which the nucleus is the largest and most important. It lies near the center of the cell and controls all of the cell's activities.

The nucleus also contains the chromosomes. Every cell (except for reproductive cells) contains 46 chromosomes, arranged in 23 pairs. Chromosomes are tiny threads made from strands of a chemical called deoxyribonucleic acid (DNA). DNA contains the genes. These minute particles contain all the instructions needed for a new human to grow and develop. Genes determine the characteristics that a person inherits, such as sex, hair and eye color, shape of nose, and intelligence. All genes are codes for proteins, most of which are enzymes needed for the many biochemical processes occurring in the cells, such as oxidation, cell respiration, and energy production.

The reproductive cells—the sperm and ova—contain only 23 chromosomes. At fertilization, a single sperm and ovum combine to form a new cell with the full number of 46 chromosomes. The genes begin to issue instructions for creating a new human, whose sex is determined by the sperm. Two of the chromosomes are sex chromosomes, which are called X or Y, depending on their shape. A woman has two X chromosomes. A man has one X chromosome and one Y chromosome. As a result, a sperm cell has either an X or a Y chromosome. If an ovum is fertilized by an X sperm, the XX combination produces a girl. If it is fertilized by a Y sperm, the XY combination produces a boy.

Cells have many functions. Some manufacture chemicals needed by the body. Others transport nourishment or protect the body against disease. Some cells live for only a few days; others live for the body's entire life. During growth, similar cells join to

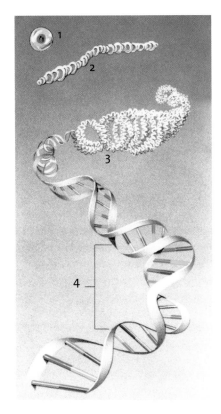

form the many tissues in the body, such as skin, bone, blood, muscle, or nerve. Tissues are collections of cells that have distinct functions in the body. Tissues join to form organs, such as the heart, liver, and lungs. Every minute, millions of cells in the body die and are replaced. New cells are produced by mitosis, a process in which cells divide to form two new and identical "daughter" cells. This is how the body grows and develops from the original fertilized egg into a baby and then into an adult; mitosis is also the way in which old cells are replaced. During cell division, the chromosomes become shorter and thicker and then split in half lengthwise. The double chromosomes then pull apart, the cytoplasm halves, and a new membrane develops around the two new cells, each of which has 46 chromosomes.

Things sometimes go wrong during the complicated process of cell replication. Chromosomal or genetic damage before birth can cause birth defects. Children with Down syndrome, for example, are born with one extra chromosome. Diseases such as sickle-cell anemia are genetic disorders that can be inherited. Cancer is also caused by abnormal cell growth but it is not inherited. However, there seems to be a genetic predisposition to certain cancers. Chemical errors in genes are called mutations.

Above: The body is made of trillions of microscopic cells (1), each with a nucleus containing chromosomes. The chromosomes (2) are shaped like coiled threads. The coiled threads are made of DNA, which has a structure like a spiral ladder (3). Sections of the ladder are called genes (4), and they contain the genetic information. When the cell divides, the genes also divide.

Right: The cell is made up of several parts. At the center of the cell is the nucleus, which controls the cell's ceaseless activities.

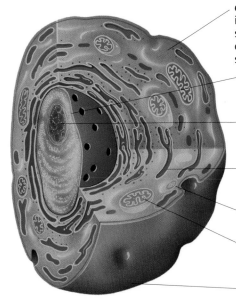

cytoplasm (gel in which other structures, called organelles, are suspended)

nucleus (control center, with chromosomes)

nucleolus (makes proteins needed for cell division)

ribosomes (makes proteins for use inside the cell)

lysosomes (store digestive juices)

mitochondria (produce energy for the cell)

cell membrane

> **SEE ALSO**
>
> BIRTH DEFECTS • CANCER • DOWN SYNDROME • GENES •
> GENETIC DISEASES AND DISORDERS

Cerebral Palsy

Cerebral palsy is a medical term that covers a range of conditions in which the nerve centers of part of the brain fail to develop properly or are damaged. That situation leads to spastic paralysis, in which the sufferer is unable to control properly the movements of certain muscles. One or more limbs may be stiff and immobile, or movements may be weak and jerky. The person may walk in an awkward and uncoordinated manner and have difficulty balancing. The muscles of the face, neck, and torso may be involved. People with cerebral palsy may also have problems with speech, sight, and hearing. Many have normal intelligence, but some have learning difficulties and some have epilepsy.

Causes of cerebral palsy

Cerebral palsy can occur because the brain does not develop properly or is damaged during pregnancy or birth. That may happen if the baby is deprived of oxygen during birth, suffers severe rhesus problems, has prolonged convulsions, or goes into a coma, or if the mother takes certain drugs.

The most common causes of cerebral palsy are thought to be due to events prior to the onset of labor. These events include prenatal stroke, infections, brain malformations, and genetic disorders. Oxygen starvation at birth may also be a factor. That may happen during a very long or difficult labor; a baby's delicate brain tissues rapidly deteriorate if they do not receive enough oxygen. Head injuries can also cause cerebral palsy.

The symptoms of cerebral palsy will probably not be noticeable until a child is about six months old. No two people with cerebral palsy are affected in exactly the same way. Some people with cerebral palsy have such mild damage that there is no obvious disability. Others are much more severely handicapped. The part of the body affected depends on the malfunctioning area of the brain.

Palliative therapy

There is no way of rebuilding damaged brain cells, so there is no cure for cerebral palsy. Proper treatment can help with many of the problems, and physical therapy can help improve the muscles in spastic limbs, develop movement, and prevent limbs from becoming deformed. Speech therapists can improve speech. Many aids are being developed to help people with cerebral palsy lead as normal a life as possible.

Q & A

Why can't some people with cerebral palsy speak properly?

Several factors can cause speech difficulties for someone with cerebral palsy. First, the speech center of the brain may be damaged. Second, a lack of good muscle control makes it hard to regulate breathing and form words. Third, people who find it difficult to control their speech may become tense when they try to speak, and this anxiety exacerbates the problem.

My brother suffers from cerebral palsy and has regular physical therapy. Will he ever be able to manage without it?

A child with cerebral palsy has to learn to sit up, walk, and control bodily movements until he or she gains independence. This learning requires an intensive course of treatment during the child's early years. As the child becomes more able to fend for him- or herself, the physical therapist will teach the parents how to encourage the child further, and gradually there will be no need for continuous treatment.

> ### SEE ALSO
> ENCEPHALITIS • EPILEPSY • MENINGITIS • NERVOUS SYSTEM

Chicken Pox

Chicken pox is an infectious disease that is common in children. Its most obvious symptom is an itchy rash. It does not last long and hardly ever has serious complications. Chicken pox is caused by a herpes virus. This virus is present in the chicken pox spots, but it is spread chiefly by droplet infection. Someone with the disease breathes out minute droplets of water containing the virus, which are breathed in by the next victim. Once inside the body, the virus needs an incubation period of 10 days to three weeks, during which it grows and spreads. The first sign of illness is a 24-hour period of feeling generally unwell, with a headache, possibly a slight fever, and perhaps a blotchy red rash that quickly fades. Within a day or so, the first spots appear in the mouth and throat, and they are painful. Then, spots appear on the trunk and face, and later, they may spread to the arms and legs. The spots start as pink pimples, which soon form tiny blisters of clear fluid. Within a day, these "teardrop" spots turn milky, form a crust, and then scab over. As soon as the crust forms, the spots begin to itch, and this itching can last for one to two weeks until the scabs drop off. New spots appear each day for three or four days, during which time the patient may have a slight fever.

Most cases of chicken pox are mild, and a child who catches it needs to stay in bed for only a day or so. If the scabs are scratched off, the spots may become infected and permanent scars can form. Soothing lotions may help, and in severe cases a doctor may prescribe an antihistamine drug. Chicken pox in adults is more severe, with a higher temperature. Adults take longer to recover. In a few cases, the virus causes a form of pneumonia or attacks the nervous system, causing encephalitis (inflammation of the brain), but the chances of recovery are good. The disease is so infectious that most people have it when they are children and are naturally immune afterward. However, there is a vaccine against chicken pox (known as the varicella vaccine), and it can be given to infants at 12 to 15 months.

Q & A

My brother had chicken pox when we were little, and now he appears to have it again. Is this possible?

It is unlikely that your brother has a second infection. Chicken pox is usually a one-time-only infection. The first "attack" of chicken pox might have been scabies (severe itching and spots caused by a mite) or several gnat bites occurring together.

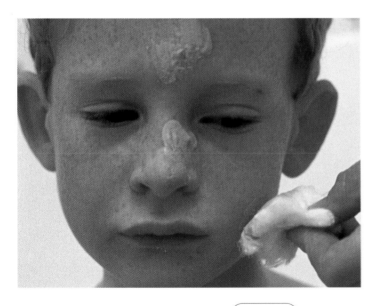

Chicken pox spots begin to itch as soon as the crusts form. Calamine lotion cools the skin and soothes the irritation.

SEE ALSO

ENCEPHALITIS • INFECTIOUS DISEASES • VIRUSES

Cholera

Q & A

My family is going on vacation to India this summer. Will I need a cholera vaccination, and will I need a certificate of proof?

Cholera vaccinations are voluntary in many countries but are strongly recommended in places such as India. People traveling from India to certain other countries will also need an International Certificate of Vaccination. The best thing to do is to get the details of all the necessary vaccinations from your travel agent, or directly from the country's embassy.

Cholera is an extremely serious and often fatal disease. It is caused by bacteria present in water that has been contaminated by the feces, urine, or vomit of an infected person. Cholera used to be widespread throughout the world, and serious epidemics broke out, killing thousands of people before it was realized that contaminated water spread the disease. The disease is now found mainly in developing countries, in places where people are crowded together in unsanitary conditions.

Cholera bacteria incubate (multiply) in the body for between 12 hours and six days before the symptoms begin. First, the patient has uncontrollable diarrhea and vomiting. The body becomes dehydrated, and the loss of salt leads to severe cramps in the arms, legs, and abdomen. The patient has an intense thirst, and drinking water leads to more cramps. A day or so later, the patient collapses. The body becomes extremely cold, the pulse can barely be felt, the kidneys or heart may fail, and the patient may die. If the patient survives to the final stages of the disease, the original symptoms may lessen, but pneumonia may set in.

Treatment includes giving a salt solution intravenously to restore the patient's fluid and salt balance, while antibiotic drugs destroy the bacteria. Anyone who is traveling to an area where cholera is present should take precautions. In such places, all water should be boiled before it is used for cooking or drinking. Food should be protected from flies and other insects, and uncooked fruit and vegetables should be avoided. Anyone who gets severe diarrhea shortly after returning from an area where cholera is present should see a doctor as soon as possible.

Cholera usually occurs in areas where hygiene and sanitation are poor. People visiting such places should avoid all contact with anyone suffering from the disease, boil water for drinking and cooking, avoid eating fruit or uncooked food that may have been washed with contaminated water, and wash their hands after using the toilet and before eating.

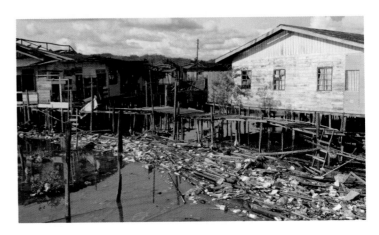

SEE ALSO

BACTERIA • DIARRHEA • EPIDEMIC • INFECTIOUS DISEASES

Chronic Fatigue Syndrome

Q & A

My brother has been diagnosed with chronic fatigue syndrome. My father thinks he is just lazy. Could my father be right?

Certain psychological states mimic chronic fatigue syndrome (CFS) outwardly, but if a doctor has diagnosed CFS in your brother, his condition will be mainly physical. However, CFS does cause some psychological depression. Support from those near him, such as his family and close friends, will help.

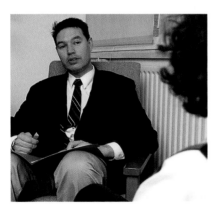

Cognitive behavior therapy has been used to treat chronic fatigue syndrome. During cognitive therapy, the patient is taught to analyze his or her thought processes, to identify negative trains of thought, and to adopt a more positive outlook.

The term *chronic fatigue syndrome* is now most commonly used for a condition that involves severe fatigue and psychological disturbance. The condition can be made worse by exercise. Chronic fatigue syndrome has had many names in the past, including myalgic encephalomyelitis, post-viral fatigue syndrome, epidemic neuromyasthenia, Otago mystery disease, and Icelandic disease. Although detailed clinical investigations into the condition have been carried out, in most cases they have failed to reveal any organic abnormality that could account for the symptoms and the disablement.

Chronic fatigue syndrome is more common in women than in men. The fatigue experienced is not simply muscle fatigue and is quite different from the weakness experienced in disorders such as muscular dystrophy. In chronic fatigue syndrome, there is often a strong psychological element, with the sufferer experiencing mild to severe depression. As a result of the accompanying depression, there has been a degree of skepticism surrounding chronic fatigue syndrome. In part, this is because doctors suspect that the symptoms mask an underlying psychological problem. However, the cause or causes of chronic fatigue syndrome have yet to be identified. Although depression is often present, it has not been established whether depression causes the disorder or arises as a result of the disorder. Other theories link chronic fatigue syndrome with viral infections or suggest that it can arise as the result of a personal trauma, such as a death, separation, or loss of work.

Critical attitudes by doctors and others in the medical field have not been helpful and have caused much distress to sufferers. Although it is important to establish whether or not the condition has a physical cause, it is also vital to acknowledge that people with the symptoms of chronic fatigue syndrome deserve help. Such a persistent disruption of normal living indicates a disorder of the whole person.

Because of the failure to discover an organic cause, doctors have not been sure how to treat the condition. In some cases, antidepressant drugs have been helpful. In others, cognitive behavior therapy has been used. This type of therapy is not concerned with the cause of the condition. Instead, cognitive therapy concentrates on persuading the sufferer to live as normal a life as possible, often with excellent results.

SEE ALSO

BODY SYSTEMS • MUSCLE • MUSCLE DISEASES AND DISORDERS • VIRUSES

Circulatory System

The circulatory system is the body's transport system. It carries food, oxygen, water, and other essential materials around the body to nourish and repair the cells; waste products are carried away and expelled from the body. The circulatory system consists of the blood, the blood vessels (veins, arteries, and capillaries) through which blood moves, and the heart (a muscular pump, which continually pushes blood through the body).

Around 2 ounces (59 ml) of blood is pumped out of the heart each time it contracts. Blood that is rich in oxygen and nutrients starts its journey from the left side of the heart, through a large artery called the aorta. The blood flows from the aorta through arteries into smaller vessels called arterioles, which supply the body's tissues. From the arterioles, blood enters a network of minute vessels called capillaries. Oxygen and nutrients are transferred to cells, and carbon dioxide and waste products are absorbed.

Deoxygenated blood then flows from the capillaries into small veins (venules) to return to the heart. The veins eventually merge into two large blood vessels, the venae cavae. From here, deoxygenated blood is delivered to the right side of the heart, pumped into the pulmonary artery, and taken to the lungs. Fresh oxygen is absorbed into the blood and the waste carbon dioxide is expelled from the body by breathing out. The now oxygen-rich blood flows through the pulmonary vein into the left side of the heart, and the journey through the body begins all over again. This complete circuit takes about 60 seconds. The heart beats on average 70 times every minute. It pumps an estimated 8,000 gallons (30,280 l) of blood around the body every 24 hours.

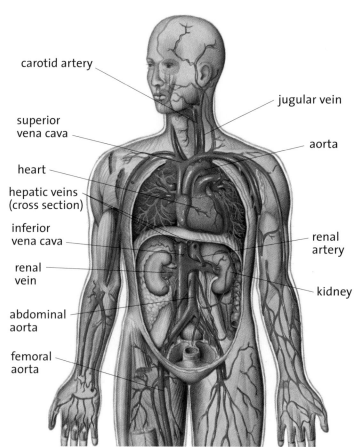

carotid artery

jugular vein

superior vena cava

aorta

heart

hepatic veins (cross section)

inferior vena cava

renal artery

renal vein

kidney

abdominal aorta

femoral aorta

The circulatory system's main arteries (red) and veins (blue) would cover many thousands of miles if they were removed from the body and laid out.

SEE ALSO

ARTERY DISEASES AND DISORDERS • BODY SYSTEMS • CIRCULATORY SYSTEM DISEASES AND DISORDERS • HEART

Circulatory System Diseases and Disorders

Q & A

I'm a teenage girl, and I keep on fainting. Do you think I might have problems with my circulation?

The most usual cause of fainting is a temporary fall in the volume of blood reaching the brain. This is a common problem in adolescents. It is often caused by emotional disturbance, which can make the arteries widen, lowering the blood pressure and preventing blood from being pumped up to the brain. People usually grow out of this sort of fainting. However, if the fainting spells increase or you are worried that you really may be ill, it is best to see your doctor promptly.

My grandmother has had a pacemaker fitted that prevents her from having dizzy spells. But what will happen when the batteries in the machine eventually run out?

The pacing box will be replaced during a small operation similar to the one she had when her pacemaker was put in. The batteries in newer pacing boxes can last up to 10 years.

In the circulatory system, arteries carry blood containing oxygen and nutrients to all parts of the body. Veins return deoxygenated blood to the heart. Without a supply of freshly oxygenated blood, the body cells die, so anything that interferes with the circulation of the blood can cause serious problems.

Artery disease

The most common serious illness in the Western world is artery disease. Its medical name is atherosclerosis. Everyone's arteries become harder and less flexible with age, and fibrous tissue may build up within the walls of an artery. Smoking makes that buildup more likely. The principal feature of atherosclerosis is the buildup of fatty material called atheroma inside the walls of the arteries, forming hard masses called plaques. The deposits of fatty material include cholesterol.

When deposits of fat and fiber build up on the wall of an artery, its central channel becomes narrower, so less blood flows through. Thus, any cut or sore is likely to become infected. This condition usually affects small arteries, particularly those in the legs and feet. Narrowing of the arteries leading to the brain can cause dizziness and even brief loss of sight. Sometimes, major arteries become narrowed. This condition is particularly serious in the coronary arteries that supply the heart muscles. Although the arteries may be able to supply enough blood and oxygen for the heart's normal workload, any extra work such as exercise deprives the heart muscle of oxygen. The result is angina: chest pain, which can vary from mild to cripplingly severe.

The wall of an artery may sometimes bulge out in a saclike swelling, particularly if the artery is already weakened by atherosclerosis. In time, this swelling, or aneurysm, starts to leak blood. Aneurysms are found in the aorta, the major artery carrying oxygenated blood from the heart through the chest and abdomen. They require emergency surgery. They also occur in brain arteries (where they are often fatal) and in the arteries of the arms and legs (where they are less serious).

Hypertension and diabetes increase the risk of developing artery problems, and both conditions tend to run in families. The level of cholesterol in the blood may also play a significant part in atherosclerosis. To help prevent illness, people with hypertension and diabetes should eat a diet that is low in cholesterol and salt. Above all, they should not smoke, as smoking certainly makes hardening of the arteries worse. Surgeons have learned how to bypass badly narrowed parts of coronary artery by grafting in sections of the patient's leg vein. This technique is particularly effective in relieving angina.

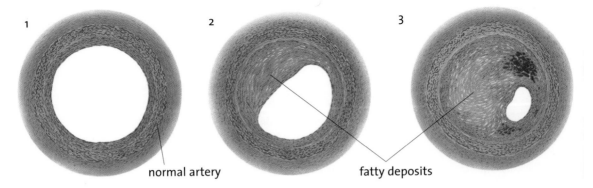

normal artery   fatty deposits

The normal artery (1) has thick walls consisting of three layers. In a moderate case of atherosclerosis (2), fatty deposits build up inside the artery. In a severe case (3), the deposit is almost total and only a narrow channel remains for the blood.

Heart attacks and strokes

Blood flows more slowly through narrowed arteries and may therefore form a clot called a thrombus, which may block the blood flow. Sometimes, part of a clot or plaque breaks away and is carried along in the bloodstream until it blocks a vessel, causing an embolism. Thrombi and embolisms are extremely dangerous. A clot in a coronary artery causes a heart attack, or coronary thrombosis, which can be fatal. A clot in one of the arteries supplying the brain causes cerebral thrombosis; a piece of a clot that breaks away causes a cerebral embolism. Both kinds of blockage cause a stroke. Strokes are also caused by a cerebral hemorrhage, when an artery leaks blood into the brain. Part of the brain's blood supply becomes cut off, so the brain is unable to control its normal range of activities.

Disorders in veins

Sometimes, a thrombosis forms in a vein deep in the leg or lower abdomen and then partly or completely breaks away. It is carried along the vein, through the heart, to the lungs, where it can block one of the arteries and cause a pulmonary embolism. The patient becomes breathless, because part of the lung is not working, and experiences chest pain. If a large part of the lung is affected, the patient can soon die. The main problems associated with veins are thromboses in deep veins; varicose veins, which form when faulty valves in the veins cause stretching and twisting of veins under the skin's surface; and an inflammation called phlebitis.

Shock

When shock occurs, the blood pressure drops and the circulation stops working because a lot of blood or fluid has been lost in an injury or because the heart fails to pump blood around the body properly. The patient is pale, cold, and often clammy to the touch; he or she may have difficulty breathing; and the blood pressure

COMMON DISEASES OF THE CIRCULATORY SYSTEM

DISEASE	SYMPTOMS	ACTION
ANEURYSM Weakening of an artery causing it to balloon outward	Pain in the back, chest, or abdomen, depending on the position of the affected artery	Consult a doctor. Surgery is needed to remove or reinforce the diseased part.
ATHEROSCLEROSIS Buildup of fat in arteries	Few symptoms; blood pressure may be raised; can lead to heart attack or stroke	A special diet may help by reducing fat and cholesterol levels. Preventive measures will be recommended.
HYPERTENSION High blood pressure	No symptoms until a dangerously late stage; routine checks are necessary	A doctor will prescribe drugs to treat the condition and recommend preventive lifestyle measures.
PERIPHERAL VASCULAR DISEASE Severe narrowing and formation of clots (thrombi) in arteries and veins, usually of the legs	Cramps in legs during exercise; feet redden when lowered, turn white when raised; toes and fingers are pale and cold	Consult a doctor. Surgery may be needed to bypass affected vessels. Foot infections should be avoided. The patient should stop smoking.
PHLEBITIS Inflammation in a vein, most commonly in a varicose vein of the leg. Often leads to the formation of a clot.	Leg is pale, painful, and swollen, and feels heavy	Consult a doctor. Bed rest is required, with legs elevated. Drug treatment may be necessary. Additional support to the area with an elastic bandage is needed.
PULMONARY EMBOLISM Blockage in one of the arteries of a lung	Pain in the legs and chest; coughing, short breath, skin looks blue; sputum may contain blood	Medical emergency; hospital care is needed, with the use of anticoagulants and possibly surgery.
SHOCK Collapse of circulation due to blood loss, burns, heart failure, or other causes	Fast, weak pulse, clammy skin, short breath, low blood pressure	Medical emergency; immediate treatment is needed.
STROKE Clot of blood in a brain artery (cerebral thrombosis) or breaking of a blood vessel in the brain (cerebral hemorrhage)	Sudden loss of function, usually on one side of the body; may be preceded by headaches, vomiting, and drowsiness.	Medical emergency; hospital treatment is needed, followed by convalescence and rehabilitation.
VARICOSE VEINS Abnormally swollen veins	Dilation of veins, usually in legs, causing them to ache	If painful, consult a doctor, who will inject the veins or advise surgery. Support hose may be recommended.

falls dangerously. This type of shock is physiological and should not be confused with the psychological shock experienced by a person who has undergone an emotional trauma. Physiological shock needs immediate medical treatment—often a fluid or blood transfusion—and treatment of the underlying cause.

SEE ALSO

ARTERY DISEASES AND DISORDERS • HEART ATTACK • HEART DISEASES AND DISORDERS • STROKE • VEIN DISORDERS

Cold

VITAMIN C

Some people feel that taking large quantities of vitamin C, which is present in citrus fruit and ascorbic acid preparations, helps get rid of a cold. For this reason, vitamin C pills and preparations are popular. To produce a useful antioxidant effect, about 0.035 ounce (1,000 mg) of vitamin C must be taken daily.

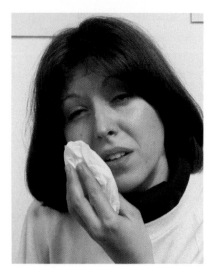

It is difficult to avoid catching colds or giving a cold to others. People who have a cold should cover their nose and mouth when coughing and sneezing. They should also wash their hands, because the virus is passed more easily by hand-to-hand contact than in the air.

The common cold is a widespread viral infection that can be caused by any one of several hundred viruses, all of which produce similar symptoms. It is impossible to immunize people against colds. Almost everyone has at least one cold a year, and some people have many more. A great deal of research has been done on the common cold, but as yet there is no way of preventing it and no cure has been found. Colds are caught from a virus spread by people who have a cold. When they cough or sneeze, they spray out tiny droplets of moisture containing the virus. A person catches the cold by breathing in the droplets or by touching hands that are contaminated with the virus. The cold virus can also enter the body via the eyelid linings (conjunctivae).

Coughs, sneezes, and cold "cures"

The first symptoms are a general ill feeling, often with aching joints and a chill. At this stage, the body temperature is often below normal and then rises. The sufferer may also have a sore throat and streaming eyes and nose, and may sneeze repeatedly. The head may feel stuffed up as the lining of the nasal passages inflames, swells, and produces extra mucus, which makes the nose congested. The sufferer may also start to cough. The symptoms depend on the virus and on which parts of the respiratory system are involved. Upper respiratory tract infection causes sneezing, a runny nose, and a stuffy feeling. Infection of the larynx results in a sore throat and hoarseness. Coughs are caused by infection of the windpipe.

A cold usually clears up in a few days, although people who smoke find that it takes longer. Spending a day in bed helps, and it prevents the virus from being spread. People who have bronchitis should see a doctor when they have a cold. Colds can lead to other infections, and a doctor should be consulted if an earache develops or if the cold lasts for more than 10 days.

There is no medication to cure a cold, but its symptoms can be relieved. Antihistamines may keep the nose and eyes from running, and decongestant sprays or inhalers clear the head. Aspirin brings down a fever, but this drug could be dangerous for children, because a disease called Reye's syndrome, which occurs mainly in children under 10, may be related to taking aspirin for a viral infection. Reye's syndrome is a rare disorder that causes brain and liver damage following an infection.

SEE ALSO

INFLUENZA • RESPIRATORY SYSTEM • RESPIRATORY SYSTEM DISEASES AND DISORDERS • REYE'S SYNDROME • VIRUSES

Colon and Colon Diseases

The colon is the main part of the large intestine. The function of the colon is to move solid material from the small intestine to the anus and to absorb salt and water delivered to it from the small intestine. The most common disorder of the colon is constipation, but this is seldom serious. Inflammation of the colon is known as colitis. That causes a bad pain in the abdomen, followed by watery diarrhea containing mucus, pus, and sometimes blood. The patient may vomit and have a high fever. Acute colitis lasts a short time and is usually the result of an infection or a food allergy. It clears up quickly once the cause is addressed. Bed rest is advisable, and doses of a kaolin and morphine mixture stop diarrhea.

Chronic colitis
Chronic colitis can lead to ulcers in the colon, resulting from infection by bacteria or amoebas, or from an immune system defect. In chronic cholitis, there may be as many as 15 to 20 bowel movements each day. In more severe cases, there may be dehydration, anemia, loss of appetite and weight, vomiting, and high fever. Aalazopyrin is the main treatment for chronic colitis. It is a combination of antibiotic and aspirin-like drugs, taken three times a day. A liquid preparation of hydrocortisone can be given as a suppository, which has a marked soothing effect. Bland, high-protein food should be eaten, with only a small amount of fruit and roughage.

Stress
Stress may cause painful abdominal spasms, known as an irritable colon, and the lining of the colon may become infected and develop abscesses. Bulges in the colon wall may fill with waste and become infected; that is known as diverticular disease.

Cancer of the colon is one of the most common forms of cancers, but it is usually slow-growing and can be removed successfully. Early detection and treatment help recovery.

COLOSTOMY

Before a colon operation, or if the colon is blocked, an operation called a colostomy is carried out. This procedure makes an opening in the abdomen through which waste material from the colon can pass to be collected in a bag. This operation may be reversed so that waste passes along the colon and out in the normal way, but some people have to live with the colostomy all their life. Once used to the colostomy, they can lead an almost normal life. The bags are easy to change and do not show under clothing.

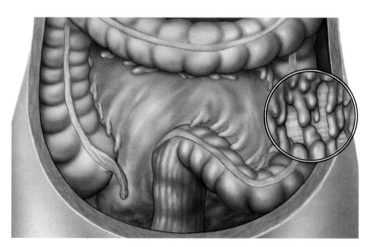

Colitis is severe inflammation of the colon. The mucous membrane that lines the colon becomes ulcerated (inset), causing pain and diarrhea.

> **SEE ALSO**
> ALLERGIES • ANEMIA • DIARRHEA • DIGESTIVE SYSTEM •
> DIGESTIVE SYSTEM DISEASES AND DISORDERS • DYSENTERY

Communicable Diseases

Communicable diseases are infectious illnesses that are passed directly or indirectly from one person to another. Those that are passed directly from person to person by close contact are called contagious diseases. They are caught by touching infected people or things they have used, by breathing in microorganisms they have spread around, or by contact with their blood or other body fluids. Communicable diseases that are passed indirectly include malaria and Rocky Mountain spotted fever (which are passed on by insects) and typhoid fever (which is spread by infected food or water). Communicable diseases are most common in places where people live close together. Refugee camps are at risk from food-borne typhoid or cholera. Other infections such as colds and influenza spread quickly through schools and offices. The spread of disease can be checked by good hygiene and sanitation, by practicing safe sex, by killing carrier insects, and by immunizing people against disease. Those with a contagious disease should be quarantined from other people, and things they have handled should be sterilized.

Q & A

Can people catch malaria in the United States? Also, can people catch it on a vacation?

There is no threat of malaria in the United States, mainly because few of the mosquito species present are able to carry malaria. However, it is possible to be bitten when traveling in a malarial area, even during a short airplane stop for refueling. Just one bite can put you at risk.

ISOLATION

Patients with highly communicable diseases are kept in strict isolation in hospitals. Private rooms, with an independent air supply, are provided. Doors are kept shut, and people who have a reason to enter must wear masks, gloves, and protective gowns. On leaving, they must wash their hands in disinfectant, and all articles removed from the room are similarly disinfected or disposed of. Less strict isolation is provided for those with diseases that are not as infectious, but hand washing after every contact with an infected patient is strictly enforced.

SOME COMMUNICABLE DISEASES

BACTERIAL DISEASES
Bacillary dysentery, brucellosis, conjunctivitis, cholera, diphtheria, food poisoning, gastroenteritis, Hansen's disease, impetigo, Legionnaires' disease, meningitis, pharyngitis, plague, pneumonia, scarlet fever, tuberculosis, tularemia, typhoid, whooping cough

FUNGAL AND YEAST INFECTONS
Athlete's foot, candidiasis, jock itch, ringworm

PARASITIC INFECTIONS
Amebic dysentery, fluke infection, hookworm disease, malaria, psittacosis, roundworm infection, schistosomiasis, tapeworm infection

RICKETTSIAL DISEASES
Q fever, Rocky Mountain spotted fever, rickettsial pox, trench fever, typhus

SEXUALLY TRANSMITTED DISEASES
AIDS, chlamydial infections, genital candidiasis, gonorrhea, herpes, syphilis

VIRAL DISEASES
Chicken pox, cold sores, common cold, conjunctivitis, dengue fever, gastroenteritis, hepatitis, herpes, infectious mononucleosis, influenza, measles, meningitis, mumps, poliomyelitis, rubella, smallpox

SEE ALSO

BACTERIA • BACTERIAL DISEASES • EPIDEMIC • FUNGAL INFECTIONS • INFECTIOUS DISEASES • RICKETTSIAL DISEASES • SEXUALLY TRANSMITTED DISEASES • VIRUSES

Creutzfeldt-Jakob Disease

Creutzfeldt-Jakob disease (CJD) is a rare and deadly condition that affects the human brain. It is one of a group of brain conditions called spongiform encephalopathies. These conditions include animal diseases such as scrapie, which affects sheep, and bovine spongiform encephalopathy (BSE), or mad cow disease, which affects cattle.

Spongiform encephalopathies are thought to be caused by tiny particles called prions. In CJD, the prions stop certain proteins in the body from working properly. The defective proteins gather in microscopic holes in the brain. The word *spongiform* refers to these tiny holes.

In 1995, a new form of CJD hit the headlines in Britain. This new variant CJD (vCJD) occurs in young people and was originally linked to people who ate beef from cattle infected with mad cow disease. The World Health Organization (WHO) has now decided there is no link between mad cow disease and vCJD. No one really knows why people develop CJD or vCJD.

Symptoms, diagnosis, and treatment

People with CJD, which may be mistaken for mild depression at first, suffer many symptoms. These symptoms include memory loss, speech problems, and personality changes. Later, the symptoms may develop into hallucinations, jerky movements, and seizures. CJD can be fatal within months or even weeks, but in some cases people survive for a year or more.

The only way to diagnose CJD is to slice through the brain and use a microscope to look for the tiny holes. That can be done only after the patient has died. While the patient is still alive, doctors perform tests such as computed axial tomography (CAT) and magnetic resonance imaging (MRI) to rule out other brain diseases.

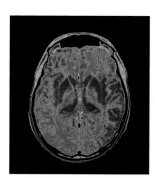

There is no known cure for CJD, so treatment is designed to make the patient as comfortable as possible. In the later stages of CJD, patients need around-the-clock care. Doctors usually prescribe a range of drugs to help patients cope with some of the symptoms.

An MRI scan of a human brain, showing areas of the thalamus diseased with CJD.

Q & A

My friend's dad has Creutzfeldt-Jakob disease. Can I catch it from him?

No. Creutzfeldt-Jakob disease (CJD) cannot be caught by touching a person who has the disease or by breathing the same air. People who nurse CJD patients or who eat with the patients are no more likely to get the disease than anyone else.

Do animals suffer from Creutzfeldt-Jakob disease?

Creutzfeldt-Jakob disease affects animals and humans. The brain becomes riddled with tiny holes and protein deposits. Sheep have a related disease called scrapie, so called because affected sheep scrape against trees and other objects. Cattle have a related disease called bovine spongiform encephalopathy (BSE), or mad cow disease, first described in Britain in 1986. Such cattle may become aggressive or anxious. British cattle may have become infected after eating feed containing sheep remains infected with scrapie or after eating feed containing the remains of cattle that had spontaneous BSE.

SEE ALSO

BRAIN • BRAIN DAMAGE AND DISORDERS • ENCEPHALITIS

Crohn's Disease

Crohn's disease is an inflammation of the digestive tract. The disease usually attacks the walls of the small intestines, but it may affect any part of the digestive system, from the mouth to the anus.

No one really knows what causes Crohn's disease. Some physicians think that the body's own immune system is to blame. Immune cells usually attack invaders such as bacteria and viruses. However, sometimes these immune cells attack the body's own cells. Diet could also play a part in causing Crohn's disease, although no direct link has been proved.

Spotting the symptoms

The first signs of Crohn's disease are diarrhea and stomach pains, which may be accompanied by weight loss, fever, and loss of appetite. Gradually, the abdomen may become swollen, and the internal inflamed areas may develop fibrous scar tissue. Cracks may form in the walls of the digestive tract, which sometimes tear open. Blood may then leak through the tiny holes into the digestive tract and out through the anus. Some people develop channels, called fistulas, that run from the bowel to the anus or skin surface.

Disease diagnosis

At first, doctors test the blood and feces to rule out other bowel diseases. Then an instrument called an endoscope is used to look inside the digestive tract. The endoscope is inserted through the mouth or anus, and the doctor examines the intestinal wall for signs of cracking and fibrous thickening. During the examination, a biopsy is usually performed to remove a small amount of tissue for examination under a microscope.

Treatment options

There is no cure for Crohn's disease, so the treatment helps relieve the symptoms. Drugs such as immunosuppressants, steroids, and sulfasalazine help reduce the inflammation, but they have side effects.

Sometimes, surgery to remove areas of damaged tissue in the digestive tract is the only option. That provides some short-lived relief, but the disease usually flares up again.

Q & A

If a person has Crohn's disease, is he or she more likely to get cancer?

Cancer of the colon and rectum is becoming more common in general, but cancer of the small intestine is still extremely rare. Some scientists believe that people with Crohn's disease, especially those who have had it for a long time and in whom it has affected the entire colon, are more likely to get cancer in this region than people who have never had Crohn's disease.

Can people with Crohn's disease lead a normal life?

People with Crohn's disease usually have periods when they are ill followed by times when they feel well. They may become depressed because they know the disease will flare up periodically. However, disease-free periods can last for months or even years, so it is possible for someone with this condition to lead a normal life. On the other hand, children with Crohn's disease may fail to develop properly because they suffer from malnutrition.

SEE ALSO

COLON AND COLON DISEASES • DIARRHEA • DIGESTIVE SYSTEM • DIGESTIVE SYSTEM DISEASES AND DISORDERS • IMMUNE SYSTEM

Cystic Fibrosis

Cystic fibrosis is a hereditary disease in which the glands produce an unusually sticky mucus. The mucus blocks the internal organs, such as the lungs, the liver, the pancreas, and the intestines, and stops them from working properly. There is no known cure for the disease, but because of advances in treatment, people with cystic fibrosis are now able to lead a more normal life, and the life expectancy of children with this condition has increased.

Q & A

Is it possible for me to be a carrier of cystic fibrosis without ever knowing it?

Yes, if there is a history of the disease in your family. Your being a carrier will matter only if you have a child with someone who is also a carrier. The effects of the disease are so serious that it is unlikely you would not know if the disease was in your family. Cystic fibrosis is the most common inherited disease among white people. A carrier of the disease does not show any symptoms.

Is there a test that I can have to find out if I am a carrier of cystic fibrosis?

Yes. Both men and women can be tested for the presence of the gene that causes cystic fibrosis.

My cousin died of cystic fibrosis when he was in his teens. I am now 18. Does this mean that I won't get it?

If you were going to get cystic fibrosis, you probably would have gotten it by now. However, the symptoms can occasionally appear in adults.

Signs, symptoms, and treatment

A baby with cystic fibrosis usually shows signs of the illness soon after it is born. Its pancreas cannot make the enzymes needed to digest food, so the baby gains little or no weight. Sticky mucus stops food from passing normally through the intestines, which may become blocked. The baby will have unusually salty sweat, which is a key symptom of the illness.

The most serious problems develop in the lungs. The sticky mucus blocks the bronchial tubes and hinders breathing. Germs are trapped in the mucus and cause many lung infections that are hard to cure. If a doctor suspects that a baby has cystic fibrosis, he or she will carry out a "sweat test" to measure the amount of salt present in sweat. An early diagnosis is important so that treatment can be given as soon as possible to prevent damage to the lungs.

Patients with cystic fibrosis are given extracts of animal pancreas to help them digest food. They should follow a special diet and may take vitamin supplements and salt tablets to replace the salt they lose in sweat. Inhalants can loosen the sticky mucus blocking the lungs, and daily exercises help keep the lungs clear. Antibiotics can treat lung infections.

Support and genetic counseling

Despite difficulties, patients with this disease may manage to lead a fairly normal life, although they need the support of doctors, nurses, physical therapists, social workers, and counselors. Because cystic fibrosis is an inherited disease that is passed down to children by their parents, anyone with a history of the condition in the family will probably be offered genetic testing before deciding to have a child. If the results are positive, genetic counseling will be offered.

SEE ALSO

BIRTH DEFECTS • BODY SYSTEMS • DIGESTIVE SYSTEM • GENES • GENETIC DISEASES AND DISORDERS • GLANDS • LUNG • LUNG DISEASES AND DISORDERS • PNEUMONIA

Deafness

Someone who is deaf cannot hear perfectly. Deafness may be extremely slight or it may be so bad that the person cannot hear anything at all. Some people are deaf in one ear; others are affected in both ears. Many people experience gradual hearing loss as they get older. In all, around 15 million Americans suffer from some form of hearing disability.

Types of deafness

There are two main types of deafness—conductive deafness and sensorineural (or nerve) deafness. In conductive deafness, sound waves cannot reach the inner ear. They may be blocked by wax in the ear, or the tiny bones in the middle ear called the ossicles may have seized up. These bones are the malleus, incus, and stapes. Infections such as colds may cause the ear passages to become inflamed and blocked. Other infections may be caused by scratching the ear or by swimming in polluted water. In addition, the eardrum may be punctured by poking something sharp into the ear, by a blow to the head, or as the result of an explosion. In each case, the sound waves are prevented from reaching the inner ear.

In sensorineural deafness, sound waves can reach the inner ear, but the delicate mechanism in the inner ear that converts sound to nerve impulses is damaged. The mechanism may be damaged by a head injury, a brain tumor, an extremely loud noise, or an illness—such as a stroke, measles, or Ménière's disease. Ménière's disease is caused by rising pressure within the cochlea of the inner ear—which causes dizziness, ringing in the ear, vomiting, and gradual deafness.

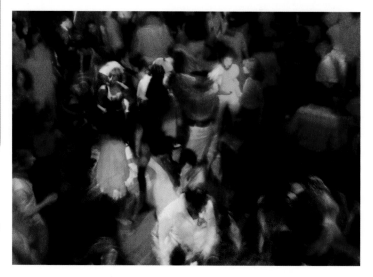

Q & A

My three-year-old brother is just learning to talk. When I call him, he sometimes does not hear. Could he be partially deaf?

A child who is slow to talk and appears deaf definitely needs a hearing test. At least that will reassure you and your parents that all is normal.

Why is deafness associated with loss of balance? My great-aunt has to wear a hearing aid, but she still loses her balance a lot.

There is a close connection between balance and hearing. The organ of hearing, the cochlea of the inner ear, is also part of the organs of balance, the semicircular canals of the inner ear. Both organs send information to the brain along the same auditory nerve. Therefore, conditions that affect one sensation easily affect the other. In old age, the amount of information carried by the auditory nerve is reduced.

Both modern musicians and their audiences are liable to suffer from some loss of hearing because even those groups that are considered quiet can produce sound levels that are dangerously high.

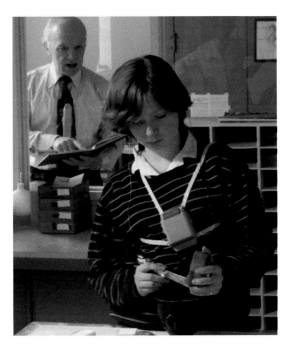

This deaf girl is using a phonic ear. The man, who is some distance away, speaks into a microphone, and the sound is transmitted to the girl's ears via a receiver.

Some babies are born with congenital deafness as a result of an abnormality of the growth of the hearing apparatus or damage to the cochlea from rubella. Congenital deafness is also caused by a shortage of oxygen at birth or by congenital syphilis.

When conductive deafness and sensorineural deafness occur together, the condition is called composite or mixed deafness.

Treating deafness

Ear infections can often be treated with antibiotics. Delicate operations, carried out under a microscope, can repair damage to the ear chambers, and the tiny ear bones can be replaced with metal substitutes. When surgery cannot help, hearing aids often allow deaf people to hear at least some of the sounds around them.

Children who are born deaf and who cannot be helped with a hearing aid are unable to learn speech by imitating other people. Devices called cochlear implants may be inserted in the inner ear at an early age to minimize the problem. These implants do not produce normal hearing, but they can be extremely helpful.

Deaf children need special teaching. Deaf people often learn to read lips and can tell what someone is saying simply by watching the lips move. Most deaf people, their families, and therapists learn a special hand sign language to communicate.

Preventing deafness

To lessen the chances of deafness, some guidelines should be followed. Hard objects should never be put into the ears. The ears should be cleaned extremely gently and carefully. People should never hit others on the side of the head, because that could rupture the eardrum. Continuous loud noises should be avoided, such as aircraft noise and loud music. Any noise that results in ringing in the ears (tinnitus) is a danger to long-term hearing. Someone who has a painful or discharging ear should consult a doctor. It is also advisable to have ears tested regularly.

SEE ALSO

BIRTH DEFECTS • EAR AND HEARING • EAR DISEASES AND DISORDERS • INFECTIOUS DISEASES • MEASLES • NERVOUS SYSTEM • STROKE • VIRUSES

Dermatitis

Q & A

I've just learned that my best friend has dermatitis. I don't want to offend her by not hanging out with her. However, I am still afraid that I will catch the dermatitis from her and that it might leave me with scars. Is this possible?

Dermatitis does not cause scarring. Nor is it infectious, so you will not catch it from your friend.

I've heard that more females than males suffer from contact dermatitis. Why would that be? Does contact dermatitis affect men and women differently?

No, but some contact allergies are more common in one sex because members of that sex tend to be more exposed to the allergen. More females than males develop an allergy to nickel, for example, because nickel has been used in fasteners on women's underwear. Chrome allergy dermatitis is generally more common in males because chrome is present in cement, which males usually handle more often than females.

Dermatitis is inflammation of the skin. The symptoms are patches of redness and tiny blisters that may ooze and form crusts. Areas of skin become dry and cracked, and the skin may scale off, leaving red, oozing patches. It is extremely irritating and itches badly, but scratching makes it worse. Dermatitis may occur first on the face or the head as dandruff, or on the hands, and spread to other parts of the body. Alternatively, dermatitis may begin anywhere.

Dermatitis is often caused by allergies or contact with irritants such as soap or chemicals. It can also be brought on by stress and emotional problems, especially in the middle-aged. Sometimes, however, there is no obvious cause. Contact dermatitis can be caused by any number of things, including poisonous plants, hair dyes, cosmetics, metal, jewelry, shoes, clothing, and common drugs such as penicillin. It can also be caused by sunlight reacting with chemicals on the skin. Perfumes, aftershaves, and sunscreens may contain ingredients that cause a reaction.

Many people who get dermatitis belong to families with a history of asthma, hay fever, or other allergies. This type of dermatitis is often called eczema.

The tendency to dermatitis cannot be cured, but a doctor can suggest taking medication to control the inflammation and itching of the skin. It is usually best to keep the skin moist with aqueous creams or barrier creams.

In many cases, the condition will clear up completely; in severe cases, however, the patient may have to be hospitalized to undergo treatment.

People should avoid harsh substances such as certain chemicals and keep irritating materials such as wool away from the skin. People who use irritating substances at work, or wash dishes, or use cleaning agents should wear protective gloves.

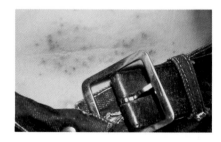

These red weals and blisters are an example of contact dermatitis. They have been caused by the metal buckle reacting with the skin.

SEE ALSO

ALLERGIES • ASTHMA • ECZEMA • SKIN • SKIN DISEASES AND DISORDERS

Diabetes

Diabetes mellitus is a disease in which the body does not produce sufficient amounts of the hormone insulin. This hormone directs the body's sugar into the cells, where it is used as fuel. Without insulin, the cells cannot work properly. Insulin-dependent diabetes, or type 1 diabetes, is quite a common illness. It used to be fatal, but modern treatments allow diabetics (people with diabetes) to lead normal lives.

Symptoms of diabetes

Diabetes can start at any age. It often begins abruptly in children but progresses more gradually in adults. The body either stops producing insulin or makes so little that it is unable to work properly. The most obvious symptom is a great thirst, causing people with diabetes to drink a large amount and produce a lot of urine. They also feel tired and weak because their body is not getting enough fuel. They may have blurred vision and itching skin, and because their resistance is low, they are vulnerable to all kinds of infections.

People with diabetes lose weight quickly, as their body uses up their fat as a fuel to replace sugar. This in turn produces harmful waste products that can cause a diabetic to go into a coma and to die. A doctor can easily tell when someone has diabetes, because the blood and urine both contain unusually large amounts of sugar.

Treatment of diabetes

People with severe diabetes treat themselves with daily injections of insulin. Diabetics are shown how to administer this themselves. Even young children are able to inject themselves. Doctors figure out how much insulin each person needs to function properly. The dose must be balanced with the person's intake of sugar and carbohydrates, so a diabetic must eat carefully and at regular times.

Getting the balance right is extremely important; if the blood sugar falls too low, the diabetic can go into insulin shock, known as hypoglycemia. The patient feels hungry, then dizzy, and soon loses consciousness. Someone who feels an attack coming on should eat something sweet as quickly as possible to raise the blood sugar. Diabetics should carry sugar lumps, candy, or other sweet foods with them at all times to counter such an attack.

People with mild diabetes may be able to control the condition by eating carefully and keeping their weight within a reasonable range. They must be particularly careful not to eat too much sugar or food containing sugar. They may also need tablets to make their bodies produce more insulin.

Q & A

I think my little brother eats far too much candy. All that sugar can't be good for him. Won't it cause him to develop diabetes—either now or later in life?

No. If a child is going to get diabetes, it will be the type caused by the failure to produce insulin (a hormone produced in the pancreas). Being overweight or eating sweet things has nothing to do with whether the insulin-producing cells in the pancreas are functioning properly or not.

My father has recently been diagnosed as having diabetes. I am afraid the illness may change his personality, by making him bad-tempered, for example. Am I right to worry about this?

Not really. Obviously, diabetes, like any illness, can put the patient under strain, but it does not cause personality changes. There is certainly nothing to suggest that diabetic children develop inadequate personalities because of their diabetes as they grow up.

CAUTION

Diabetics can lead a comparatively normal life. However, they should watch what they eat and talk to a doctor about vigorous exercise, which uses up blood sugar quickly. Diabetics need regular checkups and should always tell a dentist or doctor about their condition before undergoing any kind of treatment. When someone has had diabetes for a number of years, it can cause problems in other body systems. The eyes, nervous system, kidneys, and arterial system can be affected. Since diabetics may have poor circulation, they should always take particularly good care of their feet.

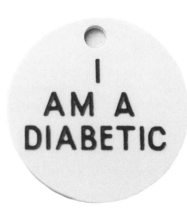

It is a good idea for people with diabetes to wear a tag such as this. If they were to slip into a diabetic coma, the emergency medical service would know immediately that they were diabetic, and precious time would be saved.

Checking urine and blood

Diabetics check their urine or blood regularly to make sure that the sugar level is correct. The only really effective way to control blood sugar is to check the levels in the blood at regular intervals. That is done using a small monitoring device that can determine blood sugar levels in blood taken from a small prick in the finger. Careful diabetic control reduces the risk of later complications.

Noninsulin-dependent diabetes

Not all diabetics need insulin injections, but for those not taking insulin it is essential to ensure that the body's own insulin production is adequate. Noninsulin-dependent diabetes (NIDD)—also known as type 2 diabetes or maturity-onset diabetes—can have serious complications. Insulin is still produced by the pancreas, but in quantities insufficient for the body's overall needs.

Noninsulin-dependent diabetes usually starts between the ages of 50 and 65, although it can affect people as young as 15. It may occur in people older than 65, and it may also have a genetic factor and run in families; of every three people with NIDD, approximately one has a relative who is also affected with the disorder. This type of diabetes usually starts with insulin resistance, a condition in which the cells cannot use insulin properly. At first, more insulin is made to compensate, but eventually the pancreas loses the ability to secrete insulin.

A principal, but not the sole, cause of NIDD is obesity. About 80 percent of people with NIDD are obese. For reasons that are not fully understood, obesity is associated with a state known as insulin resistance. It may simply be that the number of insulin receptor sites is inadequate, or it may be that the mechanisms triggered in the cell by insulin locking are adversely affected. It is known that people in wealthier societies tend to eat more food, which leads to a rise in obesity and hence a rise in NIDD.

Controlling NIDD

The object of treatment is to keep blood sugar levels within normal limits so that complications do not occur. Exercise and a healthy diet to maintain an appropriate weight are important in controlling blood sugar levels. In many cases, NIDD can be completely controlled by diet alone. What is eaten is just as important as how much is eaten. The aim is to control the blood sugar without drugs, but if necessary, production of insulin can be boosted by sulfonylurea drugs such as tolbutamide, chlorpropamide, or other drugs. If these drugs fail, insulin injections will then become necessary.

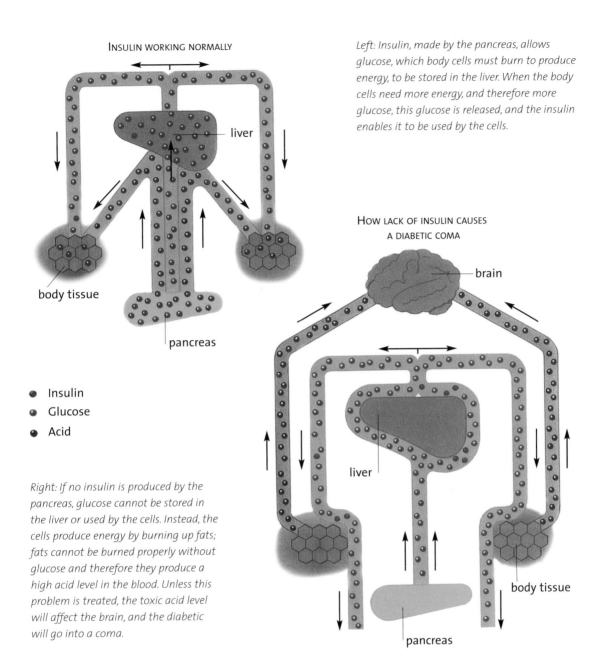

INSULIN WORKING NORMALLY

liver

body tissue

pancreas

Left: Insulin, made by the pancreas, allows glucose, which body cells must burn to produce energy, to be stored in the liver. When the body cells need more energy, and therefore more glucose, this glucose is released, and the insulin enables it to be used by the cells.

HOW LACK OF INSULIN CAUSES A DIABETIC COMA

brain

liver

body tissue

pancreas

- Insulin
- Glucose
- Acid

Right: If no insulin is produced by the pancreas, glucose cannot be stored in the liver or used by the cells. Instead, the cells produce energy by burning up fats; fats cannot be burned properly without glucose and therefore they produce a high acid level in the blood. Unless this problem is treated, the toxic acid level will affect the brain, and the diabetic will go into a coma.

SEE ALSO

CIRCULATORY SYSTEM DISEASES AND DISORDERS • EYE AND SIGHT • GLANDS • HORMONES AND HORMONAL DISORDERS • LIVER • OBESITY

Diarrhea

When someone has diarrhea, the bowel movements are more frequent than usual, often greater in volume, and very liquid. Diarrhea is not an illness but a symptom of many different infections and illnesses. It is caused by something that irritates the lining of the intestines. As a result, the intestines become inflamed and push the food through so quickly that there is no time for fluid to be absorbed in the usual way. Diarrhea may be accompanied by vomiting, cramps, and generalized weakness.

An extremely common cause of diarrhea is food poisoning, which can happen when a person eats food contaminated by bacteria. Viruses can also cause diarrhea. Certain foods, such as extremely rich or spicy foods, can bring on a bout of diarrhea if a person is not used to them. Feeling nervous can also make the intestines overactive and hurry the food through.

Having diarrhea for a day or two is unpleasant but not serious. If the diarrhea is severe and the person is also vomiting, or if it goes on for several days, a doctor should be called. He or she may want to have the feces analyzed to identify the underlying disorder. Diarrhea can be serious in babies and small children, so a doctor should be called if a child becomes dehydrated.

Chronic diarrhea is due not to infections but to other medical problems, such as Crohn's disease and ulcerative colitis. Crohn's disease is a condition that causes inflammation of any part of the gastrointestinal tract. However, it most commonly occurs at the lower end of the small intestine, the ileum. Typical symptoms include pain, ulcers, and diarrhea. Ulcerative colitis is a long-term inflammatory disease of the lining of the rectum. Sometimes it spreads to the lower part of the colon (large bowel), and in a few people it spreads to the entire colon (pancolitis). No single cause has been found to contribute to ulcerative colitis; possibilities range from an allergic reaction to an emotional upset.

Diarrhea also occurs when other diseases of the intestinal wall prevent the proper absorption of food. These conditions include celiac disease, in which the intestines cannot absorb gluten. They result in diarrhea and undernourishment.

Q & A

My mother is breast-feeding and refuses to eat grapes because she says they will give the baby diarrhea. Is this true?

Some foods, including fruit, onions, and spicy foods, can certainly affect a baby's intestines. The wise thing for your mother to do is to eat a bland diet when the baby is very young.

Whenever I eat cheese, I get diarrhea. Am I allergic to it?

Perhaps. Food allergies are more common than was previously thought. When you are allergic to certain foods, you get problems, such as rashes or wheezing, in other areas besides the intestines. To find out, stop eating cheese and see if the symptoms disappear.

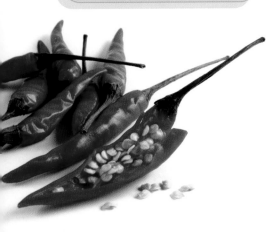

Some rich or spicy foods, such as these hot chilies, can result in a bout of diarrhea, especially if the person is not used to eating them.

SEE ALSO

BACTERIA • CELIAC DISEASE • CHOLERA • CROHN'S DISEASE • DIGESTIVE SYSTEM DISEASES AND DISORDERS • DYSENTERY • IRRITABLE BOWEL SYNDROME • SALMONELLA • TYPHOID FEVER

Digestive System

The digestive system is the part of the body that breaks down food into a form that can be absorbed by the cells. The digestive tract is sometimes called the alimentary canal. It consists of the mouth, throat, esophagus, stomach, and intestines.

From mouth to stomach

In the digestive system, digestive juices called enzymes act on the food that is eaten. Organs connected with the digestive tract produce these enzymes. Digestion begins in the mouth. As food is chewed, glands beneath the tongue increase the production of saliva, which contains the enzyme ptyalin. This enzyme starts breaking down some of the carbohydrates in the food into glucose and maltose, which are simple sugars.

From the mouth, the food travels through the throat and down the esophagus, or gullet. There, the gastric juices—a mixture of secretions composed of mucus, hydrochloric acid, and another enzyme, pepsin—are mixed with the food. The gastric juices in the stomach start to work on the proteins (foods such as eggs, cheese, chicken, and meat). The muscles in the walls of the stomach knead and churn the food around to aid digestion.

The small intestine, pancreas, and gallbladder

About four and a half hours after swallowing food, the partially digested mixture leaves the stomach in the form of a thickish, acidic liquid called chyme. This liquid passes into the duodenum, the first part of the small intestine, which is a coiled tube about 20 feet (6 m) long. The duodenum is the first part of the small intestine, which is about 10 inches (25 cm) long. Chyme contains a quantity of acid and enzymes that could damage the duodenum, but the duodenum plays a vital part in digestion by making and releasing large quantities of mucus, which protect the lining. The alkaline duodenal juices are produced under the influence of the hormone secretin, which helps neutralize the acids in the chyme.

The pancreas and the gallbladder also help with digestion. In response to the presence of food in the upper digestive tract, the gallbladder adds more enzymes that break down fats, nucleic acids, proteins, and carbohydrates. Bile is released via the bile ducts from the gallbladder, where it is stored. Bile is a yellowish fluid secreted by the liver, which helps digest fats.

From the duodenum, the partially digested food passes into the rest of the small intestine. The food takes nearly three hours to pass through the long, narrow tube of the small intestine. During its passage, the food is broken down completely by a series of enzymes. Amylase converts starch into maltose; lipase converts fats into glycerin and fatty acids; and trypsin reduces

Q & A

Is it true that babies can't digest cow's milk?

Compared with human breast milk, cow's milk contains large amounts of a protein called casein, which babies do not have the equipment to digest properly. The many powdered formula milks for babies are made from cow's milk and thus contain more casein than breast milk, but the formula milks are specially treated to make the casein more digestible. However, breast-feeding is better for a baby's digestive system, and in other ways, too.

My three-year-old sister loves spicy foods. However, won't they upset her stomach and her digestion?

There is no reason why spicy foods should cause her any problems. By the age of three, a child's digestive system can cope with an extremely mixed diet, and the degree of tolerance to spicy foods will vary, just as it does in adults. As long as these foods do not give her diarrhea or make her vomit, let her have foods that she likes.

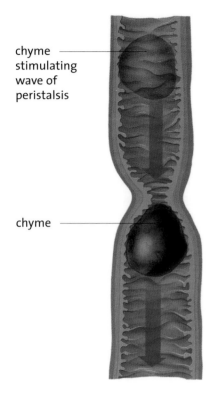

chyme
stimulating
wave of
peristalsis

chyme

Partially digested food (chyme) is moved through the intestine in waves, as the walls of the intestine contract and then relax. This wave movement is called peristalsis. It is stimulated by the presence of food in the esophagus.

proteins to amino acids. More enzymes are released from the walls of the small intestine to complete digestion. The broken-down food is now ready to be absorbed into the bloodstream.

Absorbing nutrients

The lining of the small intestine contains millions of minute projections called villi. Each villus is covered by a cell layer that absorbs nutrients. These cells have projections called microvilli. Both the villi and the microvilli increase the surface area of the small intestine to enable the efficient absorption of nutrients. The central core of each villus contains a capillary (a small blood vessel) and lacteals, which are branches of the lymphatic system. This system is a network of tiny tubes (the lymph vessels) carrying lymph, which is normally a colorless fluid. After a fatty meal, the lymph in the lacteals is milky white, owing to the presence of tiny fat globules. The function of the lymphatic system is to return liquid to the bloodstream. When digested food comes into contact with the villi, the glycerols, fatty acids, and dissolved vitamins enter the lacteals and travel through the lymphatic system to enter the bloodstream.

Other substances are absorbed directly into the capillaries in the villi. These substances include amino acids from protein digestion; sugars from carbohydrates; vitamins; and important minerals such as calcium, iodine, and iron. From the capillaries, these substances go to the liver, which extracts some of them. The rest go into the general blood circulation and are taken to the cells to provide them with energy.

The large intestine

When the digested food has gone through the small intestine, the remainder passes into the large intestine, or colon, as waste. The colon extracts water from the waste, which collects in the rectum and passes out through the anus as feces.

The surface of the small intestine is covered with small, fingerlike projections called villi. They increase the surface area and allow food to be absorbed quickly into the capillaries (blood vessels).

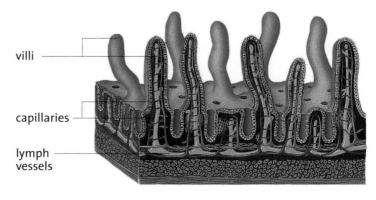

villi

capillaries

lymph
vessels

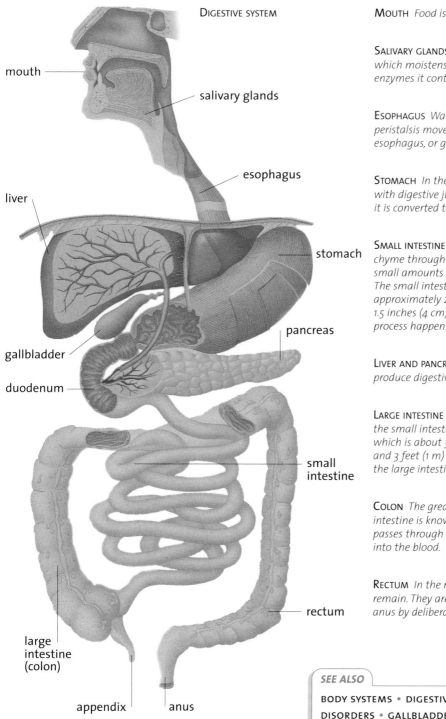

DIGESTIVE SYSTEM

mouth

salivary glands

esophagus

liver

stomach

gallbladder

pancreas

duodenum

small intestine

large intestine (colon)

rectum

appendix

anus

MOUTH *Food is taken into the mouth.*

SALIVARY GLANDS *They produce saliva, which moistens the food while the enzymes it contains start digestion.*

ESOPHAGUS *Waves of muscle action called peristalsis move the food down the esophagus, or gullet, and into the stomach.*

STOMACH *In the stomach, the food is mixed with digestive juices. After two to six hours, it is converted to a liquid called chyme.*

SMALL INTESTINE *Waves of peristalsis push chyme through the stomach and out in small amounts into the small intestine. The small intestine of an adult measures approximately 20 feet (6 m) long and 1.5 inches (4 cm) wide. Most of the digestive process happens here.*

LIVER AND PANCREAS *The liver and pancreas produce digestive juices.*

LARGE INTESTINE *Chyme passes from the small intestine into the large intestine, which is about 3 inches (7.5 cm) in diameter and 3 feet (1 m) long. The appendix leads off the large intestine.*

COLON *The greater part of the large intestine is known as the colon. As chyme passes through the colon, water is absorbed into the blood.*

RECTUM *In the rectum, only solid feces remain. They are pushed out through the anus by deliberate muscle contractions.*

SEE ALSO

BODY SYSTEMS • DIGESTIVE SYSTEM DISEASES AND DISORDERS • GALLBLADDER AND GALLSTONES

Digestive System Diseases and Disorders

Q & A

My mother says that laxatives are dangerous and that you should always treat constipation naturally. Is she right, and what does she mean by "naturally"?

Yes, your mother is right. Too many laxatives can harm your digestive system. The best natural remedies for constipation are bran, fresh fruits, and vegetables. These foods contain the naturally occurring substances, especially fiber, that encourage the bowels to move regularly, without harming them.

My grandmother got very sick when she was at our house and she had symptoms of diarrhea. However, when the doctor came, he said it was really constipation. How could this be?

This is a rather common ailment in the elderly, called spurious diarrhea. The lower intestine gets clogged with feces, yet some liquid matter manages to get past the blockage, appearing as diarrhea, and may cause the older person to lose control of the bowels and become incontinent. However, this problem can be easily treated.

Many digestive disorders are caused by the food people eat. The digestive system works best when people eat a diet containing a good deal of fiber and not too much fat. A low-fiber diet can cause constipation (infrequent bowel movements, with small, hard stools), and eating extremely spicy food can cause diarrhea, if people are not accustomed to such food. Indigestion, or dyspepsia, can be caused by nervousness, eating too fast, and emotional stress. It results in discomfort, belching, and heartburn. Also associated with indigestion is flatulence, which is a buildup of gas in the intestines. Sensible eating habits and relaxation are the most common treatments.

Contaminated food and appendicitis

Some painful and dangerous illnesses are caused by eating food contaminated by bacteria, including staphylococcal poisoning, salmonella poisoning, amebic and bacillary dysentery, botulism, cholera, and typhoid fever. These illnesses cause many symptoms, inlcuding vomiting, abdominal pain, and diarrhea. Foods may be contaminated by chemicals, which cause vomiting, or be poisonous themselves, as are some fungi.

Appendicitis is inflammation of the appendix, normally as a result of bacterial infection. It is most common between the ages of 15 and 24 years. The symptoms include pain in the lower right abdomen and sometimes nausea and vomiting. Treatment involves surgery to remove the appendix.

Ulcers and inflammation

Ulcers are small, open sores that form when the mucous membrane lining the digestive tract is damaged. Small ulcers often form in the mouth but heal quickly. Ulcers in the stomach and duodenum are more serious. Although the exact cause is unclear, the bacterium *Helicobacter pylori* may cause inflammation and ulceration by increasing stomach acid. Ulcers are more common in people who eat hurried and irregular meals, who drink heavily, who smoke, or who are nervous and under stress. Inflammation, thickening, and ulceration of the colon or another region of the digestive tract can cause Crohn's disease, with cramps and pains after eating. There may be persistent diarrhea, abdominal pain, fever, loss of weight, and bleeding, leading to anemia. Drugs can relieve the anemia, but surgery may be needed. Inflammations and ulcerations of the colon are called colitis. Some inflammations are caused by an infection or an allergy and last a short time, but others are chronic conditions. Symptoms are abdominal pain and diarrhea. Chronic colitis may never clear up completely.

GASTROINTESTINAL DISORDERS

Disorder	Symptoms	Treatment
Bad breath (halitosis): Unpleasant odor due to swallowed food or drink, dental disease, or sometimes disorders of the respiratory or digestive systems	Bad breath	Removal of cause, change of diet, and good dental hygiene
Foreign bodies: Fish bones, toothpicks, buttons, coins, and so on, swallowed by children and the unwary	Choking, or severe pain in colon	Small round objects can pass through the digestive tract with no problem. Sharper ones may require surgery.
Gastritis: Inflammation of the stomach lining, caused by drugs, food poisoning, infection, alcohol, or eating the wrong type of food (acute); inflammation of the lining of the stomach, leading to ulceration and hemorrhage, caused by poor diet, alcoholism, enzyme deficiency, hiatus hernia, diabetes, cancer, or emotional stress (chronic)	Pain in abdomen, loss of appetite, nausea, vomiting, and diarrhea (acute gastritis); pain on eating, pain in back, rapid feeling of fullness, nausea, and blood in vomit (chronic gastritis)	Usually corrects itself when the cause has been eliminated by vomiting or diarrhea; bed rest and bland diet are recommended (acute). Treatment for specific diseases and avoidance of alcohol, tobacco, and very spicy food; bland diet with small meals eaten frequently; removal of causes of stress, or prescription of tranquilizers (chronic)
Gastroenteritis: Inflammation of the lining of the stomach and the intestines	Pain in abdomen, loss of appetite, nausea, vomiting, and diarrhea	As for acute gastritis (above)
Hemorrhoids (piles): Swollen and twisted veins that are located in the anal canal, hemorrhoids may become ulcerated or thrombosed and may eventually protrude from the anus; they occur in most adults.	Pain and bleeding during defecation, constipation	May regress naturally with high-fiber diet; hemorrhoids may be injected, or removed surgically.
Infection and infestation: Bacteria, viruses, and various types of parasites may live in the human digestive tract over a period of time and cause a variety of problems.	Various	Various
Malabsorption: Failure of absorption of nutrients from the digestive tract due to various disorders	Weight loss, increased excretion of protein and fat, diarrhea, and anemia	Various specific diets and treatments
Nausea and vomiting: Vomiting is usually a natural response to harmful substances that must be expelled undigested from the body. Some feelings of nausea and vomiting are psychological in origin.	Nausea due to real or imagined cause; deliberate vomiting during temper tantrums, or on eating wholesome but unpalatable food, or because of an eating disorder	Treatment of physical disorder, if present; reassurance and psychotherapy if not
Peritonitis: Inflammation of the lining of the abdominal cavity and the organs (peritoneum), which is most commonly caused by the perforation or the rupture of an organ such as the appendix, or perforation of an ulcer	Mostly sudden, severe, localized pain in the abdomen, spreading, and leading to shock	Emergency operation, or occasionally medication
Polyps and benign tumors: A growth of protruding tissue that can arise anywhere in the digestive tract	Bleeding, cramps, abdominal pains, or no symptoms	Polyps should be removed by surgery, because some do become cancerous.

One problem of the large intestine is irritable bowel syndrome. Its cause is not really known, but attacks may be triggered by stress. The main symptoms are spasmodic lower abdominal pain and bouts of diarrhea and constipation. A high-fiber diet and antispasmodic drugs may help, but people with irritable bowel syndrome may find it recurs after long gaps, usually when they are nervous or under stress.

Hernias and diverticular disease

The lining of the esophagus is seldom damaged. Sometimes, however, a hiatal hernia forms at the point where the esophagus passes through a gap in the diaphragm and into the abdomen. Part of the esophagus and the upper stomach then bulges back into the chest, and acid from the stomach may make its way back into the esophagus, causing a burning sensation called heartburn. The lining of the esophagus can also be damaged by swallowing acid or a strong alkali.

Sometimes, bulges called diverticula form in the colon, which is the major part of the large intestine. These bulges develop with age, and waste matter may fill them and become infected, causing diverticulitis. The condition can cause bleeding. Alternatively, an inflamed diverticulum may bulge into the abdominal cavity. This extremely serious condition needs immediate surgical treatment. However, rest, a healthy diet, and antibiotics help control diverticulitis.

Cancer of the digestive system

Cancer is unusual in the small intestine but common in the stomach and colon. Treatment may include a combination of surgery, radiotherapy, and chemotherapy. If the disease is diagnosed and treated early enough, patients can live a normal life.

The symptoms are similar for mild or serious cases, so people should consult a doctor if they have long-lasting pain or nausea, if they lose their appetite for more than a few days, if their normal pattern of bowel movements changes, or if they have bleeding.

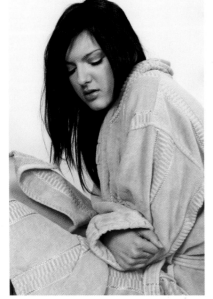

Irritable bowel syndrome results in spasmodic lower abdominal pain and bouts of diarrhea and constipation. Stress and nervousness make it worse.

> **SEE ALSO**
>
> ANEMIA • APPENDICITIS • BACTERIA • BOTULISM • CANCER • CHOLERA • COLON AND COLON DISEASES • CROHN'S DISEASE • DIARRHEA • DIGESTIVE SYSTEM • DYSENTERY • GASTROENTERITIS • HEMORRHOIDS • HERNIA • IRRITABLE BOWEL SYNDROME • SALMONELLA • TYPHOID FEVER • ULCERS

Diphtheria

Q & A

I thought diphtheria had been wiped out a long time ago, but my mother says that the vaccinations are still being given. Is it really necessary for babies to be vaccinated against the disease?

Yes. Because many countries now carry out immunizations, death from diphtheria is rare. However, there are always minor outbreaks of diphtheria, even with immunization.

Once a person has been vaccinated, can that person's immunity to diphtheria wear off?

No. However, booster doses of diptheria vaccine may be required if there is an epidemic.

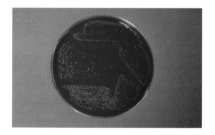

This blood agar plate culture shows Corynebacterium diphtheriae, *the bacterium that causes diphtheria.*

Diphtheria is an extremely serious infection of the throat and nose, caused by the bacterium *Corynebacterium diphtheriae*. Diphtheria occurs mainly in children under the age of 10 and can be fatal if untreated or if treatment is delayed. Children in many countries, including the United States, are now immunized against diphtheria, so in these countries the infection is rare.

The bacteria causing diphtheria produce poisons, or toxins, that attack the mucous membranes of the throat and nose. If antitoxin is not administered promptly, the toxins can affect the nervous system, the kidneys, and the heart. The disease can be contracted by contact with an infected person, through airborne droplets from coughs and sneezes. Sometimes, it is transmitted through infected milk or by a carrier—someone who has the bacteria in his or her system but who is symptomless.

Symptoms, treatment, and prevention

After an incubation period lasting from two days to one week, the infected person develops a sore throat, a headache, and a fever. A soft, grayish membrane forms in the throat and may spread into the mouth and nose. Swallowing and breathing become extremely painful, and the glands at the sides of the neck swell. The membrane can make it so difficult to breathe that a tracheotomy (surgery to the throat to access the airway) may need to be performed to allow the patient to breathe.

Diphtheria is treated with antibiotics to fight the bacteria and antitoxins to counteract the toxins. The disease is so infectious that the patient must be isolated in a hospital and kept in bed for several weeks or even months. That period is followed by a very gradual return to normal life. However, if the infection is treated in time, the patient should recover completely.

Immunization for children and boosters for adults protect against diphtheria. Children who are immunized produce antitoxins after an infection. Immunization consists of an initial injection, then two more, and a booster a year later. Another booster can be given before the child starts school. Before a child has the vaccination, a test called the Schick test may be given. A small amount of diphtheria toxin is injected into the skin. The reaction shows if a child is naturally immune before having the vaccination. If large numbers of children remain unvaccinated, there is always the possibility of an epidemic.

SEE ALSO

BACTERIA • BACTERIAL DISEASES • INFECTIOUS DISEASES

Down Syndrome

Q & A

I have a younger sibling who has Down syndrome. I am extremely worried. Is it likely that I could have a child with Down syndrome when I grow up and get married?

It would be wise to discuss this concern with your doctor to rule out the possibility that you carry the familial type of Down syndrome. However, this type is very rare.

Is it possible for a child with Down syndrome ever to improve his or her mental ability?

There is not much that can be done to improve the intelligence, as such, of a child with Down syndrome. However, researchers who have given large doses of vitamins to Down syndrome children have reported improvements. On the other hand, this effect has not been proved scientifically; therefore, it would be wrong to take such reports as fact. However, it is also true that if children with Down syndrome are properly trained and taught, then it can seem that their ability is improved; in fact, they are simply realizing their potential.

Down syndrome is the name given to the collection of birth defects caused by an extra chromosome. Normally, people are born with 46 chromosomes, 23 inherited from each parent. These chromosomes carry the genes, which are the chemical messages that determine how each individual will develop. Some babies are born with an extra chromosome, a condition known as trisomy 21. As a result, they develop abnormally in several ways.

Features of Down syndrome

The most noticeable feature of Down syndrome babies is their slanted eyes, round face, flattened head, and small features. Their hands and feet are short and broad. Many Down syndrome babies are born with a heart defect, and their digestive system may also be faulty. All children with Down syndrome have learning difficulties to some extent.

People with Down syndrome are usually exceptionally happy, gentle, and loving. As children, they need loving care and extra attention to make sure the mind is stimulated. They need special teaching to make sure that they develop as much as possible. There is a large variation in handicaps. Some Down syndrome children may be only a little below average and will grow up able to live an ordinary life and work at a normal job. Others are much more severely handicapped physically and mentally. These people may need to live in a special home.

NORMAL CELL

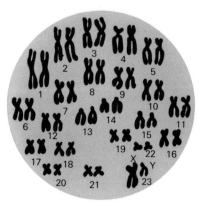

DOWN SYNDROME CELL

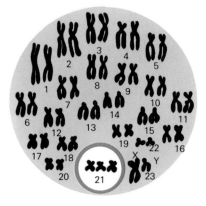

In Down syndrome, there are three of chromosome 21 (circled right) in each body cell instead of two.

This little girl has Down syndrome. She will need special care for all her life.

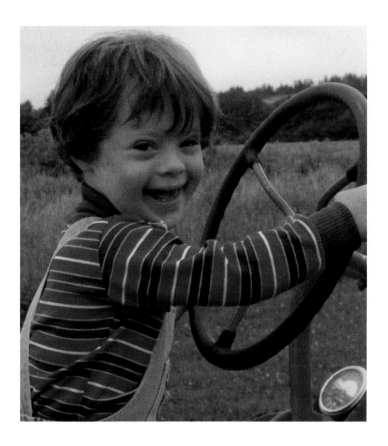

Older mothers and Down syndrome

People with Down syndrome probably inherit their extra chromosome from the mother. It is not known why that should be the case. However, older mothers, particularly those who are over the age of 35, have a much greater chance of producing a Down syndrome baby.

For this reason, older women are often given a quick and painless test called an amniocentesis when they are pregnant. In this procedure, doctors draw off a tiny quantity of the amniotic fluid that surrounds the developing baby in the uterus. They can tell from cells in this fluid whether or not the baby has an extra chromosome.

SEE ALSO

BIRTH DEFECTS • CELLS AND CHROMOSOMES • DIGESTIVE SYSTEM DISEASES AND DISORDERS • GENES • GENETIC DISEASES AND DISORDERS • HEART DISEASES AND DISORDERS

Dysentery

Q & A

I am going to South America this summer on a student-exchange program. Is there a drug I can take with me in case I get dysentery?

It would be better to try to prevent the disease in the first place. Avoid food prepared with local water, such as salad or washed fruit; drink bottled water or canned drinks; and eat only canned meat and vegetables and fruits that can be peeled or boiled. Do not take any drug for a stomach upset until you know the cause, because the drug may interfere with the diagnosis and result in the wrong treatment.

Is typhoid the same as dysentery?

No, although there are some similarities between the two diseases. Both are transmitted by contaminated food and water, but typhoid is a form of gastroenteritis (inflammation of the intestines), caused by bacteria from the *Salmonella* genus. The incubation period for typhoid is longer than that for dysentery, usually one to two weeks.

Dysentery is an infection of the intestines characterized by severe diarrhea, often containing mucus and blood, and abdominal pain. There are two types: amebic dysentery and bacillary dysentery (shigellosis). Both diseases are spread from infected people to others through food or water that is contaminated by feces. Amebic dysentery is common in underdeveloped countries and is also present in the United States. Bacillary dysentery is present all over the world where people are crowded together in unhygienic conditions.

Amebic dysentery is an infection of the inner lining of the large intestine and the liver caused by a microscopic parasitic amoeba, *Entamoeba histolytica*. The symptoms are blood-stained diarrhea, stomach pains, nausea, and vomiting. These symptoms may last for a few weeks and then die down but will come back from time to time. The amoebas make their way to the colon, where they multiply and form abscesses. Sometimes, amoebas move through the bloodstream to the liver, where they form abscesses. They may even spread to the lungs and the membrane enclosing the heart. Once the organism has been recognized, it is easily killed by taking drugs for about 10 days. Afterward, the patient will need monthly checkups for a while to make sure that all the amoebas have been destroyed.

Bacillary dysentery, or shigellosis, is caused by *Shigella* bacteria. Bacillary dysentery begins between 12 hours and three days after infection. The symptoms include fever, cramps, and severe diarrhea, which may contain blood and mucus. The disease lasts from four to seven days. The symptoms are similar to those of amebic dysentery, cholera, typhoid fever, and salmonella, so it is important to see a doctor.

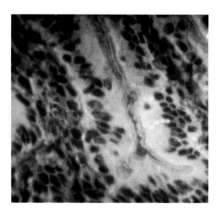

In bacillary dysentery, Shigella *bacteria penetrate the lining of the intestines.*

SEE ALSO

BACTERIAL DISEASES • CHOLERA • DIARRHEA • GASTROENTERITIS • INFECTIOUS DISEASES • SALMONELLA • TYPHOID FEVER

Ear and Hearing

Q & A

My sister was recently blinded in an accident. Will her hearing improve to compensate?

No, but blind people train themselves to be more discerning in picking out sounds, because they must rely more on their sense of hearing.

Can a person with hearing in only one ear identify the direction from which a sound is coming?

To some degree, yes. However, such a person will be much less accurate in pinpointing the direction of the sound than a person with hearing in both ears.

Why can I pick out one sound from many others when I concentrate hard?

This is the result of selective interpretation by the brain. By making a special effort, your brain can screen out all the unwanted sounds and tune itself to notice one particular frequency.

The ears are delicate, complicated organs that provide a sense of balance and enable people to hear. Each ear is divided into the outer ear (which receives sound waves), the middle ear (which acts as an amplifier), and the inner ear (which transmits sound waves to the brain). The outer ear, or pinna, is the fleshy part that can be seen. At the center of the pinna is a bony canal leading to the tympanic membrane, or eardrum. The eardrum is a thin sheet of membrane that separates the outer and middle ear. The membrane vibrates when sound waves reach it.

Inside the middle ear are three linked bones: the malleus, the incus, and the stapes, commonly called the hammer, anvil, and stirrup. These three bones act as levers, matching the free movement of the eardrum to the stiff movement of an opening between the middle ear and inner ear called the oval window. The malleus is attached to the eardrum and picks up its vibrations. It transmits them through the anvil to the stirrup, which is attached to the inner ear through the oval window. Another opening, the round window, is covered by a membrane and allows free vibration of the fluid in a structure called the cochlea. Sound waves reach the inner ear through the skull bones.

A narrow tube, the eustachian tube, connects the middle ear to the back of the throat. This tube helps equalize the air pressure on either side of the eardrum. The popping in the ears that occurs when someone goes down quickly in an elevator is caused by small movements of the eardrum, which result from changes of pressure in the middle ear.

The hearing part of the inner ear is the cochlea. This name means "snail shell," which is what the structure resembles. The cochlea is filled with fluid. Thousands of tiny, hairlike sensors

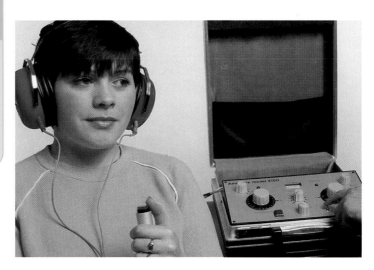

This girl is having her hearing tested by an audiometer. Sounds are emitted; she listens through earphones, and if she can hear them, she signals by pressing the button.

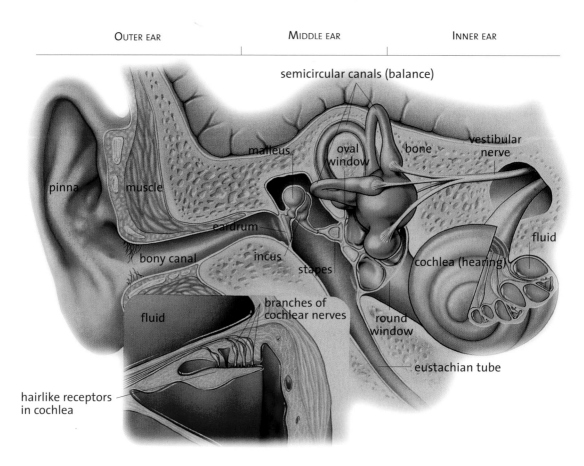

OUTER EAR   MIDDLE EAR   INNER EAR

semicircular canals (balance)

malleus   oval window   bone   vestibular nerve

pinna   muscle

eardrum

bony canal   incus   stapes   cochlea (hearing)   fluid

fluid   branches of cochlear nerves   round window

eustachian tube

hairlike receptors in cochlea

The outer ear receives sounds, the bones of the middle ear link the drum to the inner ear, and the inner ear transmits messages to the brain. Hairlike receptors in the cochlea send messages along nearby nerves to the brain, in response to the vibrations of the fluid inside.

convert the vibrations in the fluid into nerve impulses and then pass these impulses to the brain via the auditory nerve.

The balancing part of the inner ear is attached to the cochlea. It consists of three semicircular canals, two placed vertically and one horizontally. Sensitive hairs inside these canals detect the position of the head. They then pass on this information to the cerebellum, a part of the brain. The cerebellum also receives information from the joints and the eyes about the position of other parts of the body. The cerebellum processes these messages and sends out instructions to the rest of the body that keep it balanced. When people spin around rapidly or are rocked to and fro when traveling, they feel dizzy because at least one of the semicircular canals has been overstimulated.

SEE ALSO

BONE • DEAFNESS • EAR DISEASES AND DISORDERS

Ear Diseases and Disorders

Q & A

Can earwax cause deafness?

Yes, earwax can cause temporary deafness. A small amount does no harm, but if the canal is blocked completely over a period of time, or if the wax swells suddenly because water enters the ear canal, moderate hearing loss, discomfort, and pain may result.

My ears ring after I go to a rock concert. Could the noise damage my ears?

Prolonged exposure to very loud noises can cause irreversible ear damage. It starts with deafness in the highest frequencies and moves on to the lower ones, but avoiding prolonged exposure to loud noises can stop its progress.

Is it true that measles can cause deafness?

Yes, but rarely. Measles can be complicated by an inflammation of the middle part of the ear, which contains the bones that transmit sound from the eardrum to the inner ear. If the infection is not treated properly, this part of the conducting system may become damaged.

Everyone should take good care of his or her ears; damage to them can lead to permanent deafness. If people experience pain, discharge from the ears, ringing noises, or loss of hearing, they should tell their doctor. Early treatment and advice can often prevent more serious harm.

The most common problem with the outer ear is infection of the skin lining it. This can be a local infection (such as a boil) or the whole lining of the ear may become inflamed (otitis externa). Swimming in polluted water is a common cause of ear infection. Infection may also spread to the ear from infected skin on the face; this is particularly common in people who have very greasy skin and a tendency toward dandruff. The infection can cause swelling and a discharge of pus, and even loss of hearing if the ear becomes blocked. Treatment with antibiotics clears up the problem. It is important to take antibiotics fairly promptly, before the infection spreads to the middle ear.

Earwax

Everyone produces earwax. The purpose of earwax is to clean the ear canal and to keep it moist. However, earwax can build up externally and cause discomfort. If that happens, it should be cleaned away carefully with a damp facecloth. If the wax gets packed down against the eardrum, it can cause earache, loss of hearing, and ringing noises in the ear. In this case, the wax should be syringed out professionally by a doctor or nurse. The ears should never be cleaned with sharp objects or even cotton swabs, because such cleaning can lead to a buildup of wax and could also damage or infect the eardrum.

The eardrum may be damaged by loud noises, a change in pressure caused by a high dive or a trip in an unpressurized aircraft, an explosion, or a sharp blow to the head. The eardrum will heal in a week or so, but a doctor should be consulted if a problem is suspected.

Middle-ear problems

Middle-ear infections are often caused by viruses or bacteria traveling along the eustachian tube, from the back of the nose and throat. Pus builds up in the middle-ear chamber, and as it cannot drain away, the ear becomes extremely painful. In a particularly severe infection, the pressure of the pus may rupture the eardrum, allowing the pus to drain from the outer ear.

Unless the infection is treated, it may spread to the mastoid bone behind the ear. A mastoidectomy may then be necessary; this is an operation in which the surgeon drains the pus in the mastoid bone to the exterior.

COMMON EAR DISORDERS

Condition	Cause	Symptoms	Treatment
Congenital deafness	Abnormality of the ear or damage to the auditory nerve from rubella or shortage of oxygen at birth	Extreme or total deafness, speech difficulties	Special education, hearing aid, speech therapy
Damage to the auditory nerve (three types)	Severe loud noise, for example from aircraft, loud machinery, and gun or bomb explosions Large dosages of streptomycin, quinine, or aspirin Growth on nerve between ear and brain (acoustic neuroma)	Gradual deafness Deafness occurs during or after course of drug Progressive deafness	Wearing ear protectors to prevent damage; hearing aid if damage already present Avoid drugs concerned Surgical removal of tumor
Earwax	Excessive production of wax, sometimes from skin conditions such as dermatitis	Wax swells following a cold or after a swim, and deafness then develops	Wax is syringed out by a doctor using warm water
Eustachian congestion	Inflammation and congestion of eustachian tube after a cold or infection blocks the tube	Periods of deafness, which may clear on blowing the nose	Decongestant tablets; tube may need to be unblocked by doctor
Foreign body in outer ear	Placing a small object in the ear, usually done by a child	Discomfort and discharge of pus; deafness sometimes unnoticed	Removal of foreign body; antibiotic drugs may be necessary
Infections damaging the auditory nerves	Viral or bacterial; can follow measles, mumps, and meningitis	Progressive deafness	Hearing aid; learning to read lips and speak from memory
Injury to the eardrum, possibly puncturing it (perforation)	Skull fracture, shock from an explosion, blow on ear, or unskilled attempt to remove a foreign body or wax from ear	Often sudden pain at moment of injury; deafness, occasionally dizziness and ringing in the ear	Antibiotics from doctor; gradual return of hearing
Ménière's disease	Rising pressure within cochlea of the inner ear	Vertigo, ringing in the ear, vomiting, gradual deafness	Drug treatment to reduce the pressure of the fluid
Middle-ear inflammation (otitis media)	Viral or bacterial; follows repeated blockage of the eustachian tube from congestion; frequently occurs in children	Deafness with pain in the ear and fever; release of sticky fluid from the middle ear; possible perforation of the eardrum and pus discharge	Antibiotics and painkillers; place warm hot-water bottle near the ear to relieve earache; heals when infection is eradicated
Otosclerosis	Fusion of the stapes into the oval window; frequently occurs in young adults and gradually worsens	Slow onset of deafness and sometimes tinnitus (buzzing or ringing sound in the ear)	Surgical removal of tiny stapes bone and replacement by vein graft or plastic device
Outer-ear inflammation (otitis externa)	Often associated with dandruff; made worse by scratching or cleansing the outer ear with rough towels or hard objects	Itchy, red, swollen, painful ears; debris of swelling blocks ears; often recurs	Special eardrops and painkillers from doctor to treat initial stages; corticosteroid eardrops to prevent further skin irritations
Senile deafness (presbyacusis)	Aging	Gradual inability to hear (high-pitched sounds first)	Hearing aid; learning to lip-read and speak from memory

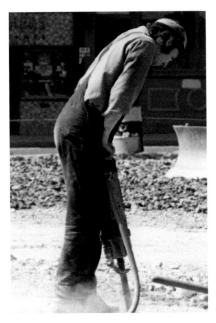

This man is using a pneumatic drill to dig up the surface of the road. Continuous loud noises can permanently damage hearing, so people who work in a noisy job should wear ear protectors.

Sometimes, the amplifier system of bones in the middle ear seizes, causing increasing deafness. This problem can be cured by an operation to replace the stapes bone with plastic.

Inner-ear problems

Inflammations of the inner ear, although uncommon, can cause deafness and may lead to problems with balance. The patient can suffer from bad attacks of dizziness, ringing in the ears, and sometimes vomiting. These inflammations usually spread from the middle ear. They may heal by themselves; if not, antibiotics help.

The same sort of symptoms are caused by the rare disorder Ménière's disease, which is thought to be caused by too much fluid in the ear's cochlea. At first, only one ear is involved, but eventually the second ear is also affected. Drugs can help reduce the symptoms, and in some cases an operation to drain excess fluid may be possible.

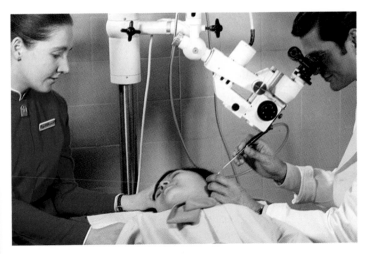

A doctor uses a magnifying microscope to examine a patient's ear for the presence of earwax or any foreign body. Anything that is causing a problem can be removed with fine forceps or a suction tube that is attached to a vacuum pump.

RINGING EARS

Tinnitus, or "ringing in the ears," is a symptom of many ear infections. The noises heard include ringing, hissing, buzzing, and roaring. Some people hear such loud noises that they cannot sleep. Tinnitus caused by infection of the outer and middle ear disappears once the infection has cleared, but tinnitus that is caused by damage to the cells of the inner ear can be extremely difficult to treat.

SEE ALSO
BIRTH DEFECTS • DEAFNESS • EAR AND HEARING

Eczema

Eczema is a condition that results in itchy, inflamed skin, which may become crusty, scaly, or covered with tiny blisters. Eczema usually appears during childhood but then disappears as the child grows older. The most familiar form of eczema develops from exposure to substances that cause an allergic reaction. This form of eczema is related to asthma and hay fever. Many people who have eczema also have asthma or hay fever, or both. Stress is another contributory factor.

Eczema itch

The most annoying symptom of eczema is the itch. Scratching the blisters creates bleeding sores, which make it easier for the infection to spread. The sores then dry out, leaving the skin dry and cracked. The inflamed skin can appear anywhere on the body. It usually starts on the face and scalp and then spreads to the hands and limbs, especially around folds of skin.

Preventing eczema

Eczema can be extremely uncomfortable, but it is important to avoid scratching the inflamed skin. Scratching makes the condition much worse. Cotton mittens prevent babies and infants from scratching the affected area. If the eczema is due to an allergy, the substance that causes the reaction should be avoided. Because some babies are allergic to cow's milk, eczema can be avoided by breast feeding or by using alternatives such as goat's milk or soy milk.

People with eczema have sensitive skin, so it is important for them to avoid contact with harsh chemicals and irritating materials such as wool. The skin should be kept clean to avoid infection, but it should not be washed too often. Many people with eczema use aqueous creams instead of soap.

Treatment options

Various medicines can be used to relieve and control the inflammation and itching. Tried and trusted remedies include zinc paste and coal tar, but doctors now prescribe steroid creams that contain hydrocortisone. Other creams may be used to increase the water content of the skin. Antihistamines often reduce the itching, although it is virtually impossible to avoid scratching the inflamed skin.

SEE ALSO

ALLERGIES • ASTHMA • DERMATITIS • SKIN • SKIN DISEASES AND DISORDERS

Q & A

Will my five-year-old sister's eczema get better as she gets older?

Half the children who suffer from eczema when they are young have grown out of it by the time they are six. In most other cases, it will clear up by their teens. However, eczema is notorious for disappearing and reappearing without obvious cause. It may return in adolescence or adulthood, especially at times of stress.

If I touch someone with eczema, will I catch it?

Definitely not. Eczema is not infectious and cannot be passed from person to person.

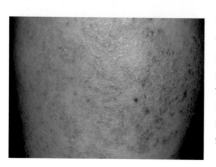

Eczematous skin rash on a man's leg. The skin becomes inflamed, crusty, and scaly, and tiny blisters may form.

Edema

Q & A

My aunt has both varicose veins and edema. Is there any connection between the two things, or is my aunt's case just a coincidence?

Yes, there is a connection. The leg veins have valves that prevent blood from moving back toward the ankles. Varicose veins are so stretched and swollen that the valves cannot stop the blood from slipping back. That blood flow causes a rise in pressure with reduced inflow of tissue fluid, causing edema.

My mother's doctor gave her potassium pills to take with her water pills. Why does she have to take these potassium pills? What exactly will they do for her?

Water pills stop the kidneys from reabsorbing the salt they filter out. The loss of salt and water reduces the volume of the blood, and the edema subsides. However, the pills remove potassium too, so it may be necessary to make up the loss to prevent the body from experiencing potassium deficiency.

The body normally contains a large quantity of water: in the blood, inside the body cells, and in the spaces between the cells (extracellular spaces). An excess of fluid, mainly water, in the extracellular spaces is called edema. There is a constant flow and interchange of fluid between the blood and the extracellular spaces and between the extracellular spaces and the interior of the cells. This interchange is important, because it allows vital nutrients to pass from the blood to the cells and waste material to pass out of the cells and into the blood for disposal.

Causes of edema

The amount of fluid present in the blood is affected by how much a person drinks. An excess of water in the blood is usually quickly corrected by an increase in the amount of fluid passed by the kidneys. The loss of larger quantities of dilute urine ensures that no excess of fluid occurs in the tissue spaces, and edema is avoided. For efficient loss of excess fluid, the kidneys should be working properly. Kidney disease is one of the causes of edema.

For fluid to be carried efficiently in the blood from the tissues to the kidneys, an efficient circulation is needed. Heart failure is defined as the inability of the heart to maintain adequate blood circulation. One of the main signs of heart failure is edema. If the right side of the heart is weakened, blood stagnates in the body, and edema occurs in the lowest parts, causing swelling of the ankles and lower back. If a finger is pressed into such edema, it leaves a hollow that slowly fills. That is called pitting edema. Failure of the left side of the heart causes edema in the lungs, with congestion, coughing, and breathing problems.

Another important cause of edema is inadequate quantities of proteins dissolved in the blood. These proteins thicken the blood and cause it to draw water from extracellular spaces. This process is called osmosis. Protein loss may be due to kidney disease or to starvation.

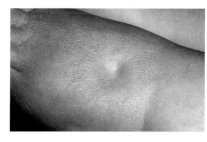

This picture shows pitting edema: a finger pressed into the swelling has left a hollow that slowly fills with extracellular fluid.

SEE ALSO

ALLERGIES • BLOOD • HEART • KIDNEY • LYMPHATIC SYSTEM • MALNUTRITION • VEIN DISORDERS

Emphysema

Emphysema is a serious disease of the lungs. The tiny air sacs (alveoli) become damaged and the lung tissues become less elastic. Many alveoli burst and merge with one another, so the internal surface area of the lungs becomes smaller. The lungs become less efficient at supplying the blood with oxygen. The most obvious symptom of emphysema is breathlessness and then coughing, which is brought on by any effort—even by talking or laughing. The breathlessness may make chewing and swallowing difficult. Lack of oxygen in the blood gives the skin a bluish tinge. People who suffer from emphysema catch lung infections easily. In time, the strain of breathing damages the heart. They become more and more disabled and eventually die.

Emphysema has nothing to do with increased air pressure in the lungs. It is not caused by playing wind instruments, for example. The delicate lung tissue is damaged mainly by smoking and persistent bronchitis; it is unable to withstand the normal pressures during breathing and coughing and breaks down. Emphysema cannot be cured, but the progress of the disease can be slowed down. The most important thing is to stop smoking. Patients should avoid dusty or polluted places and keep away from anyone with a chest infection. Bronchodilator drugs help clear air passages, and breathing pure oxygen from a cylinder allows more oxygen to enter the blood.

Q & A

Some people who have never smoked still have emphysema. How is this possible?

Smokers are much more likely to get emphysema than nonsmokers, but because only a minority of smokers develop severe emphysema and a few people with emphysema have never smoked, additional factors are involved. In nonsmokers, the factor is thought to be a lack of alpha-1 antitrypsin, a substance in the blood that helps protect the lungs from damage done by the accidental release of harmful enzymes.

My sister had whooping cough and now has emphysema. Why?

She has interstitial emphysema, in which air bubbles appear in the chest. These bubbles result from the sharp intake of breath before each cough, rupturing alveoli in the lungs and causing a release of air. Your sister should make a full recovery.

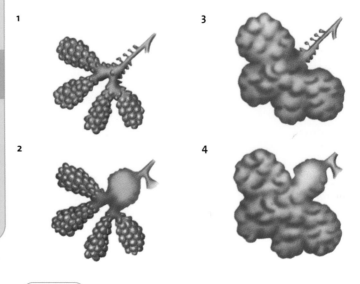

Normal bronchioles and alveoli (1). In pulmonary emphysema, a disease that can affect miners, the bronchioles may be distended (2); so may the alveoli (3). Sometimes, both are swollen (4).

SEE ALSO

BLOOD • HEART • LUNG • LUNG DISEASES AND DISORDERS • RESPIRATORY SYSTEM

Encephalitis

Encephalitis is inflammation of the brain caused by a virus. Mild encephalitis is quite common, but severe encephalitis is a rare and serious disease that can be fatal. If the condition is the main disease, it is known as primary encephalitis. However, if encephalitis occurs as a complication of another illness, it is called secondary encephalitis.

Primary encephalitis is caused by a virus transmitted from animals to humans by insects, such as ticks and mosquitoes. Eastern and Western equine encephalitis, St. Louis encephalitis, West Nile virus, and California encephalitis are all present in the United States. These diseases are carried by mosquitoes and mainly infect humans during periods of warm weather. Secondary encephalitis can follow a number of illnesses caused by viruses or bacteria. These illnesses include measles, chicken pox, rubella, meningitis, and influenza.

The symptoms of encephalitis are fever, headache, and sometimes vomiting. The symptoms may be so slight that the patient hardly notices them or they may be severe. In serious cases, the patient soon becomes drowsy or confused and may have difficulty speaking or may go into convulsions. The drowsiness may deepen into a coma. Antiviral drugs are the mainstay of treatment, but other supportive measures are also necessary. Encephalitis occasionally develops as the result of vaccination, particularly against rabies and, until it was discontinued, against smallpox.

Q & A

My little brother has measles. Is there any way for us to make sure that he does not also get encephalitis?

Encephalitis is an extremely rare complication of measles, but there is no way to predict who will get it. If you and your parents are worried, keep a close eye on him; if he is very drowsy, has a high fever, or has convulsions, your parents should call the doctor immediately.

Can a vaccination cause encephalitis?

Encephalitis can occur as a result of a vaccination, but this effect is rare and the risk is much less than that of getting the disease for which the vaccination was given. Vaccinations are usually not given to people who have an abnormal immune system— such as those who have many allergies or who are on drugs that suppress the immune system—because they are more likely to contract encephalitis.

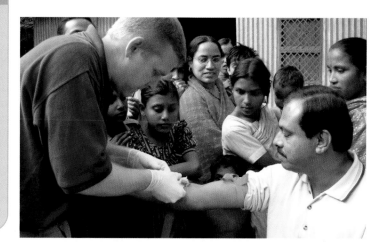

A doctor from the Centers for Disease Control takes a blood sample from a patient in a Bangladeshi village after an outbreak of Nipah virus encephalitis.

SEE ALSO

BACTERIA • BRAIN • BRAIN DAMAGE AND DISORDERS • VIRUSES • WEST NILE VIRUS

Endometriosis

The female uterus, or womb, is a muscular organ with a specialized lining called the endometrium. The endometrium is a membrane that is continuously changing throughout the menstrual cycle. It gradually thickens, and its blood vessels and mucous glands increase up to the time of the menstrual period, when the endometrium is cast off in menstruation.

Misplaced lining
Endometriosis is a condition in which patches of endometrium develop in areas of the body other than on the inside of the uterus. These patches may occur anywhere in the body, but the most common sites for misplaced endometrium are in the ovaries or on the outside of the lower part of the large intestine near the uterus. It is rare for such tissue to penetrate to the inside of the bowel. Endometrial tissue is thought to spread via either the bloodstream or the lymphatic system.

Unusual locations
Endometrium may also occur on the outside of the fallopian tubes, on the bladder, deep within the muscular wall of the uterus itself, or scattered around the interior of the pelvis. Rarely, endometrium occurs at a site remote from the uterus, and it has even been found on the lining of the nose and the lungs. Strange cases of what is known as vicarious menstruation (bleeding from abnormal locations at the time of menstruation) have been attributed to endometriosis.

Controlled by sex hormones
Endometriosis never occurs before the onset of menstruation and it is rare below the age of 20. It most often affects women between the ages of 30 and 40 and always settles down after menopause. Endometrial tissue is under the control of the sex hormones; the same changes therefore occur in the endometrium wherever the tissue may occur within the body, and all endometrial tissue, wherever it is located, undergoes menstruation. Therefore, bleeding and the casting off of thick, mucous-secreting tissue occurs from all the remote patches.

Ovarian cysts and infertility
Unlike the endometrium that is cast off during menstruation, this material cannot usually escape; instead, it accumulates within the body and can cause problems. When the ovaries are affected by endometriosis, there is a tendency for ovarian cysts to develop. These cysts can become so large that affected women sometimes believe they are pregnant. Ovarian cysts

Q & A

Could endometriosis be the cause of frequent nosebleeds?

It is unlikely; endometriosis of the lining of the nose is extremely rare. If the nosebleeds coincide with a woman's monthly period, however, she should check with her doctor.

I overheard my aunt telling my mother that she has had a fertility drug for endometriosis and is now worried that she is likely to have more than one baby. Is she?

It would be unlikely, because the dose your aunt was given would have been very small. Even when the drug is given for infertility, only between 8 and 10 percent of women have multiple births.

I've heard that it is possible for a hysterectomy to cure endometriosis. Why would that happen?

The growth of endometrial tissue is governed by hormones that are controlled by the ovaries. If the ovaries are removed (as in a complete hysterectomy), the endometrial tissue does not grow.

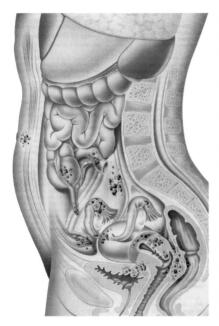

A cross section of the female abdomen shows some of the most likely sites (colored blue) where endometriosis may occur.

caused in this way are full of a dark chocolate-colored fluid. Endometriosis is a common cause of female infertility. Up to half of all infertile women have this disease.

Symptoms of endometriosis
The bleeding causes a local buildup of pressure, and pain occurs with each menstrual period. Symptoms of endometriosis include severe abdominal pain with each period, excessive menstrual bleeding (menorrhagia), irritation where patches of endometrial tissue occur, and pelvic pain and backache between periods.

Infertility is common. When the patches are on the large intestine, there may be cyclic pains in the rectum and, occasionally, mild diarrhea and a sense of incompletion when emptying the bowels (tenesmus). Endometrium in the small intestine can cause obstruction of feces or can lead to a twisting of the bowel (volvulus). These symptoms can be caused by another condition; for example, in women with endometriosis, intestinal symptoms are more likely to be due to irritable bowel syndrome than to the endometriosis.

Diagnosis and treatment
Endometriosis is diagnosed by gynecological investigation. Although patches can be seen by scanning, these cannot always be distinguished from cancer. The only sure method of diagnosis is taking a biopsy for microscopic examination. Laparoscopy can be useful, and biopsies can be taken during this procedure.

Women with endometriosis find that they are much better when they are pregnant; during pregnancy there is no menstruation. This fact suggested a method of treatment. The symptoms of endometriosis can be effectively controlled by the continuous use of oral contraceptives or by any other drug treatment that suppresses the function of the ovaries. Hormone therapy, with drugs designed to block the action of the pituitary ovary-stimulating hormones (gonadotropins), is effective. The drugs danazole (Danol) and florizel (Dimetriose), for example, block the release of gonadotropin. For a complete cure, however, surgical removal of the patches of endometrial tissue, wherever they might be, is necessary.

> **SEE ALSO**
> BODY SYSTEMS • GLANDS • HORMONES AND HORMONAL DISORDERS • IRRITABLE BOWEL SYNDROME • LYMPHATIC SYSTEM • MENSTRUAL DISORDERS

Epidemic

An epidemic is an outbreak of a disease that affects an unusually large number of people in the same area and at the same time. Infections spread fastest when people live in crowded and unsanitary conditions. Cleanliness, modern immunization techniques, and public health programs have made epidemics of serious diseases quite rare in developed countries. People who study the distribution of diseases and how these diseases spread are called epidemiologists.

Epidemics and pandemics

In earlier times and in developing countries, epidemics have killed thousands or even millions of people. The first recorded epidemic of plague spread through Asia and Europe in the fifth century CE and killed some 100 million people. About 50 million people died in the influenza pandemic (worldwide epidemic) of 1918–1919.

One of the latest epidemics is acquired immunodeficiency syndrome (AIDS), which has spread to nearly every country of the world and now affects many millions of people.

Another example is severe acute respiratory syndrome (SARS), a disease caused by a virus and spread by coughing, sneezing, and hand contact. It began in 2002 in southern China, spreading quickly to other countries and killing a number of people. People with SARS have to be isolated and cared for by protected medical personnel. Antibiotics are of no value, but the antiviral drug ribavirin is effective against the SARS virus. A high proportion of patients need lengthy periods in intensive care before they are out of danger.

Avian influenza

Avian influenza, or bird flu, is an infection caused by type A influenza viruses that are common among birds. One of the most contagious subtypes is the H5N1 virus. The risk from avian influenza is low for most people, but cases of human infection have been reported since 1997. Some limited human-to-human spread of H5N1 has occurred. Because all influenza viruses can change, the H5N1 virus might one day be able to infect humans and spread easily from one person to another. If that happened, an influenza pandemic could begin.

Classing outbreaks as epidemics

There is no set number for an outbreak of disease to be classed as an epidemic; it all depends on the disease. Every winter, an average number of people are expected to have influenza. Approximately every third winter, however, many more people than usual catch influenza at around the same time. That

Q & A

I would rather avoid all shots if possible. Are influenza (flu) shots truly effective against influenza epidemics?

There is a good deal of evidence to suggest that people who have been vaccinated against influenza are less likely to get it and that if they do get it, the illness is less severe than it is in unvaccinated people. Influenza is still regarded as a fairly trivial disease in healthy people; but for those who are elderly or sick, especially those with severe bronchitis, it is wise to have an influenza injection before the start of winter.

BLACK DEATH

One of the most famous epidemics in history was the black death. This was the medieval name for plague, a killer bacterium called *Yersinia pestis*, which is spread to people by fleas that have bitten infected rats. In the fourteenth century, rats carried the plague to Europe. In the next few years, the disease spread across the continent, killing one person in every four.

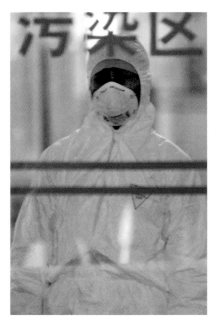

Health workers caring for people with severe acute respiratory syndrome (SARS) have to wear protective clothing.

CHILDHOOD PLAGUES

Epidemics of the infectious diseases of childhood used to be common. These diseases include measles, mumps, diphtheria, and whooping cough. They are all extremely infectious, so before immunization was common, one infected child could start an epidemic that would quickly spread through a school and even a whole neighborhood. To prevent that, children who had been in contact with an infectious disease used to be put in quarantine. Children in many countries are now immunized against all of these diseases. As a result, only isolated cases are now found.

situation constitutes an influenza epidemic. However, if only a dozen or so people develop Legionnaires' disease (a bacterial infection of the lungs), the outbreak can be classed as an epidemic because the disease is not very common.

New germs and germs that change

An epidemic may begin when a disease-causing organism or agent, such as a virus or bacterium, is introduced into a community of people who have never encountered it before. As a result, none of them will have built up any immunity to the disease, and many of them will quickly succumb. That used to happen often when explorers and traders took illnesses such as measles to new lands. It can happen now when travelers catch a disease such as typhoid fever in one country and develop it in another. When U.S. construction workers went to Panama to build the canal in 1904, they came across the yellow fever organism for the first time, and thousands died from the disease.

Some epidemics occur because the organism causing a disease has mutated (changed) to form a new strain and no one has become immune to it. Influenza epidemics are impossible to prevent, because the flu virus is continually changing.

Endemic diseases

Epidemics are likely to break out in disaster areas where people are crowded together in camps. Famines and other disasters also cause epidemics by lowering people's general health and resistance to disease. They are then likely to get endemic diseases—diseases that are always around in the region but that normally affect only a few people.

Stopping the spread

When an epidemic breaks out, public health personnel take action to stop it from spreading. They trace those who may have been in contact with the disease and who may be at risk of catching it. If possible, the health workers immunize them, ensure they get proper treatment, and stop them from spreading the disease. To do this, they must trace all contacts of people with the illness, and they must find out how it started.

SEE ALSO

AIDS AND HIV • AVIAN INFLUENZA • BACTERIAL DISEASES • INFECTIOUS DISEASES • INFLUENZA • LEGIONNAIRES' DISEASE • PLAGUE • SARS • VIRUSES • YELLOW FEVER

Epilepsy

Tiny electric signals in the brain pass messages from one cell to another. These signals control the functions of the body. In epilepsy, the signals in one group of nerves suddenly become unusually strong and the result is a convulsive seizure. Epilepsy can now be kept under control by taking regular medication. People with the illness can lead a normal life. Epilepsy does not usually make people mentally disabled.

Types of seizures

There are two main types of epileptic attack, depending on the part of the brain that is affected. A mild form goes by the French name *petit mal* ("little illness"), or absence attacks. It appears in some children, and they usually grow out of it. In this form of epilepsy, the child loses touch with his or her surroundings for up to 30 seconds and perhaps jerks his or her hands and head slightly. The seizures may be so slight that no one notices what is happening and the child may just seem to be daydreaming.

The second main type of seizure is called *grand mal* ("great illness"). This form usually lasts for one or two minutes. Many people who suffer from epilepsy can tell a few seconds in advance that an attack is coming. They may have a headache or see spots; smell an odd, unreal odor; or have the feeling that everything has happened before. Then they lose consciousness and fall to the ground, the body becoming rigid. They may twitch or go into convulsions and possibly urinate. Next comes drowsiness, and they will probably fall asleep. When they wake up after an attack, they remember nothing about it.

Q & A

I have epilepsy, and my doctor has me on medications for it. However, is there anything else that I should be doing to help prevent my epileptic attacks in the future?

The only thing that keeps seizures at bay is regular medication. Modern drug therapy is very effective, and most people with epilepsy lead a full and active life. However, it can be helpful to avoid hunger, fatigue, and stress.

My little brother, who has epileptic attacks, wants a bicycle. Should our parents buy him one?

A bicycle would not be safe for him at present. Your parents should explain this to him, dealing with the situation as a nuisance, not a tragedy. If the seizures disappear entirely for a long time, your parents can think again about giving your brother a bicycle, but they should ask his doctor's advice first.

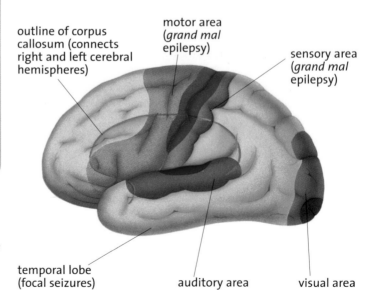

outline of corpus callosum (connects right and left cerebral hemispheres)

motor area (*grand mal* epilepsy)

sensory area (*grand mal* epilepsy)

temporal lobe (focal seizures)

auditory area

visual area

Grand mal seizures are associated with both the motor and the sensory areas of the brain. In a focal seizure, the disordered electrical activity is often located in just the temporal lobe.

After a person has an epileptic seizure, helpers should ensure that his or her clothing is loose and that breathing is unrestricted. Someone should stay nearby and reassure the person when he or she recovers.

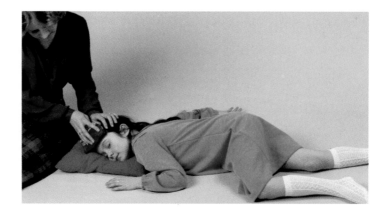

After an epileptic seizure, a person should be placed gently in the recovery position. He or she may take anything from a few minutes to half an hour to recover consciousness and may then sleep for a couple of hours.

Anticonvulsant drugs

People with epilepsy are given anticonvulsant drugs, which bring their unusual brain signals under control. Taking these drugs regularly ensures that there will be few or no epileptic attacks, although regular checkups with a doctor are necessary.

Anticonvulsants produce unwanted side effects, however. One of the most common side effects is drowsiness. People with epilepsy should not swim unless they have a good, sensible swimmer with them, and cycling can also be dangerous. Some states place restrictions on drivers with epilepsy.

Causes of epilepsy

In most cases, doctors cannot tell what makes a person have epileptic attacks, although the condition does run in families. Sometimes, epilepsy is the sign of some disease of the brain, such as a brain tumor. It may also be the result of a head injury, poisoning, alcoholism, or (in older people) narrowing of the arteries to the brain. Babies born with brain damage caused by rubella or brain damage suffered during birth have a much higher than normal chance of epilepsy.

FIRST AID FOR A CONVULSION

Nothing will stop epileptic seizures. The only help that can be given is to stop sufferers from injuring themselves.

1. Move hard furniture away from the person and move him or her clear of fire.
2. Do not push anything into the mouth or force open the jaws.
3. If the seizure occurs in a dangerous place, such as the middle of the road, get the person to a safer place and call an ambulance.
4. If a person has a convulsion for the first time, call a doctor. Stay with the person until the attack is over. When the fit is over, turn the person on his or her side and loosen any tight clothing. Reassure the person and check his or her breathing.

SEE ALSO

ARTERY DISEASES AND DISORDERS • BRAIN • BRAIN DAMAGE AND DISORDERS • GENETIC DISEASES AND DISORDERS • NERVOUS SYSTEM • NERVOUS SYSTEM DISORDERS • RUBELLA

Eye and Sight

Q & A

My little sister has measles. She loves to read, but I've heard that it's dangerous for people to read while they have measles, and for a while after. Is this true?

No. Although measles causes inflammation of the eyes and photophobia (discomfort in strong light), there is no danger to the sight. It is simply an old wives' tale.

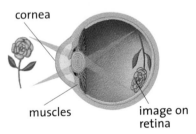

cornea

muscles

image on retina

lens

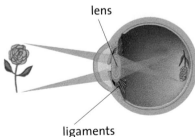

ligaments

Light rays from a nearby object (top) diverge, and the surface of the lens curves more to focus them. Light rays from a distant object (bottom) are almost parallel, so the lens has less focusing to do.

The eye is a marvelously accurate, self-repairing video camera. It can give a lifetime's service with the minimum of attention, and it suffers from relatively few diseases. Its purpose is to receive the rays of light that are all around and transform them into signals that the brain can interpret. People see things because light has bounced off them into the eyes.

There is one thing about light that needs to be known before someone can understand how the eye works: although light usually travels in a straight line, it can be bent if it passes through certain substances, such as the lens of a camera or the lens of the eye. It can also be bent inward to form tiny but perfectly formed images of much larger objects.

How people see

When light strikes the eye, it passes through a round, transparent window, called the cornea. This window is the first of two lenses in the eye. The cornea is surrounded by the white of the eye, which admits no light. Behind the cornea is a chamber filled with watery fluid, which constantly drains away.

At the back of this chamber is the iris, which is a disk of muscle with a hole in the center called the pupil. The iris has muscles that can make the pupil larger or smaller. The purpose of that is to admit more or less light, just like a shutter in a camera. The color of the iris gives the eye its distinctive color. Behind the iris is the fine focusing lens, which focuses the light rays on the back of the eye. A muscle around the lens changes its shape to adjust the focus as required.

Behind the lens is the main chamber of the eye. It is filled with a delicate gel consisting of 99.9 percent water, called the vitreous humor. At the back of the eyeball is a layer called the retina. The retina consists of two types of light-sensitive cells, called cones and rods because of their shapes. Cones pick up color and provide clear vision. Rods do not detect color but they enable people to see in dim light. A main nerve from the retina, called the optic nerve, carries messages from the eye to the brain. Where the optic nerve leaves the retina, there is a small area where a person is blind. People do not notice this blind spot, because the eyes overlap their fields of vision.

What happens in the brain

Messages from the optic nerve of each eye are passed to an area of the brain called the visual cortex, where they are processed and understood. At an area called the optic chiasma, which is situated at the base of the brain, the nerve fibers from the inner half of the retina cross over to the optic nerve from the other eye,

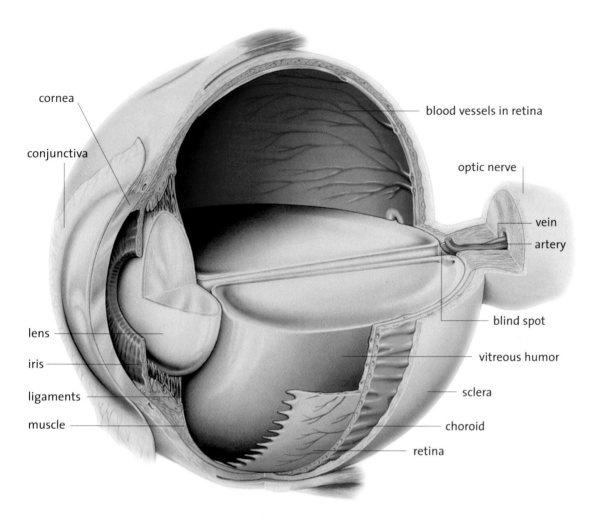

cornea

conjunctiva

blood vessels in retina

optic nerve

vein

artery

lens

iris

ligaments

muscle

blind spot

vitreous humor

sclera

choroid

retina

A cross section of an eyeball showing its different parts.

while those from the outer half continue directly into the brain. The visual cortex has two halves, one in each hemisphere, or side, of the brain. Each hemisphere has its own separate blood supply. As a result, it is rare for a stroke—in which the normal blood supply to part of the brain via an artery is interrupted by a blood clot or hemorrhage—to cause complete blindness. However, severe damage to one half of the visual cortex always causes the loss of part of the field of peripheral vision.

SEE ALSO

BRAIN • EYE DISEASES AND DISORDERS • GLAUCOMA • RETINA AND RETINAL DISORDERS • STY

Eye Diseases and Disorders

Most eye problems arise because the eyes are not perfectly shaped and therefore have difficulty focusing, or because the muscles that control them are not working properly.

Common eye disorders

The most common eye problem is nearsightedness (myopia). That happens when the eyeball is too long or the corneal curvature is too great, or both. Light rays entering the eye focus before they reach the retina at the back; as a result, the viewer can see objects clearly when they are close, but any object that is far away appears out of focus or blurred.

Farsightedness (hyperopia) is exactly the opposite. The eyeball is too short or the cornea is too flat; the rays have not yet come to a focus when they meet the retina. Thus, distant objects are clear, but objects close to the eye are blurred. Hyperopia is often concealed in young people because the lenses are more flexible and they can more easily focus the image. As focusing power diminishes with age, the hyperopia becomes apparent.

Sometimes, the cornea is unevenly curved. As a result, objects appear distorted. That is called astigmatism. These three eye problems are hereditary, and they appear in childhood. Myopia usually appears around puberty and progresses while the body is growing. Hyperopia becomes more manifest with the loss of focusing power and is always obvious before middle age. The greater the optical effect, the earlier it becomes manifest. Astigmatism is usually stable by late adolescence.

Wandering eyes

Some eye problems occur because the muscles controlling the eyes are not working properly. A person may find it impossible to align both eyes on the same spot at once. Instead, one eye wanders inward (a convergent squint) or outward (a divergent squint). Other people's eyes cross, causing double vision (seeing two images of an object).

Q & A

I have always been extremely nearsighted, but the problem seems to be getting worse as I get older. Will my sight continue to deteriorate until I go blind?

Neither nearsightedness nor farsightedness leads to blindness. Nearsightedness usually progresses during body growth and then stabilizes in adulthood.

My grandfather recently suffered from cataracts and had to have them removed. I'm worried now that my father and I will eventually have the same problem. Are cataracts hereditary?

There is no need to worry; cataracts are neither hereditary nor contagious. Cataracts are usually a result of advancing age, but ultraviolet light may cause cataracts, so wear sunglasses on bright days.

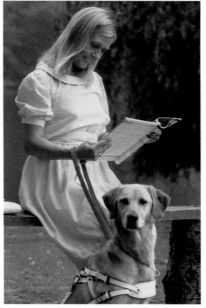

Why should anyone who can read a book need a guide dog? This woman has tunnel vision; she can see only through the central part of her eyes and can read just a few words at a time. She cannot see things left or right, or up or down, without moving her head, so she could not move around safely without her dog.

A common cause of nearsightedness (1) is an eyeball that is too long. As a result, light rays form an image in front of the retina. Objects close by may appear in focus, but those farther away will be fuzzy. Nearsightedness is corrected by a concave eyeglass lens (2). In farsightedness (3), the eyeball is short, so the image cannot form within the eye. Close objects appear blurred, but those farther away are clear. A convex eyeglass lens (4) focuses the image on the retina. (The image on the retina is always upside-down.)

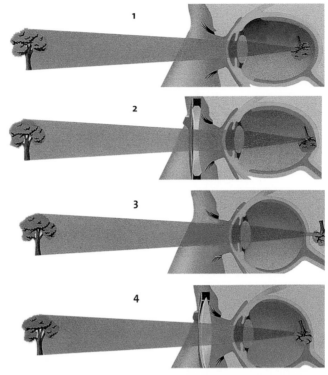

EYE DISORDERS

Disease	Symptoms	Cause	Treatment
Astigmatism	Distorted vision	Uneven curvature of the cornea	Corrective eyeglasses
Blindness	Loss of vision	Disease or injury	Usually none
Cataract	Gradual loss of vision	Clouding of lens due to age, injury, or illness	Surgery to replace lens
Conjunctivitis	White of eye reddens and is sore; discharge of pus from eye	Viral or bacterial infection; allergy	Antibiotics
Cross-eyes	Eyes do not align on one single object; each appears to look across the other's line of sight	Weak or unbalanced eye muscles	Corrective eyeglasses; surgery to balance muscles
Detached retina	Flashes of light; floating black shapes; black curtain over the eye	Hole in retina, leading to lifting of retina from underlying surface	Surgery to seal hole or reattach retina
Double vision	Seeing two images of an object	Many causes, among them brain injury, high blood pressure, nerve and muscle disorders	Medical attention to treat underlying cause

(continued)

EYE DISORDERS *(continued)*

DISEASE	SYMPTOMS	CAUSE	TREATMENT
Farsightedness	Inability to see near objects clearly	Eye too short from front to back	Corrective eyeglasses or contact lenses
Glaucoma	Blurred vision; halos around lights; headache; loss of vision	Increased pressure of fluid in eyeball caused by faulty drainage	Reduction of pressure by surgery to improve drainage of fluid
Keratitis	Painful, red eye; irritation; loss of vision	Damage to the cornea by injury, ultraviolet light, infection, too few tears	Antibiotics; rest; sometimes surgery
Macular degeneration	Blurring and loss of central vision	Reduction of blood supply to macula (part of retina)	Early laser treatment to try to halt degeneration
Nearsightedness	Inability to see distant objects clearly	Eye too long from front to back	Corrective eyeglasses or contact lenses
Optic neuritis	Blurring of vision	Inflammation of optic nerve	Steroid injections
Retinitis pigmentosa	Gradual loss of vision	Genetic	None
Squint	Failure of both eyes to focus on the same object at once	Uncoordinated muscles of eyeball; *see also* causes of double vision	Patch over strong eye to stimulate lazy eye to work; operation to adjust muscles of the eyeball
Sty	Painful red swelling on the eyelid	Bacterial infection of hair follicle	Hot compresses; antibiotic ointment
Trachoma	Eyelids swell, tears flow, granules form; eyelids become scarred; cornea ulcerates; gradual loss of vision	Chlamydia infection	Antibiotic drugs; surgery to remove scarring of eyelids
Tunnel vision	Loss of all but central field of vision	Damage to outer area of retina due to glaucoma or retinitis pigmentosa	None

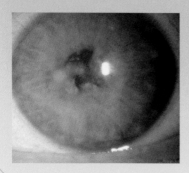
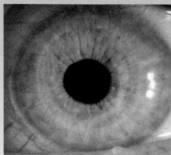

This diseased cornea (far left) has lost its transparent quality. Five weeks later (left), after a new cornea has been grafted, the eye looks clear. The very fine zigzag line of stitches holds the grafted cornea in place.

GO TO THE DOCTOR IF

- Your eyes are red and inflamed
- You have blurred vision
- You have double vision
- You see flashing lights
- You see rainbow-colored halos around objects
- Your eyes hurt
- You lose vision, even for a very short time

Any of these symptoms could mean that there is something seriously wrong with your eyes.

People with poor sight who wear glasses or contact lenses should have their eyes tested regularly throughout their life, in case the lenses need adjustments.

Normally, the eyes move together, but in these cases, the muscles do not move the eyes at the same time. This problem is quite normal in babies but should stop around the age of about six months.

Any fixed deviation of one or both eyes in a small baby calls for attention by an eye expert, known as an ophthalmologist, without delay, as does any obvious limitation of eye movement. Squinting in toddlers or older children also requires immediate ophthalmic attention. Failure to treat such cases can lead to a permanent defect.

If an adolescent or adult suddenly develops double vision, it may be a symptom of some serious illness such as diabetes, brain injury, or hypertension. The person should see a doctor.

Eyesight and aging

The internal focusing lenses of the eye lose their elasticity progressively from infancy onward. When people reach the age of around 45 years, the lenses of their eyes have become less elastic, so that reading without glasses may be impossible. This condition is called presbyopia. Other disorders include the gradual misting over of the lens, called cataract, and loss of vision caused by the disease known as glaucoma. Sometimes, the area near the optic nerve does not get a good enough supply of blood, and sight in the center is lost.

The retina, the layer of light-sensitive cells in the eye, can lift away from the blood vessels beneath. This condition is called a detached retina. A hole or tear can appear in the retina. Symptoms include flashes of light and cobwebby shapes in front of the eye. The hole or tear can be sealed with a laser, and the retina can be reattached by freezing in a simple operation. A sudden loss of sight may indicate a serious disorder, and a doctor should be consulted as a matter of urgency.

Eye infections

If the cornea is scratched, it can become infected and may develop an ulcer. Vision becomes blurred and the eye is red and painful. This problem needs medical attention because a scar may form. If the cornea is very badly damaged, it may be possible to carry out a transplant operation to replace it. Other infections include trachoma, conjunctivitis, and sties.

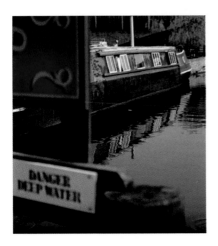

With farsightedness, the boat is in sharper focus than the sign. With nearsightedness, the sign in the foreground would be clear but the boat would look blurred.

> ### SEE ALSO
> BLINDNESS • EYE AND SIGHT • GLAUCOMA • RETINA AND RETINAL DISORDERS • STY

Fibroids

Fibroids, or leiomyomas, are abnormal but benign (noncancerous) tumors in the uterus that consist of muscle and fibrous tissue. They are solid and white and grow in the muscular wall of the uterus. They can vary in size from as small as a pea to as large as a grapefruit. Fibroids are common in middle-aged women but may shrink or disappear after the menopause, when estrogen levels fall. Fibroids are the most common tumor of the uterus; one in five women under the age of 40 has fibroids. Many more above this age have them.

Small fibroids may not cause problems, although in women of childbearing age, they can cause heavy menstrual bleeding or prevent conception. Large fibroids may feel uncomfortable, because they exert pressure on the bowel and bladder.

Sometimes, fibroids are removed by surgery, but often those causing no problem are left alone. In women who want more children, fibroids can be removed surgically from the uterus, which is left intact. Women who do not want more children can have a hysterectomy, in which the uterus is removed.

Q & A

I have heard some people refer to fibroids and other people refer to polyps. This is confusing. Is there any difference between a fibroid and a polyp?

Both fibroids and polyps are benign tumors in the reproductive organs. Fibroids occur in the wall of the uterus; polyps can appear either inside the uterus or along the cervical canal. Both may cause excessive bleeding during periods or at mid-cycle; in a few cases, fibroids may prevent conception. If difficulties arise, fibroids or polyps can be removed surgically.

How long does a woman have to wait after having a fibroid removed before she can try to have a baby? Is there a minimum time that should pass first?

It is sensible for the woman to wait until the scars from the removal surgery have healed. The recommended time differs among obstetricians, but it is usually six months to one year.

Fibroids form in the walls of the uterus and along the cervical canal.

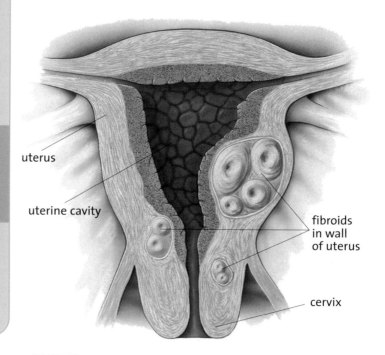

uterus

uterine cavity

fibroids in wall of uterus

cervix

SEE ALSO

BODY SYSTEMS • CANCER • HORMONES AND HORMONAL DISORDERS • MENSTRUAL DISORDERS • MUSCLE

Fibromyalgia

Fibromyalgia is a chronic condition that causes fatigue and pain in muscle tendons, ligaments, and other so-called "white" connective tissue. It also causes tenderness in particular areas of the body, especially around the shoulder blades, the upper back, and at the base of the skull. Often, the symptoms of fibromyalgia include stiffness as well as pain.

Formerly called fibrositis, fibromyalgia can be caused by straining a muscle or a joint and is common in people with rheumatoid arthritis, whose deformed joints stress the surrounding muscles. Another extremely common cause is tension. Many people who have been sitting hunched over textbooks or over a keyboard get stiff, painful shoulders.

Q & A

My older sister complains of muscle pain and fatigue. What is wrong with her, and can anything be done to help her?

She may have fibromyalgia, a muscle disorder that causes tender, painful muscles. Your doctor can arrange blood tests to eliminate other disorders, and the pain can be helped by ultrasound treatment and deep tissue massage.

Since his hip surgery a few months ago, my grandfather has experienced a bad case of fibromyalgia. Could the surgery be the problem?

Most likely the anesthesia, the emotional and physical stress associated with undergoing surgery, or his body mechanics following the surgery caused fibromyalgia to flare up.

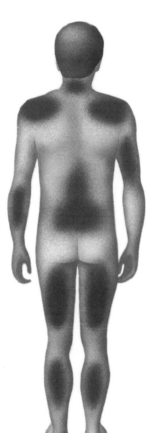

The red areas show typical sites where fibromyalgia occurs.

Sometimes, the muscles go into spasm, so that small knots can be felt in the tissue. Whatever is the underlying cause of the problem, fibromyalgia is usually made worse by cold and dampness.

Fibromyalgia often comes on suddenly; the sufferer feels pain when moving, and certain areas are tender to touch. It usually clears up in a few days; taking hot baths and aspirin or muscle-relaxant pills should relieve the pain. If it lasts, a doctor may give a pain-relieving injection, and skilled massage or manipulation may also help.

Research has shown that exercise can greatly improve the symptoms of fibromyalgia for most people, reducing pain, boosting energy levels, and helping to make sleep patterns regular. Low-impact aerobic exercises—such as walking, cycling, and swimming—are better than harder exercises such as weight training. A physiotherapist may also recommend gentle exercises that include stretches.

SEE ALSO

ARTHRITIS • JOINT DISORDERS • MUSCLE • MUSCLE DISEASES AND DISORDERS • SPRAINS AND STRAINS

Fractures and Dislocations

Q & A

My parents and I are planning our first skiing vacation. I don't want a broken leg. What can I do to minimize the risk?

You can make sure that you are physically fit before you go. Start toning up your muscles for a few weeks before you leave. Jogging, in-line skating, and bicycle exercises are very good for the leg muscles. Better still, take a ski class, which will certainly save you from a few unnecessary falls.

A few months ago, my mother slipped on ice and dislocated her shoulder. She had it put back in place but has had a lot of aches and stiffness since then. Is there anything she can do about it?

Pain and stiffness after a dislocation are common. Physiotherapy will improve joint mobility and aspirin may help relieve the pain. Occasionally, an injection of a steroid drug into surrounding tissues is required.

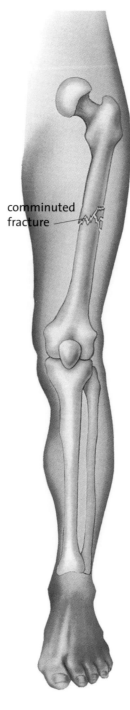

comminuted fracture

In this comminuted fracture of the femur (thighbone), the bone has shattered into small pieces. Treatment involves operating to remove fragments, joining the bone ends with a metal plate, and immobilizing the limb in plaster.

A fracture is a break in one of the bones of the body. Some fractures are simple breaks that heal quickly and easily; in other, more serious fractures, the bones may be broken into several pieces. This type of break requires skilled treatment and takes time to heal properly. A dislocation is the displacement of a bone from its socket or from an associated bone.

A simple (closed) fracture is one in which a bone is broken but the skin is intact and the tissues around the break are virtually unharmed. In a compound (open) fracture, the skin is broken by the bone. This type is more serious because there is a much greater risk of infection. When the bone has broken into several pieces, the fracture is described as comminuted. When one end of the broken bone has been driven into another bone, it is an impacted fracture. A depressed fracture is one in which the broken bone is pressing down on the structure underneath. Sometimes, the bone is not broken right through but is simply cracked. Such fractures are known as greenstick fractures. That type of injury is most common in children, whose bones are still growing and are relatively supple.

It takes a great deal of force to break a healthy bone. Fractures are most often caused by accidents such as falls. Elderly people, whose balance is poor, fall more often, and their bones tend to break more easily than those of younger people. Some diseases, including osteoporosis, make the bones so brittle that they break for little or no apparent reason. These types of fractures are known as pathological fractures.

FIRST AID FOR FRACTURES

Do
• Call for an ambulance
• Make patients comfortable (moving them as little as possible)

Do not
• Give the patient anything to eat or drink, or a painkiller, in case an anesthetic has to be given when the bone is set
• Try to realign the fracture yourself; you could cause damage

Symptoms and treatment

The most obvious symptom of a broken bone is pain, and damaged tissues in the area around the break may cause the area to swell and look deformed. Movement and pressure may make the pain worse. Broken bones in the hands and feet and broken ribs may be mistaken for sprains or torn muscles, but a limb that is broken cannot be used. The chief danger from a fracture is shock, caused by pain and blood loss. Bone, like any other tissue of the body, has a rich blood supply; the bigger the bone that breaks, the greater the loss of blood. Broken bones may also damage the tissues around them.

Broken bones need medical treatment. A doctor should be called, or the person should be taken to the hospital by ambulance. The victim should be moved as little as possible, particularly if there is any danger of a back injury. When the patient reaches the hospital, he or she will be treated for pain and shock and given an X-ray to assess the damage. The broken bones will then be put in the correct position. A shattered or awkwardly broken bone may need to be repaired with a metal plate screwed along the bone. Some breaks, such as rib fractures, can be left to heal by themselves, but most fractured bones need to be held in position as they heal. This is often done by encasing the area in a plaster cast; a leg may have to be in a cast for 12 weeks or more before it is strong enough to take the body's weight. Bones usually heal extremely well, and in many cases, the fracture leaves no outward sign once it has healed. It may even be difficult to see on a later X-ray.

The supple bones of babies and children may bend and crack rather than break completely. This sort of injury is known as a greenstick fracture (top). The limb should be immobilized in a plaster cast. In a compound fracture (bottom), the broken bone pierces the skin. Damaged tissue and bone fragments must be removed, the bone must be realigned, and the limb must be set in plaster.

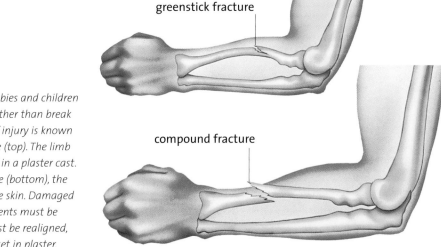

greenstick fracture

compound fracture

The shoulder normally has a rounded contour. If the humerus (armbone) slips out of the scapula (shoulder blade) socket and becomes dislocated, it makes the shoulder take on a square shape (inset).

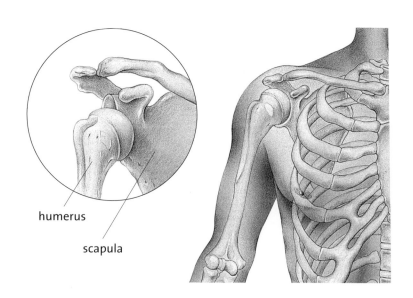

humerus

scapula

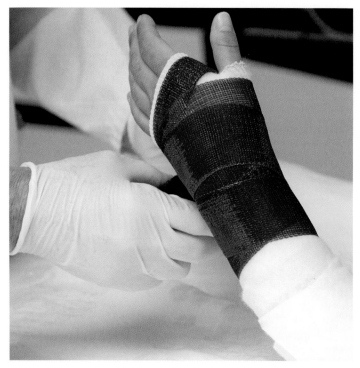

This person has suffered a broken wrist and has had the injury set in a plaster cast that holds together the broken bones to allow them to heal properly.

Dislocation

Another type of bone injury is a dislocation, in which the bone of a joint is wrenched out of its socket. A dislocated bone is extremely painful because the force of the injury damages the tissues, nerves, and blood vessels around it. The joint swells and needs treatment as quickly as possible. A skilled therapist may be able to put the bone back in position if it is treated immediately, but after 15 minutes or so, the swelling is so great that a general anesthetic is necessary. The shoulders, thumbs, and fingers are the joints most often affected; others include the jaws, elbows, knees, and hips. Some babies are born with dislocation of the hip, which is usually cured by putting the hip in a stabilizing sling for a few months.

SEE ALSO
BONE • BONE DISEASES AND DISORDERS • OSTEOPOROSIS

Frostbite

Frostbite is the damage that occurs when part of the body freezes. It harms and sometimes kills the tissues beneath the skin. Anyone living or working in very low temperatures can get frostbite. People may even get frostbite in their own homes if they are not properly dressed and do not move around to keep their circulation going. Vulnerable parts of the body include the ears, nose, chin, fingers, and toes because they are difficult to cover and have relatively poor circulation.

As freezing begins, the blood starts to thicken. It blocks the tiny vessels that carry it around the body. The surrounding tissues cannot get oxygen from the blood and become damaged. Further damage is caused by ice crystals that form in the cells. As an area freezes, it becomes white and stiff. It feels painful, but victims will not feel a pinprick, because the nerve supply is frozen. When the area is warmed, it becomes red and swollen and the skin blisters. Normal feeling will not come back for several weeks. Sometimes, frostbitten fingers and toes have to be amputated when the tissues die and rot away.

Q & A

After my hands have been very cold, I get terrible pain if I warm them in front of the fire. Is this anything to do with frostbite?

Not usually. When your hands are very cold, the blood vessels constrict. That reduces the supply of oxygen-bearing blood to the surface tissues, including the nerves, impairing sensation. When you warm up your hands quickly, those tissues demand oxygen as they come back to life. However, the blood vessels in the lower layers of skin respond more slowly to the warmth and cannot meet the demand immediately. The temporary lack of oxygen is felt as pain.

FIRST AID FOR FROSTBITE

Frostbitten people should be sheltered and given something hot to eat or drink. Frozen areas must be warmed slowly and not by direct heat. Frostbite on the face can be covered with a dry, gloved hand. If possible, frostbitten areas should be soaked in warm water and bandaged with dry, sterile dressings. Gauze should be placed between fingers and toes. Medical help should be sought quickly.

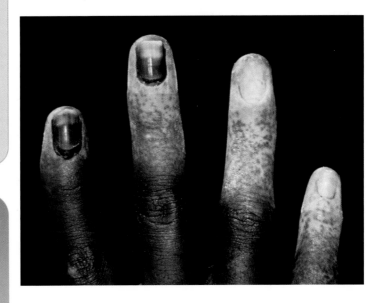

These frostbitten fingers have turned white and stiff. Frostbitten areas of the body should never be rubbed in an attempt to restore the circulation, because that can cause permanent damage to the tissues.

SEE ALSO

BLOOD • CIRCULATORY SYSTEM • GANGRENE • SKIN

Fungal Infections

Q & A

I have athlete's foot, which I'm told is due to a fungus. Is this the fungus that causes thrush?

Athlete's foot can occasionally be caused by *Candida albicansis*, a yeast fungus that is responsible for thrush. However, most cases of athlete's foot are caused by one of the filamentous (threadlike) fungi, which are best known for causing the various forms of ringworm.

Can babies get yeast infections in areas other than the mouth?

Yes, young babies can often get an infection on top of a diaper rash. Candida fungi tend to grow in warm, moist places such as the diaper area.

A fungus is an organism that cannot make its own food. Instead, it lives by digesting the tissues of other plants or animals. Fungi live mainly in the air and the soil, especially in warm, damp places. They also live in animal excrement and in water supplies. There are hundreds of different types of fungi; some, like the mold that produces the antibiotic penicillin, are extremely useful to people. A few types of fungi can infect humans and animals.

The most common fungal infections affect people's skin. These include the ringworm fungi. When they infect the scalp, they cause scaly patches and broken, lifeless hair. They also cause barber's itch, in which lumps and sores appear on the bearded area of a man's face and neck. In jock itch, raised, itchy patches appear on the groin. Athlete's foot causes red, oozing patches between the toes. These infections are often passed from one person to another by sharing towels. Another fungus, the yeast candida, causes candidiasis, in which sore white patches appear in the mouth or genital area and vagina. The mold aspergillus can infect the skin of the outer ear canal.

Sometimes, fungi enter the body through injured skin or punctures. The sporotrichosis fungus lives in the soil and in decaying plant material. It may enter the skin on a thorn or splinter and produce a wartlike sore. Inflammation spreads to the lymph nodes above the sore, and a small line of sores appears. Madura foot, a tropical disease, is caused by a variety of fungi. Again, the infection may enter via a thorn or splinter, or it may be picked up by walking barefoot with an open sore on the foot. Months or even years later, a small inflamed lump appears and oozes pus. This sore eats through the foot and destroys muscles and tendons until the foot is deformed and useless.

Internal infections

Other serious fungal infections destroy tissues deep in the body. Some infections affect the lungs. They can be caught by breathing in fungus spores. Lung infections such as this are slow to develop and difficult to diagnose. Their symptoms are similar to those of influenza and include a headache, chills, fever, night sweating, a cough, and loss of weight. Fungal lung infections

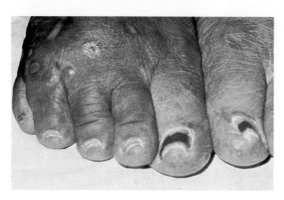

Madura foot is a serious and disabling tropical disease that can be caused by various fungi. The infection enters through a wound from a thorn or splinter, and the first symptom—an inflamed lump—appears months or even years later. People visiting tropical countries should not walk barefoot.

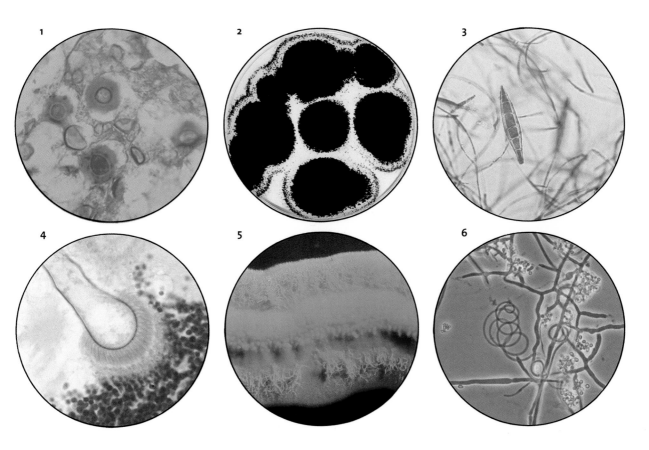

These fungi cause infections in different parts of the body. (1) Cryptococcosus may lead to a type of meningitis in the brain. (2) The mold Aspergillus niger *can infect the skin of the outer ear canal. (3)* Microsporum canis *affects the scalp and produces ringworm. (4)* Aspergillus fumigatus *may infect the lungs and cause asthma. (5)* Candida albicans *is a yeastlike fungus that causes a common vaginal infection. (6)* Trichophyton mentagrophytes *produces athlete's foot.*

include histoplasmosis, which is spread by bird and bat droppings; coccidioidomycosis (valley fever), which is common in dusty areas; aspergillosis; and blastomycosis. Although such infections are usually mild, severe forms can occur and may spread to other parts of the system. Internal fungal infections are rare except in people with immune deficiency.

Another serious fungal-like condition is called actinomycosis. This disease attacks deep skin tissues and mucous membranes in the chest, neck, and abdomen. Occasionally, it affects the brain and heart. Actinomycosis is now recognized as a bacterial disease with colonies that resemble fungi. It is treated with antibiotics.

Fungal skin infections are treated with creams and lotions. The treatment of fungal infections has been revolutionized by the development of highly effective antifungal drugs.

SEE ALSO

ATHLETE'S FOOT • HAIR AND SCALP DISORDERS • RINGWORM • SKIN DISEASES AND DISORDERS

Gallbladder and Gallstones

The gallbladder is a small, muscular sac that acts as a reservoir for bile, a substance produced by the liver. Bile is a green fluid that helps break down fats during digestion. Whenever fatty foods arrive in the intestine from the stomach, the gallbladder releases bile to help digest them. The gallbladder is attached to the bile duct, a tube that takes bile from the liver to the duodenum, which is the first section of the small intestine.

Gallstones are hard, stonelike objects that can form in the gallbladder. They build up, like crystals, from chemicals in the bile and vary from the size of a tiny bead to a pigeon's egg. Gallstones may cause no trouble and people may not even know that they have them. Sometimes, they go away without treatment, but in other cases the gallbladder can become inflamed by them. Sufferers experience fever, vomiting, and pain in the upper right part of the abdomen. If stones block the bile duct, the pain is severe and the condition is called

Q & A

My father has a gallstone, and his doctor thinks it may have developed years ago. How can he have had it for so long without having problems?

Around half of the people with a gallstone have no trouble at all, no matter how long they have had it, and many doctors prefer to leave the stones alone. The stones grow very slowly, so it may be many years before they cause any trouble.

My mother and my older brother both have gallstones. Does this mean that the condition runs in families, and that I am likely to get them, too?

Your chances of developing gallstones are increased, but you will not necessarily get them.

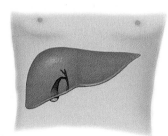

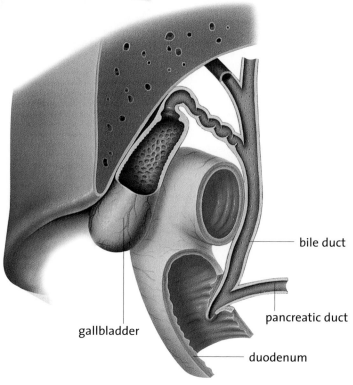

bile duct

pancreatic duct

gallbladder

duodenum

The gallbladder is a pear-shaped sac that lies on the underside of the liver. Bile is concentrated and stored in it. When fatty foods pass into the intestine from the stomach, the gallbladder empties its bile into the duodenum through the bile duct. The bile acts to break down fat during the digestive process.

Two types of gallstones are shown here. Those on the right are formed largely from cholesterol. Such stones can grow up to 0.5 inch (1.2 cm) in diameter; only a few form, but they are large enough to block the bile duct. On the far right are mixed stones, formed by a mixture of cholesterol and bile. They may occur in large numbers.

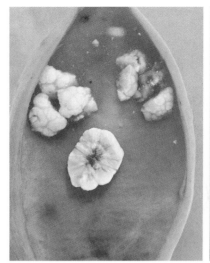 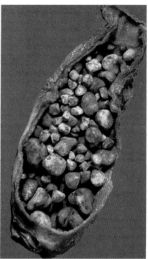

cholecystitis. Bile is prevented from reaching the intestines, and the patient therefore becomes jaundiced, with yellowish skin, urine discolored by bile, and pale feces. In severe cases, the cure is to remove the stones and sometimes the gallbladder. If the stones are not causing any problems, they can be left alone or they can be dissolved in the gallbladder with drug therapy or shattered by ultrasound treatment.

Other gallbladder problems

Cholangitis is an inflammation of the bile ducts, which lead from the liver and gallbladder to the small intestine. The condition is usually caused by bacterial infection of the duct and bile, as a result of a blockage in the duct, often by a gallstone. Antibiotics are prescribed to treat mild episodes. In more serious cases, surgery is needed to drain infected material from the bile duct.

A rare condition called sclerosing cholangitis results in a narrowing of all the bile ducts in and around the liver. Drugs may help, but a liver transplant may be needed.

Biliary colic, a severe pain in the upper right area of the abdomen, is caused by the gallbladder trying to rid itself of gallstones or by the movement of gallstones in the bile duct. Surgery may be performed to remove the gallbladder. Removal of the gallbladder causes no ill effects; one can get along without it.

SEE ALSO

DIGESTIVE SYSTEM • DIGESTIVE SYSTEM DISEASES AND DISORDERS • JAUNDICE • LIVER

Gangrene

Gangrene is the death and decay of body tissue. It happens when the blood supply to the tissues is blocked or reduced. The most common cause of gangrene is blockage of the arteries, particularly in the legs. Gangrene usually starts in the toes, because the blood has to travel farther to get there and the blood vessels are smaller. Severe frostbite or injury can cause gangrene if the blood supply is cut off. So can poor circulation caused by diabetes.

At first, the skin becomes red and shiny. When pressed, it turns white and remains so for a few seconds. Later, the gangrenous area turns purple and finally goes black. If the dead tissues become infected, they will swell up and produce pus, a condition known as wet gangrene. Sometimes, the injured tissue is infected with bacteria called clostridia. They produce toxins and gas, causing a condition called gas gangrene, which will make the patient extremely ill. Gangrenous areas are very painful while the tissues are dying, but then they become numb. Affected areas may have to be amputated, and some of the surrounding tissues may also be removed to prevent the infection from spreading. People with poor circulation should protect themselves against injuries to their legs or feet, which could turn gangrenous.

Peripheral vascular disease

Peripheral vascular disease is a narrowing of the arteries in the legs and sometimes in the arms. That results in a restricted blood flow and causes pain. Gangrene may develop in severe cases. In most cases, the disease is caused by atherosclerosis, in which fatty deposits form on the inner surfaces of the arteries. Smoking causes atherosclerosis, as can hypertension (high blood pressure), diabetes that is not controlled properly, and a diet that is high in fat.

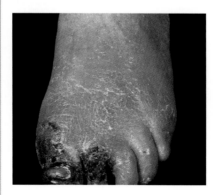

These gangrenous toes have turned black. As the blood supply cannot be restored, they must be amputated to stop the spread of infection.

SEE ALSO

BACTERIA • BLOOD • CIRCULATORY SYSTEM • DIABETES • FROSTBITE • SKIN DISEASES AND DISORDERS

Q & A

I am a diabetic. Is it inevitable that one day I will get gangrene because of this?

No. Artery disease in the legs is more common in diabetics than in nondiabetics, but it is still rare. To avoid gangrene, take good care of your feet, with a podiatrist's advice if necessary, and don't smoke. Remember that any compression of the feet tends to impede blood supply to the toes and encourage gangrene. Above all, careful control of your diabetes will ensure the lowest possible risk of gangrene and other diabetic complications.

When I had my appendix removed, the surgeon told me that it was gangrenous. Doesn't gangrene happen only in the feet or legs?

Gangrene is most likely to occur in the legs or feet, but it can also affect any organ or tissue in the body that has been deprived of its blood supply. That may happen in organs in the abdomen when arteries become blocked by artery disease, by inflammation, or by twisting of the intestines.

Gastroenteritis

Gastroenteritis is an infection causing inflammation of the stomach and intestine. The prefix *gastro-* refers to the stomach, and the *enteron* is the intestine. The ending *-itis* implies inflammation. Gastroenteritis is a common complaint and in a normally healthy adult usually clears up after a few days, leaving no lasting effects. However, the infection can be far from trivial, especially in people who are either very old or very young. Every year, at least 10 million people, mostly babies and infants, die from severe gastroenteritis. Most of these deaths occur in tropical and developing parts of the world and are caused by severe loss of fluid (dehydration) as a result of persistent vomiting and by malnutrition. In developed countries, deaths from gastroenteritis are rare. If adequate medical resources are available, death from this cause is usually preventable.

Causes of gastroenteritis

Gastroenteritis is caused by infecting organisms that live in the intestine. They include *Escherichia coli* (E. coli); salmonella organisms, of which there are more than 1,500 different species; a range of viruses (enteroviruses); and the protozoan organism *Giardia lamblia*. Such infections can be avoided by good hygiene, but in the developing world this is often difficult, and sometimes almost impossible, to achieve. Most cases in developed countries

Q & A

My father had gastritis and now has enteritis. What is the difference between the two?

Gastritis is an inflammation of the stomach, whereas enteritis affects the intestines. The two may be part of an infection of the intestinal tract, and the symptoms of gastric upset may be combined with diarrhea. Gastritis is often the result of eating or drinking something that irritates the stomach lining, whereas enteritis can result from food poisoning, food allergies, and sometimes adverse reactions to certain drugs.

My older brother is a trainee chef. How soon can he return to work after an attack of gastroenteritis?

Since he is involved in the preparation of food, he must not return to work until his doctor tells him it is safe to do so; his intestine may still carry the bacteria after the symptoms have subsided. Even if he is extremely careful about hygiene, there is still a chance that he could pass on the infection. Simple tests will show when he is free of infection.

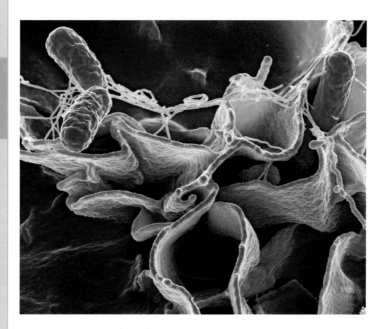

Salmonella bacteria (green) are a common causes of gastroenteritis. The organisms are particularly likely to be present in eggs and poultry.

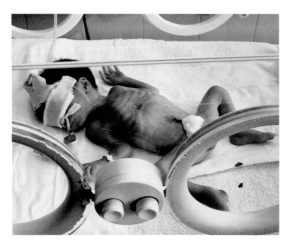

This baby is suffering from gastroenteritis and is being rehydrated in a hospital.

AVOIDING GASTROENTERITIS

People can reduce their risk of acquiring gastrointestinal infections by taking a few simple precautions in the home:

- Hands should be washed after every visit to the toilet and before handling food. People who handle raw meat should wash their hands again before touching any other food.
- Raw meats should not come into contact with other foods.
- Frozen meat and poultry should be thoroughly defrosted before cooking and never refrozen.
- All food, especially meat and chicken, should be cooked through before it is eaten.
- Cooked food should not be reheated more than once.
- Surfaces and appliances in the kitchen and bathroom should be kept scrupulously clean.

occur in bottle-fed babies. Breast-fed babies seldom suffer from gastroenteritis. Gastroenteritis in bottle-fed babies is encouraged by the absence of antibodies present in breast milk; the ease with which a bottle, the teat, or the milk itself can be contaminated; and the fact that milk at feeding temperature is an excellent culture medium for bacteria. This risk is greater if the milk is not used immediately but is kept artificially warm.

Symptoms and treatment

Gastroenteritis causes fever, cramping pains in the abdomen, diarrhea, and vomiting. The great majority of attacks are mild and clear up without treatment. If diarrhea and vomiting are severe, however, death can occur in a day or two. In severe cases, there is little urinary output, and any urine produced is dark and strong. The skin is dry, inelastic, and flushed; the eyes are sunken; and the mouth is dry, with a furred tongue. As the condition worsens, the patient shows irritability, lethargy, and mental confusion. These symptoms indicate dehydration, which leads to an alteration in the balance of the chemicals in the blood and tissue fluids, especially sodium and potassium. That can seriously interfere with the function of body cells.

A baby's life can often be saved by adequate fluid intake by mouth. Special rehydration fluids have been designed for this purpose and are available in many clinics. However, in many cases, sick babies are too weak to swallow, and their only chance of survival is to receive fluids by infusion into a vein. This procedure is called intravenous rehydration. These fluids must be sterile and may consist of a solution of salt and glucose. World Health Organization enterprises to train "barefoot" doctors in the skills of inserting a tiny infusion needle, under sterile conditions, into a vein in a baby's scalp and setting up a glucose-saline drip have led to the saving of hundreds of lives.

Even in developed countries, dehydration in babies is dangerous. Diarrhea should never be treated casually. If the feces are extremely watery and the infant is showing signs of general upset, such as fever, vomiting, or failure to feed, then medical attention is urgently required.

SEE ALSO

BACTERIAL DISEASES • DIARRHEA • DIGESTIVE SYSTEM DISEASES AND DISORDERS • MALNUTRITION • SALMONELLA • VIRUSES

Genes

A gene is the unit that passes hereditary characteristics to the next generation. Thousands of genes are present on each chromosome of plant and animal cells; genes determine what each organism will look like and how it will react to its environment.

Genes consist of lengths of DNA that contain a code specifying the construction of proteins, many of which are enzymes, that activate biochemical cell reactions. Each cell contains a full set of genes, but not all of these genes are active. Genes control each other and are switched on and off depending on their function. The gene code is a sequence of chemical groups called bases. An absence of one or more bases is a mutation, and genetic diseases and disorders are caused by mutations.

Each cell has two sets of chromosomes, one set inherited from each parent. There are therefore two instructions for every characteristic, such as eye color. The color of the eyes depends on which gene is dominant. For example, brown is dominant over blue. If one parent has blue eyes and the other has brown eyes, a child who inherits a brown-eye gene from one parent will have brown eyes. If both parents have brown eyes and each has one gene for brown eyes and one for blue eyes, then each of their children has a one-in-four chance of having blue eyes and a three-in-four chance of having brown eyes.

Q & A

How many genes are there?

Humans are estimated to have between 30,000 and 35,000 genes. The average gene has 3,000 bases; the largest has 2.4 million bases. Geneticists have isolated several thousand genes. The Human Genome Project has sequenced the whole of the human genome and the genomes of some bacteria.

If I have too many X-rays, will the radiation cause abnormalities in my genes that may affect my future children?

The radiation dose that people absorb from X-rays is extremely small. In women of childbearing age, X-rays of the lower abdomen are taken only during the 10 days after the first day of the menstrual period to keep X-rays from affecting an embryo.

Do genes determine personality?

Personality is decided by genetic inheritance, upbringing, and environmental influences.

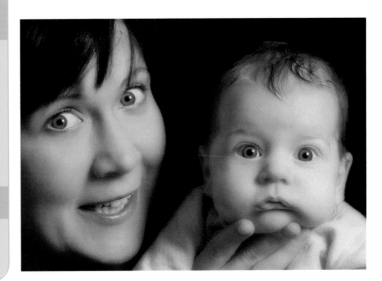

The color of a child's eyes is determined by the genes it inherits from both the mother and the father.

SEE ALSO

BIRTH DEFECTS • CELLS AND CHROMOSOMES • DOWN SYNDROME • GENETIC DISEASES AND DISORDERS • HEMOPHILIA

Genetic Diseases and Disorders

Q & A

I was told that blood taken from the umbilical cord of newborn babies can be used to treat genetic diseases. Is this true?

Yes, transplantation of umbilical cord blood to treat Fanconi's anemia was first carried out successfully in 1988. Cord blood banks were then set up in the United States and Europe. During the following 15 years, around 2,000 people, mainly children, received cord blood injections. Cord blood is valuable because it contains large numbers of stem cells—cells that can turn into any other kind of cell.

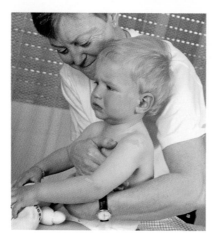

This infant is having physical therapy for cystic fibrosis, a serious genetic disorder.

Genetic diseases and disorders can be caused by inheriting whole chromosome defects, by single defective genes (mutations), by combinations of mutant genes, or by a combination of gene mutation and environmental factors.

Whole-chromosome defects are usually serious: a missing chromosome is usually lethal, and survival is rare. More than half of all spontaneous abortions are the result of whole-chromosome abnormalities. An extra chromosome is common; three copies of chromosome 21 are the cause of Down syndrome, which occurs in 1 in 700 births. Three copies of chromosomes 13 or 18 produce severe defects, and the child seldom survives infancy. One part of a chromosome may be deleted or duplicated, resulting in miscarriage or in birth defects that vary in severity. Sometimes, part of a chromosome is incorporated into another chromosome, in a process called translocation. People with a balanced translocation are unaffected, because all the genetic material is present. However, their offspring may have extremely serious abnormalities.

Genes provide instructions to cells to make enzymes and proteins that are needed for growth and other functions of the body. Abnormalities in single genes cause many disorders, but most of these are rare. More than 4,000 single gene disorders are known, and approximately 1 person in 100 has one of these disorders. They include sickle-cell anemia, hemophilia, cystic fibrosis, and Huntington's disease. There are two possible causes of abnormal genes: the defective gene may have been inherited from a parent or a normal gene could have become faulty during cell division when eggs and sperm form.

Individual gene mutations are extremely common. Sometimes, whole genes are missing or a part of the DNA molecule may be absent, changing the sequence of the gene. Stop codons, which indicate the end of a gene, may be in the wrong place or may be missing, so that adjacent genes run together. Disorders from gene mutations in the X chromosomes are called X-linked, or sex-linked, disorders. Abnormal genes on other chromosomes are called autosomal disorders. Most are inherited, but gene mutations in the ovaries or testes can occur from radiation and exposure to various toxic chemical substances.

SEE ALSO

BIRTH DEFECTS • CELLS AND CHROMOSOMES • CYSTIC FIBROSIS • DOWN SYNDROME • GENES • HEMOPHILIA • HUNTINGTON'S DISEASE • MARFAN SYNDROME • MUSCULAR DYSTROPHY • SICKLE-CELL ANEMIA

Glands

Glands are organs that manufacture and secrete substances to perform various functions in the body. There are three main groups of glands: endocrine glands, exocrine glands, and the glands of the lymphatic system. The major endocrine glands—the pituitary, adrenals, thyroid and parathyroid, pancreas, ovaries, and testes—secrete hormones directly into the bloodstream, where they are taken to their target tissues, which are then stimulated into activity. Exocrine glands, such as sweat glands, release a secretion externally, via a canal or duct, to the body's surface. Finally, the lymphatic system produces antibodies and special blood cells called lymphocytes.

The endocrine glands

The body is like a finely tuned musical instrument, with the glands of the endocrine system keeping all the parts working in harmony.

The endocrine system controls many of the vital functions of the body. In turn, the endocrine glands are controlled by a part of the brain called the hypothalamus, which is attached to a master gland called the pituitary, situated at the base of the brain. The pituitary is fed stimulating hormones by the hypothalamus; these hormones act on the other glands in a feedback system. For example, the thyroid gland produces thyroid hormone, which is essential to keep all the body systems active. If the level of thyroid hormone is too low, the pituitary releases thyroid-stimulating hormone to urge the thyroid to produce more of its hormone. Once the level rises, the feedback mechanism ensures that no more stimulating hormone is produced until it is needed. The parathyroid glands are also stimulated by the pituitary to control calcium and phosphorus levels in the blood.

The pituitary gland also controls the release of hormones from organs to ensure that bodily functions are carried out. For example, the pituitary gland stimulates the adrenals to release corticosteroid hormone, which affects metabolism; adrenaline and noradrenaline to increase heart rate and blood flow to muscles; aldosterone to regulate salt excretion; and cortisol to boost sugar levels. The ovaries and testes are stimulated to release male and female sex hormones; and the pancreas, both an endocrine and an exocrine gland, is stimulated to produce two hormones: insulin to regulate blood sugar levels and glucagon to increase blood sugar levels. Apart from its stimulatory function, the pituitary secretes growth hormone; prolactin, to help produce breast milk; a hormone to regulate water balance; and one to contract the uterus (womb) in labor.

Q & A

If glands stop working, is it possible to perform a transplant?

No, but other treatment can be given. If the endocrine glands (which form the hormone system) stop working, a hormone substitute can be given by mouth. If the pancreas stops producing insulin, diabetes results. That is treated with insulin by injection.

I had infectious mononucleosis, and my friend said it was a glandular disease. Was she right?

A common feature of infectious mononucleosis is a swelling of the lymph nodes, and people often refer to this as a swelling of the "glands." However, infectious mononucleosis is a disease that affects the whole body, rather than the lymph nodes alone.

My armpits smell. Is it possible to remove the sweat glands?

Sweat does not smell offensive until it begins to decompose. The solution is frequent washing and using a deodorant. Also, consult your doctor; he or she can recommend other treatments.

FEMALE GLANDS

MALE GLANDS

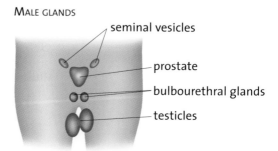

seminal vesicles

prostate

bulbourethral glands

testicles

pineal gland

pituitary gland

salivary glands

thyroid gland

parathyroid glands

thymus

mammary gland

adrenal gland

sweat glands

ovary

stomach

pancreas

small intestine

This diagram shows the location of the endocrine and exocrine glands in a woman. The yellow spots indicate lymph nodes, which are known as glands but are part of the immune system, along with the thymus. The pineal gland controls body rhythms such as waking and sleeping. A man's glands are the same, except for the reproductive glands (above right). Whereas a woman has mammary glands and ovaries, a man has testicles (which produce testosterone), seminal vesicles, bulbourethral glands, and a prostate gland (which produces seminal fluid).

The exocrine glands

The exocrine glands release secretions to the surface of the body. For example, sweat glands produce sweat, secreted through pores in the skin. Modified sweat glands in the ears produce earwax. Sebaceous glands in the skin produce sebum, which keeps the skin supple. Tear glands produce fluid to lubricate the eyes, and mammary glands produce milk. Other exocrine glands produce digestive fluids. These glands include the salivary glands, the pancreas, glands in the lining of the stomach and the intestines, and the liver.

The lymph nodes

The lymph nodes, which are commonly, but incorrectly, referred to as glands, are part of the lymphatic system. This system is a network of lymph vessels and lymph nodes. The lymph nodes contain lymphocytes, which are blood cells called white cells that help fight the spread of infection. Lymph nodes vary in size from microscopic to 1 inch (2.5 cm) in diameter.

The pineal gland

Deep within the brain, the pineal gland secretes the hormone melatonin, which affects the regulation of the day-night internal body clock. This hormone is secreted mainly during the hours of darkness and is not produced when bright light enters the eyes. If given as a drug, melatonin alters the body clock settings, so it is sometimes taken to prevent jet lag.

SEE ALSO

BLOOD • BODY SYSTEMS • BRAIN • HORMONES AND HORMONAL DISORDERS • LYMPHATIC SYSTEM • SKIN

Glaucoma

Glaucoma is a serious disorder of the eye. It happens when the fluid, or aqueous humor, constantly secreted into the front part of the eye is unable to drain away properly. As more and more fluid is produced, pressure builds in the eyeball. Unless the condition is treated, the sufferer may go blind.

The pressure in the eyeball gradually destroys the tiny blood vessels that feed the cells and nerves that enable people to see. The most common type of glaucoma—chronic simple or open-angle glaucoma—produces no symptoms and is thus potentially extremely dangerous. Regular checks of eye pressure after the age of 40 are desirable; if there is a family history of glaucoma, these checks are essential. A less common form called subacute or angle-closure glaucoma causes ocular symptoms such as blurred vision and rainbow-colored halos that appear around objects. In both types of glaucoma, the cells affecting peripheral (side) vision are the first to be destroyed. The patient may develop tunnel vision, seeing only what is straight ahead. Glaucoma develops gradually, so the patient may not notice it for some time, but eventually all of the sight may be destroyed.

Regular eye tests allow an ophthalmologist to see changes inside the eyeball. If glaucoma is treated in time, medicines can reduce the pressure in the eye. Otherwise, surgery can make a new drainage channel. However, the cells of the eye that have been lost can never be restored.

Q & A

My grandfather has glaucoma, and his eyesight has worsened over the past year. Will his eyesight ever improve?

Even when glaucoma is treated properly, eyesight may not improve. Usually, the aim of treatment is to prevent further loss of sight.

Several members of my family have suffered from glaucoma. Is this just a coincidence?

Glaucoma often runs in families. Some people are born with a tendency to glaucoma, owing to abnormalities of drainage of the anterior chamber of the eye, but the condition does not show up until adulthood. Glaucoma rarely affects people under 40.

My grandmother has had an operation for glaucoma. Will her eyesight now stay the same?

It is impossible to say. Sometimes progressive loss of sight results when glaucoma fails to respond to treatment.

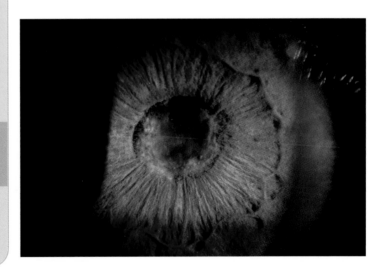

The pigment on the lens indicates glaucoma, in which the pressure inside the eye increases and causes damage.

SEE ALSO

BLINDNESS • EYE AND SIGHT • EYE DISEASES AND DISORDERS • RETINA AND RETINAL DISORDERS

Gonorrhea

Q & A

My friend says that you can contract gonorrhea without ever having had sexual intercourse. Is that true? If so, how else could you get this disease?

Gonorrhea is never passed on in any way other than by sexual contact, because the organisms responsible quickly die once outside the body. However, it is possible for an infected mother to give her daughter vulvovaginitis (an infection of the vulva and vagina), for example, by letting her use a heavily infected towel.

If a pregnant woman has gonorrhea, will it harm the baby?

Gonorrhea cannot be passed to a baby in the uterus, but it may be transmitted during the birth, in which case the baby's eyes will become inflamed. If the baby is infected, antibiotic treatment is 100 percent effective. However, if a pregnant woman suspects that she has gonorrhea, she should go to her doctor or a prenatal clinic. Unless she is allergic, she will be prescribed penicillin.

Gonorrhea is a disease caused by a gonococcal bacterium, *Neisseria gonorrhoeae*. Almost all cases are acquired during sexual intercourse, but a small number are transmitted to babies from infected mothers during birth. Such babies, if left untreated, can develop a blinding eye infection. The risk of contracting gonorrhea from an infected partner during sexual intercourse is high—the risk to females from males being greater. The male-to-female transmission rate is 80 percent; the female-to-male rate is somewhat less. Among sexually promiscuous people, gonorrhea is one of the most infectious diseases known.

Between 1997 and 2000, there was an increase of nearly 34 percent in the number of cases of gonorrhea in large cities. Millions of young people have gonorrhea, and the prevalence of the disease is higher now than it has ever been.

Symptoms

Gonorrhea shows itself quickly in men. The first symptoms appear two to five days after intercourse. There is a yellow or clear penile discharge along with severe irritation. In women, the only immediate indication may be irritation and a change in an existing vaginal discharge. In general, gonorrhea is more serious in females than in males, because in about 10 percent of cases, the gonococcal infection spreads into the uterus (womb) and along the fallopian tubes to cause inflammation and damage. This disorder, called salpingitis, can partially block the tubes, causing infertility or an increased risk of dangerous tubal (ectopic) pregnancy. In males, gonorrhea can cause a narrowing and partial obstruction of the urethra (urine outlet tube). This condition is hard to treat and requires surgery. Gonorrhea can also seriously affect other parts of the body.

Antibiotic resistance

Originally, *N. gonorrhoeae* was extremely sensitive to penicillin, and a single dose would cure the condition. However, because of the overuse of antibiotics, gonococci have become resistant to some antibiotics, especially penicillins. Such resistance is common in the United States, and it is now inadvisable to use penicillin to treat gonorrhea. The same applies to Africa and the Far East. People who contract gonorrhea should tell their partners immediately so that urgent treatment can be obtained.

SEE ALSO

BACTERIAL DISEASES • SEXUALLY TRANSMITTED DISEASES

Gout

Gout is a form of arthritis in which crystalline deposits of uric acid cause painful, inflamed swelling of the joints. People with gout have raised blood levels of uric acid; normally, this acid is excreted by the intestines and the kidneys, but that is not the case with gout. The abnormality is usually of genetic origin.

In the past, people thought that rich food and alcohol caused gout and that it was a disease of the wealthy. It is now known that anybody, rich or poor, can get gout and that it is more common in men than in women.

Symptoms

The first attack of gout usually involves a single joint, such as the big toe, which becomes red, swollen, and extremely painful and tender. The patient may have a slight fever. The attack can last for up to 10 days, and other attacks will follow at irregular intervals. These episodes may involve other joints, including the fingers or wrists. In some cases, crystals of uric acid settle in the joints, skin, and kidneys and do permanent damage.

Some foods encourage gout, so the doctor may suggest that the patient should cut down on red meat, oily fish, and alcohol. If the disease returns, patients may be given drugs to prevent the formation of uric acid and to encourage the kidneys to excrete it. They will need to take the drugs for the rest of their lives.

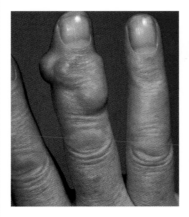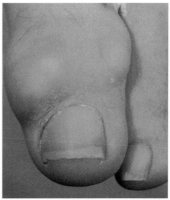

Chronic gout may cause swollen joints, as in this big toe (right); it may also cause collections of chalk stones to form on the fingers (left) or even on the ears in some individuals.

SEE ALSO

ARTHRITIS • GENETIC DISEASES AND DISORDERS • JOINT DISORDERS • KIDNEY • SKIN

Q & A

I heard that gout is connected with rich foods. Does dieting help? Which foods, if any, should be avoided?

Certain foods rich in the chemicals known as purines produce excess uric acid after digestion, which can lead to gout if the body does not excrete it efficiently. Examples of high-purine foods include liver, kidney, venison, meat extracts, legumes, goose, duck, turkey, anchovies, sardines, fish roe, and herring. These foods are best avoided in large amounts. However, if they are eaten in moderate amounts their contribution is relatively slight.

Does gout have anything to do with cancer, or is there no connection at all between the two things?

Gout does not cause cancer, but sometimes cancer can cause gout. In some cancerous growths, the creation and degeneration of tissues increase, leading to higher levels of uric acid. Therapy that destroys tumors rapidly may also raise the uric acid level and produce symptoms of gout.

Guillain-Barré Syndrome

Q & A

If, in Guillain-Barré syndrome, the insulating (myelin) sheath of the nerves is not permanently damaged, what happens to it? How is this different from what happens with multiple sclerosis?

In Guillain-Barré syndrome, once the attack by the immune system settles, remyelination occurs; the stripped areas grow new myelin to cover the bare patches on the nerve fibers. In multiple sclerosis, the areas of the insulating sheath are permanently lost.

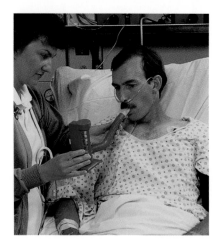

A man with Guillain-Barré syndrome receives respiratory therapy in a hospital. The plastic tube in his mouth assesses his breathing, while the smaller tube under his nose provides an oxygen supplement.

The nerve fibers outside the brain and spinal cord are covered by sheaths of a fatty insulating material called myelin. This sheath is important because it allows normal electrical nerve impulses to be passed around the body. The myelin sheath can be damaged in a process known as demyelination, which affects the ability of the nerves to transmit nerve impulses.

Guillain-Barré syndrome is a serious disorder of this type in which damage occurs to various nerves, causing them to become inflamed. Inflammation usually occurs as a result of a viral infection. The myelin sheaths themselves do not become infected, but they are attacked by cells in the immune system that are created in response to the viral infection.

The damage that occurs to the myelin sheath in Guillain-Barré syndrome can affect any of the nerves emerging from the spinal cord and often involves the roots of these nerves. Spinal nerves contain fibers that activate muscles (motor nerves) and fibers that carry sensation impulses around the body (sensory nerves). The result of failure of nerve conduction is that the muscles connected to the affected fibers are unable to contract properly and information about the various sensations (sensory impulses) cannot get through to the brain. That causes a progressive weakness in the muscles, which, in moderate cases, usually starts with a weakness in the legs. Other symptoms include tingling and numbness, which usually starts in the hands and feet and spreads inward to affect other parts of the body. In more extreme cases, muscle weakness can lead to total paralysis and difficulty in speaking. It usually takes about 10 to 14 days for these symptoms to take full effect, but in some severe cases the patient is paralyzed within 24 hours.

The most serious result in Guillain-Barré syndrome occurs when muscles that are used to maintain breathing are affected, including the diaphragm and those between the ribs (the intercostal muscles). Paralysis of these muscles is rapidly fatal unless the supply of oxygen to the brain and other organs is maintained by artificial ventilation. An air-pumping machine rhythmically inflates the lungs by way of a tube passed through an opening in the neck (tracheostomy). Even those who require this measure usually recover when the attack settles and the nerve fibers are remyelinated. In mild cases, recovery can take weeks. In serious cases, full recovery may take several months, and physical therapy may be required.

SEE ALSO

NERVOUS SYSTEM • NERVOUS SYSTEM DISORDERS • PARALYSIS

Gum Diseases

Q & A

My gums often bleed when I brush my teeth. Why?

Your gums are likely to be inflamed because of a buildup of plaque. This is a sticky substance made of bacteria that live in the mouth, food debris, and dried saliva. Plaque can be removed by brushing for several minutes each day in the correct way—a circular, up-and-down motion of the brush. If your gums still give you trouble after a week or so, visit your dentist.

Is it possible to catch gum disease from another student's silverware in the school cafeteria?

With the exception of one rare condition, gum disease is not infectious. The bacteria that usually cause gum disease are present in small numbers even in a healthy mouth. If the bacteria are not removed by brushing, their numbers increase and cause serious gum damage.

If plaque is not removed by brushing, calculus will form. Plaque can damage the bone, and deep pockets may form in the gum around the tooth. The excess gum tissue may then have to be removed.

If people do not have healthy gums, they cannot have good teeth. Gum diseases are the most common cause of tooth loss in people over the age of 35, but they are easily prevented by good dental care. People should clean their teeth carefully for several minutes at least twice a day and visit a dentist regularly.

If teeth are not cleaned properly, a sticky substance called plaque builds up on them. Plaque inflames the gums, which become red and swollen and may bleed when the teeth are brushed. This problem is called gingivitis. Proper cleaning soon clears up gingivitis. Healthy gums fit tightly around each tooth, but if gingivitis is not cured, the swollen gum forms a pocket around the neck of the tooth. Plaque builds up, and bacteria multiply, out of reach of a toothbrush. Plaque that accumulates over a long period may harden into calculus (tartar). Before long, the ligaments that hold the tooth in place (periodontal ligaments) are damaged. This damage spreads to the bony socket in which the tooth is set, which begins to break down. Pus can form, causing an unpleasant taste and bad breath. This condition is known as pyorrhea, or periodontal disease. Gradually, the tooth becomes loose and eventually falls out. Another danger is that the gums pull back from the teeth, and abscesses may form.

A dentist can remove any plaque that has built up on the teeth. If the gums have formed permanent pockets, the dentist can cut them away, and further damage can be prevented.

Gums can also become inflamed in some diseases, such as diabetes and leukemia, and from lack of vitamins. A disease called trench mouth causes painful, bleeding ulcers on the gums, particularly between the teeth. It can affect those whose physical resistance is low. It was common among soldiers fighting in the trenches in Europe in World War I (1914–1918).

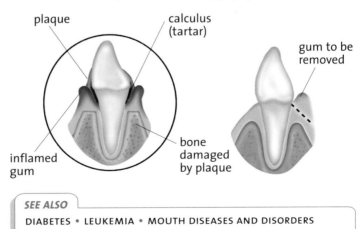

plaque

calculus (tartar)

gum to be removed

inflamed gum

bone damaged by plaque

SEE ALSO

DIABETES • LEUKEMIA • MOUTH DISEASES AND DISORDERS

Hair and Scalp Disorders

Hair and scalp disorders include hair falling out (alopecia), abnormal hair growth (hirsutism), and hair scaling. The study of the hair and scalp in healthy and diseased conditions is called trichology. Trichologists often work with medical practitioners, because increased hair loss may be the first sign of a serious disease.

Causes of excessive hair loss

A number of things can cause excessive hair loss. Stress after an illness or major surgery may result in the sudden but temporary loss of a large amount of hair.

Hormonal problems may also cause hair loss. If the thyroid gland is overactive or underactive, that can lead to hair loss. Hair loss or abnormal hair growth may occur if male or female hormones, known as androgens and estrogens, are out of balance. During pregnancy, high levels of certain hormones cause the body to keep hair that would normally fall out. When the hormones return to pre-pregnancy levels, that hair falls out and the normal cycle of hair growth and loss starts again.

Q & A

Should hair be dried with a hair dryer, or should it be left to dry naturally?

It is always better for hair to dry naturally, but sometimes that is not possible. If you use a hair dryer, do not set the temperature too high and do not hold it too near your hair. In addition, you should spend only the minimum time necessary under the hair dryer. Smooth and brushless rollers should be used. Heated rollers should not be used more than twice a week, and they should be removed before the hair becomes overdried.

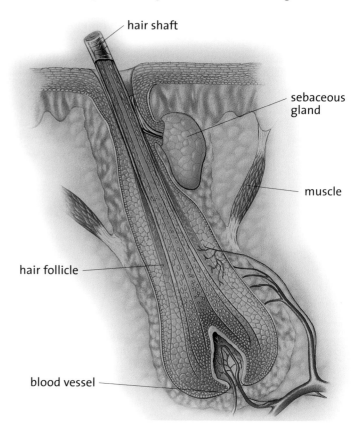

Each hair consists of a shaft, which is the visible part of the hair, and a follicle in which the shaft is rooted. The root of the hair is nourished by blood, and the sebaceous gland lubricates the follicle. When a person is cold or frightened, a muscle contracts and makes the hair stand on end.

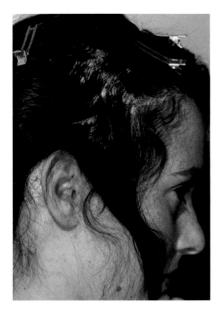

Psoriasis is a form of scaling. It can be treated with crude coal tar ointment or steroid cream, applied at night. The hair must be carefully washed in the morning, and the area must be exposed to sunlight to benefit from ultraviolet rays.

Some medicines, such as chemotherapy drugs, excess vitamin A, and antidepressants, can cause hair loss. Certain bacterial and fungal infections can also cause hair loss.

Some people have an impulse control disorder called trichotillomania that causes them to pull out hair from their scalp or face, causing noticeable bald patches and a receding hairline. This condition affects at least 2 percent of the population and usually starts around puberty or early adulthood.

Excessive use of chemical treatments for styling (such as for coloring and permanent waves), excessive heating, and tight pulling with rollers may also damage hair.

Treatment for excessive hair loss

Depending on the type of hair loss, different treatments are available. If a medicine is causing hair loss, a different one may be prescribed. Correcting a hormone imbalance may prevent further hair loss. Recognizing and treating a scalp infection can help stop the hair loss.

Certain medicines may also help slow or prevent the development of common baldness; they include minoxidil (Rogaine) and finasteride (Propecia). It may take up to six months before a difference is noticeable with these treatments.

If adequate treatment is not available for hair loss, different hairstyles or wigs, hairpieces, or hair weaves may be used. Hair transplant or artificial hair replacement is a successful but expensive remedy.

Scaling

Scaling is another common scalp disorder. The top layer of the skin of the scalp (the epidermis), like that of skin everywhere else on the body, consists of dead cells. These cells gradually wear away over time and are replaced by cells from the layers below (the dermis). This shedding of the dead cell layer is called scaling. The term *dandruff* is loosely applied to several scaling conditions.

One of the most effective antidandruff agents in current use is a compound called zinc pyrithione, which is present in some proprietary shampoos. It suppresses the bacteria present in the scalp that are responsible for scaling. If the dandruff persists after use of an antidandruff shampoo, the condition may be more complex, and a qualified trichologist or a dermatologist should be consulted.

ALOPECIA AREATA

The disease alopecia areata is a common reason for baldness. It causes round bald patches. If it occurs in childhood and is extensive, there is little hope of regrowth. If the condition starts in adulthood, there is a good chance that the hair can regrow within a few months.

SEE ALSO

FUNGAL INFECTIONS • HORMONES AND HORMONAL DISORDERS

Hamstring Injuries

Q & A

A hamstring injury has kept me away from football for a month now. I have been resting, so why should it take so long to heal?

Except in the first 24 hours, rest is not the treatment for muscle injuries. Once the bleeding into the muscle has stopped, massage, heat, and exercise are the best ways to minimize the damage done by bruising, and they will get the muscle back into shape. You really need to start a program of recovery now.

My brother has strained his hamstrings a number of times. Has he developed a weakness as a result of his injury?

Yes, probably, because an original injury was not treated properly. If your brother's hamstring muscles are treated adequately, there is no reason why they should not make a complete recovery. However, he needs to be careful to avoid over-stretching these muscles.

The hamstring muscles are a group of three muscles that form the back of the thigh (the ham area) and span the femur (thighbone). They help bend the leg at the knee and twist the leg in and out.

Hamstring injuries are common, especially among athletes, but they are not serious. The hamstrings are a group of three muscles at the back of each thigh. Individually, they help twist the leg in or out by rotating the knee. Together, the hamstring muscles help bend the leg at the knee. These muscles are long, thin, and easily damaged. A hamstring may tear or become bruised following a blow. Overstretched muscles can also tear when they are tired or are used without being warmed up. The signs of a hamstring injury range from a dull ache to a sharp shooting pain in the back of the thigh. Eventually, the muscle goes into spasm. Ruptured blood vessels can also cause swelling and tenderness in the muscle.

Prevention and treatment

The best way to avoid hamstring injuries is to warm up before exercise by stretching the muscles. Fatigue increases the risk of hamstring injuries, so it is also important to stop before getting too tired. At the first sign of pain, the area should be massaged, and the warm-up exercises should be repeated. A support bandage may be necessary. If the pain continues, all activity should be stopped and medical help should be sought.

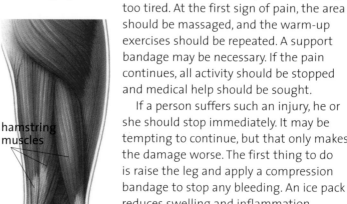

hamstring muscles

calf muscles

If a person suffers such an injury, he or she should stop immediately. It may be tempting to continue, but that only makes the damage worse. The first thing to do is raise the leg and apply a compression bandage to stop any bleeding. An ice pack reduces swelling and inflammation.

Follow-up treatments include ultrasound massage to aid recovery. Heat and conventional massage help disperse blood clots and prevent internal scarring. Stretching exercises also help the muscle recover. Severe hamstring injuries usually require pain relief. Crutches may also be needed to assist walking. Hamstring injuries can take several days to several months to heal.

SEE ALSO

MUSCLE • MUSCLE DISEASES AND DISORDERS • SPORTS INJURIES • SPRAINS AND STRAINS

Hansen's Disease

Hansen's disease, formerly called leprosy, used to be one of the most dreaded diseases. Its victims were kept away from other people and were often cruelly treated. Now, owing to increased awareness and understanding of the disease, it is known that Hansen's disease is not very infectious and can be cured.

Hansen's disease is caused by bacteria that attack the skin and the nerves. All feeling is lost in the affected areas of the body, which may become deformed. Hansen's disease is now common only in damp tropical and subtropical regions in parts of South America, Africa, and Asia. It is spread by continuous contact with an infected person over a long period of time.

There are two forms of Hansen's disease. In both cases, symptoms appear a long time, perhaps several years, after infection. The milder (tuberculoid) form affects the nerves. There is a slowly developing loss of feeling in many parts of the body, and the skin develops a rash. The sufferer does not feel minor injuries to numb areas, so infections often set in that may lead to gangrene. Eventually, the muscles waste away.

The lepromatous form of Hansen's disease is more serious. The face and ears are most often affected, but all of the skin may be involved. Numb areas of skin gradually thicken and corrugate. Soft nodules form, particularly on the ears, nose, and cheeks, and often develop gangrenous sores. The face broadens to develop a lionlike appearance. Large areas of the body may become numb and sometimes paralyzed.

Several drugs, including minocycline, rifampicin, ethionamide, and dapsone, are used to treat Hansen's disease. Some of them are given in combination to produce the best effect. Thalidomide is useful in some forms of Hansen's disease. Feeling cannot be brought back to damaged nerves, but physical therapy can strengthen wasted muscles, and surgery can improve disfigured areas.

Q & A

Are there any types of Hansen's disease that are disfiguring but not infectious?

All types are infectious, but only after prolonged contact with an infected person. Disfigurement usually results from unnoticed damage to anesthetized (numb) skin; an infection then occurs, and gangrene (decaying tissue) sets in. Such cases are no more infectious than others, although where the nose is affected, transmission may take place through tiny exhaled droplets of moisture that pass from the lungs and out through the nose.

Is it at all possible for a baby to get Hansen's disease at birth?

The bacteria that cause Hansen's disease cannot travel from the placenta to the fetus, so newborn babies cannot be infected. The disease is usually transmitted by close contact between an affected mother and her child. If the mother is treated early, the child remains unaffected.

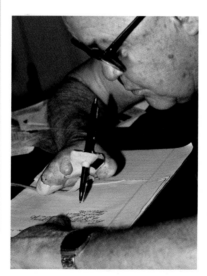

Hansen's disease in this man's fingers caused loss of feeling, infections, and gangrene—with the result that the fingers had to be amputated.

SEE ALSO

BACTERIAL DISEASES • GANGRENE • TROPICAL DISEASES

Heart

The heart is a large, muscular organ situated just above the diaphragm in the middle of the chest, although slightly more of it lies on the left side of the body than on the right. The heart's function is to pump blood around two separate circulations, or systems of blood vessels, in the body.

The body's major circulatory system is called the systemic circulation. It is a massive branching network of blood vessels—arteries, veins, and capillaries—to every part of the body and back to the heart. The heart pumps fresh blood filled with oxygen into the aorta, the central artery of the body. From there, the blood is distributed to the rest of the arteries. This blood circulates through the organs and tissues of the body, delivering nutrients and oxygen to them. When all the oxygen has been absorbed from it, the blood is described as deoxygenated. This blood returns to the heart through the veins.

The heart then pumps the deoxygenated blood through its second circuit: this time a short journey to the lungs. This is called the pulmonary circulation, from the Latin word meaning "lung." The lungs replace the used oxygen in the blood and remove the carbon dioxide that has accumulated in it. This oxygenated blood returns to the heart, and the circuit continues.

Structure and working of the heart

The pumping action of the heart is carried out by two pairs of chambers (compartments): the left and right atria (which are the upper chambers) and the left and right ventricles (which lie below the atria). Each chamber is a muscular bag, with a strong, muscular wall called the septum that divides the left and right sides of the heart. The muscular walls of the chambers contract to push the blood along, and valves between the chambers control the direction of the blood flow.

The heart powers both the pulmonary and the systemic circulations in the following way. Blood flows through pulmonary veins from the lungs into the left atrium of the heart. This blood is rich in oxygen, provided by the lungs. The left atrium contracts and pushes the blood into the left ventricle. A valve between the left atrium and left ventricle ensures that the blood cannot flow back the other way. The left ventricle then contracts and pushes the blood out through another one-way valve into the aorta, and this major artery carries fresh, oxygenated blood to all parts of the body. On its return, the used blood has now lost its oxygen and flows into the right atrium of the heart, which pushes the blood into the right ventricle. The right ventricle pumps this blood back to the lungs to pick up more oxygen, thus completing the double circulation. One-way valves ensure that

Q & A

Can healthy people strain the heart through exercise in the same way that they can pull a muscle?

No. In a healthy person, this problem would not happen. However, before people go for a long run, they should remember that "healthy" is not the same as "normal." Coronary artery disease is common and may limit the work the heart can do. People in their forties and fifties are likely to have some degree of artery disease, and it is not unknown in younger people. Everyone should build up to exertion gently to avoid putting the heart under undue stress. People should also do warm-up exercises before they start.

When I get a shock, my heart feels as if it will jump out of my chest. What causes this feeling? Is it serious?

Do not worry; your heart is quite normal. The shock makes your adrenal glands pump out adrenaline, which suddenly drives your heart to beat very fast and forcefully, causing these symptoms.

the blood flows one way only. With each heartbeat, the two atria contract, followed by the two ventricles. When the body is at rest, this process is repeated between 50 and 80 times a minute.

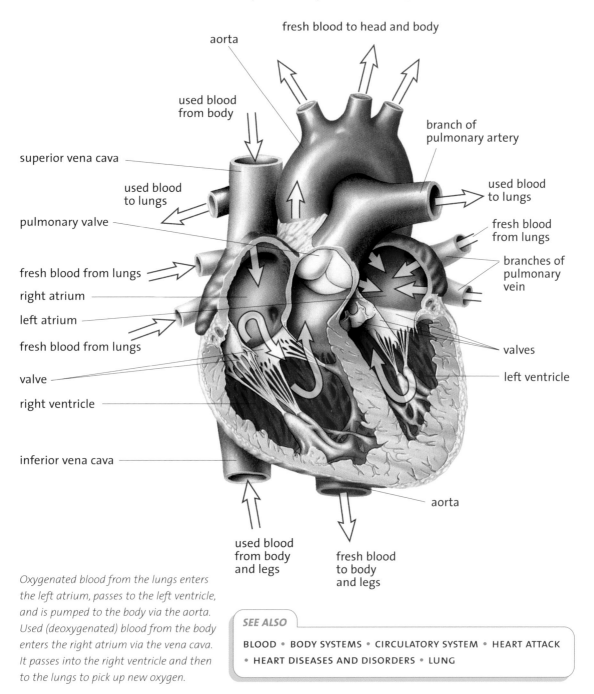

fresh blood to head and body

aorta

used blood from body

superior vena cava

used blood to lungs

pulmonary valve

fresh blood from lungs

right atrium

left atrium

fresh blood from lungs

valve

right ventricle

inferior vena cava

branch of pulmonary artery

used blood to lungs

fresh blood from lungs

branches of pulmonary vein

valves

left ventricle

aorta

used blood from body and legs

fresh blood to body and legs

Oxygenated blood from the lungs enters the left atrium, passes to the left ventricle, and is pumped to the body via the aorta. Used (deoxygenated) blood from the body enters the right atrium via the vena cava. It passes into the right ventricle and then to the lungs to pick up new oxygen.

SEE ALSO

BLOOD • BODY SYSTEMS • CIRCULATORY SYSTEM • HEART ATTACK • HEART DISEASES AND DISORDERS • LUNG

Heart Attack

A heart attack occurs when the blood supply to the heart is obstructed. The coronary arteries are vessels that supply the heart with blood rich in food and oxygen. Heart attacks occur when these arteries become clogged with fatty deposits, a condition known as atherosclerosis. Blood clots can form around the deposits and block the artery. In turn, that obstruction blocks the blood supply to the heart. The person will then feel the chest pain that indicates a heart attack.

Warning signs

A heart attack may come as a surprise, but most people get a warning. When the coronary arteries start to get blocked, the heart works harder during exercise or excitement. That may cause a crushing, suffocating pain in the chest, which may spread to the arms and neck. Anyone who experiences this pain, called angina, should consult a doctor immediately. Smokers, diabetics, and those with a family history of heart attacks are most at risk.

Often, the main symptom of a heart attack is a severe pain in the chest. The pain is usually more acute than angina; it may be so severe that the person collapses. In some cases, there is little pain and the person may mistake the heart attack for indigestion or heartburn. Other symptoms include sweating, shortness of breath, and a weak or slow pulse.

Diagnosis and treatment

A heart attack is a life-threatening condition. It requires immediate hospital treatment. In the hospital, doctors confirm the heart attack with blood tests. An electrocardiogram (ECG) may be given to monitor the electrical activity of the heart. In this procedure, the heart's tiny electric currents are recorded on a machine called an electrocardiograph, which prints out the result—the ECG—on a roll of paper. Any heart disorder, such as a heart attack, shows up as a change of pattern.

Morphine is usually given as pain relief. More drugs may be given to improve the circulation and limit damage to the heart muscle. If there are no complications, most patients can return home to rest after a week or so.

Q & A

Is there anything I can do now to prevent a heart attack from occurring in later life?

Do not smoke. Smoking significantly accelerates the pace of atherosclerosis (the hardening and thickening of the artery walls), which is the cause of coronary artery disease, and it is thus a main factor in heart attacks. There is also strong evidence that if you eat less food that contains saturated fats (which are mostly of animal origin, such as butter and cream), you can reduce the risk that your coronary arteries will become narrowed by cholesterol deposits. Aerobic exercise in the form of running, cycling, and swimming may also help.

My father, who has always led an extremely active life, has just had a heart attack. Does this mean that he will have to slow down now?

Not necessarily, unless he has been told to do so by his doctor. Your father should avoid sudden bursts of activity, however, and build up to any exertion more gradually than he did before.

SEE ALSO

ARTERY • ARTERY DISEASES AND DISORDERS • CIRCULATORY SYSTEM • CIRCULATORY SYSTEM DISEASES AND DISORDERS • HEART • HEART DISEASES AND DISORDERS • STROKE

Heart Diseases and Disorders

Q & A

I overheard my mother telling my father that my little brother has a heart murmur. I'm very worried. Will my brother need an operation?

No. Murmurs in children are extremely common; one study found a murmur in up to 80 percent of normal children. These incidents are called innocent murmurs, and no action is necessary. If your brother's doctor had thought the murmur was dangerous, he or she would have made a referral to a specialist.

My grandmother says that she needs to have one of her heart valves replaced. I'm worried about her. Is it true that there is only a 50 percent chance of surviving this type of open-heart surgery?

Do not worry. If such heart surgery were so dangerous, it would have been given up years ago. The risk depends on which valve is concerned and how many other problems there are. For uncomplicated replacements of a single valve, the chance of surviving is virtually 100 percent.

The heart is a complicated and hardworking organ. If it stops working and is not restarted, death will quickly follow. Heart problems are among the most common causes of death in the Western world.

Heart attacks and angina are not diseases of the heart itself. They are caused by problems in the coronary arteries, which supply blood to the heart muscle. When blood supply is interrupted, the heart cannot work properly. In a heart attack, or coronary thrombosis, a clot (thrombosis) in the artery cuts off the blood supply to part of the heart muscle, and this area of muscle dies. If too much muscle is damaged, the heart stops working. In angina, the heart muscle does not get enough oxygen because not enough blood reaches it, and chest pain results.

Heart defects

In the early weeks of pregnancy, a fetus's heart develops from a single straight tube into a four-chambered pump with two separate circulation systems. This complicated process does not always develop perfectly. Problems may be caused by hereditary factors or by an illness of the mother, such as rubella.

A fetus with a deformed heart often miscarries, but sometimes babies are born with heart defects. The valves controlling blood flow may not work properly or there may be holes between chambers. If used blood mixes with fresh blood in the heart, or if not enough blood gets to the lungs, the baby's skin may have a blue tinge.

A doctor detects a heart problem by listening to a baby's chest for a heart murmur. Murmurs are common, and often no action is needed. Other tests, including X-rays, electrocardiograms (ECGs), and ultrasound scans, show if a defect is serious. Many heart defects are minor, but some need surgery. Surgeons can now operate on tiny babies, but they may prefer to wait for a year or more to see if the heart repairs itself, and until the child is bigger and stronger.

Valve damage

Illness, particularly the infection called rheumatic fever, can damage the valves of the heart. These valves may become narrow, so that the heart has to strain to pump blood, causing pressure to build. This narrowing of the valves is called stenosis.

Sometimes, a valve does not close properly and blood leaks back through it. This defect is known as valve incompetence, and the heart then has to work harder to keep the blood circulating. Faulty valves can be replaced—with plastic valves, or with valves derived from another part of the patient's body, or with valves

HEART DISEASES AND TREATMENTS

DISEASE OR PROBLEM	CAUSES	SYMPTOMS	TREATMENT
Cardiomyopathy, congestive	Usually unknown. However, alcohol, metal poisoning, and some hormonal conditions can cause it.	Heart failure, problems with heart block (slow heartbeat), and possibly palpitations. Valves may become leaky	Symptoms are treated with drugs and sometimes a pacemaker is necessary.
Cardiomyopathy, hypertrophic	Cause unknown. It may run in families.	Angina and occasionally fainting attacks due to obstruction of left ventricle	Drugs may relieve the obstruction; occasionally an operation may be necessary.
Coronary artery disease	Blockage of the coronary arteries with atheroma (fatty deposits)	Angina. It may cause a heart attack and heart failure.	Treatment with drugs or by surgery can improve the heart's blood supply and end the pain. Diuretics remove excess fluid from lungs and tissues.
Endocarditis	Abnormal valve owing to preexisting heart problem. An infected valve may burst.	Fever, heart failure, and general ill health	Antibiotics. Badly damaged valves may need surgery
Heart block (very slow heartbeat)	Degenerative disease of the heart. It may be complication of a heart attack.	Dizziness and fainting	Pacemaker
Heart failure	Almost any form of heart disease	Breathlessness on exertion due to fluid in the lungs; swelling of the ankles.	It may be treated with diuretics or possibly surgery, in the case of valve disease, for example.
Palpitations	Anxiety and overactivity of the thyroid gland; abnormalities in structure; post–heart attack	Sensation of rapid heartbeat; dizziness or fainting if too little blood reaches brain	Drugs are used to suppress the abnormal heart rhythm.
Valve disease	Sometimes caused by rheumatic fever. It may be congenital (present from birth).	Heart failure. Aortic valve problems often cause angina because heart wall thickens. Fainting can occur with aortic stenosis (blocked outlet valve) when there is insufficient blood in the circulation. Mitral (inlet) valve problems usually cause palpitations.	Treatment is surgical in cases where the symptoms are sufficiently bad. Otherwise, drugs are used to control the symptoms. Surgery is often necessary for marked aortic stenosis.

created from processed animal tissue. Abnormal heart valves sometimes cause endocarditis (an infection of the heart tissues), which gradually destroys the tissues.

Too fast, too slow

The heart has its own pacemaker. This group of cells controls the rate at which the heart beats according to what an individual is doing. Heartbeats normally vary from below 70 beats a minute

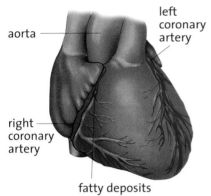

aorta

left coronary artery

right coronary artery

fatty deposits

How arteries become blocked: fatty deposits have caused a partial blockage of the right coronary artery, restricting the blood flow (above). A blood clot (thrombosis) has now caused a total blockage in the narrowed artery (above right). That prevents the artery from supplying some of the heart muscle with blood, so this area of muscle dies.

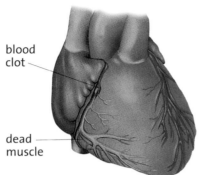

blood clot

dead muscle

at rest to more than 160 beats a minute during hard exercise.

A fast heartbeat is known as tachycardia, and it often causes the symptom known as palpitations (an uncomfortable feeling of the heart beating strongly). Sometimes, the heart beats quickly without any apparent reason. This reaction is not usually serious and is often caused by anxiety.

A more serious form of rapid heartbeat is called atrial fibrillation: the heart muscle contracts very quickly, but the heart does not have time to fill properly between beats, and very little blood moves forward. Likewise, if the heart beats too slowly (heart block), it cannot move much blood around. Both of these conditions cause dizziness and faintness, because not enough blood reaches the brain. Rapid beating can be cured with drugs, and heart block can be cured by fitting the patient with an artificial pacemaker.

Heart diseases

If the muscular walls of the heart become damaged, in a condition known as cardiomyopathy, the heart beats less efficiently, but this problem is rare. Heart problems cause severe symptoms. Coronary artery problems, including heart attack and angina, cause pain or heart failure. If blood is not pumped properly, it builds up in the vessels and forces fluid into the tissues, causing edema.

If the left ventricle is affected, fluid collects in the lungs, causing breathlessness. Usually, the right side of the heart is also affected, causing fluid to collect in other body tissues, especially the ankles.

Heart failure is treated with drugs: diuretics to get rid of fluid, a drug to stimulate the heartbeat, and possibly an anticoagulant to prevent the blood from clotting and blocking the arteries.

CARDIAC ARREST

Sometimes, when a person's normal heartbeat is disturbed, the heart contractions stop. After a few seconds, the patient loses consciousness and no pulse can be felt. Breathing then stops. This type of heart failure is known as cardiac arrest and needs immediate treatment with cardiopulmonary resuscitation (CPR) to restart circulation and breathing. Unless CPR is carried out within a few minutes, the heart and brain will be damaged beyond repair.

SEE ALSO

ARTERY DISEASES AND DISORDERS • BRAIN • CIRCULATORY SYSTEM DISEASES AND DISORDERS • EDEMA • HEART • HEART ATTACK • RHEUMATIC FEVER

Heat Sickness

The body temperature is normally about 98.4°F (37°C). If the surrounding temperature rises, the body's thermoregulation system reacts: it stops the body from overheating and protects the brain, which cannot tolerate high temperatures. The body reacts in two ways. Its main reaction is to perspire. As the sweat evaporates, the skin cools. The body can also lose heat by the dilation of blood vessels; when they widen, more blood reaches the skin, which takes on a flushed appearance, and the blood cools. Sometimes, the body is badly affected by heat. Heat cramps, which are caused by physical effort in extremely hot conditions, are an occupational hazard of miners and firefighters.

In the condition called heat exhaustion, or heat prostration, victims may collapse as a result of excessive loss of fluid and salt. Victims sweat so much that their body temperature remains normal. In very hot, damp places, however, the sweat may not evaporate and cool the body. Heatstroke—or sunstroke—may occur; in this condition the patient's temperature rises rapidly. This is a very serious condition that can lead to permanent brain damage and even death. People who move from a cool climate to a hot one are at risk of heat exhaustion or heatstroke. Outdoors, they should wear light clothes and a sun hat and should be careful not to sunbathe or exercise for too long. A lot of fluid is lost during perspiration; this fluid has to be replaced by taking extra liquids and salt. Anyone who shows signs of heat sickness should be taken to a cool place as soon as possible and given salty water to drink.

Q & A

What is the difference between sunstroke and heatstroke?

There is no difference. Both terms describe the serious and potentially fatal condition that can occur if the body is excessively heated, resulting in the total breakdown of the temperature-regulating mechanism in the body. Heatstroke is a more accurate name, because you can suffer from its effects away from the sun. If the temperature is high enough, you can get heatstroke even when not in direct sun.

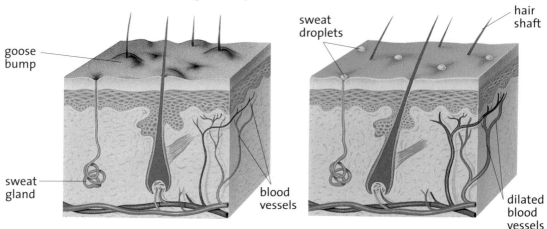

When the body is cold (left), the blood vessels narrow, less sweat is produced, the hair stands straight out from the skin, and goose bumps develop. When the skin is heated (right), the blood vessels dilate, the sweat glands work harder, and the hair lies closer to the skin.

SEE ALSO

BLOOD • BODY SYSTEMS • SKIN • SUNBURN

Hemo-chromatosis

Hemochromatosis is a genetic disorder that results in an accumulation of iron in the body. The gene defect responsible for hemochromatosis produces a molecule called a transporter protein. This protein carries iron from food across the wall of the intestines and into the bloodstream. A person with hemochromatosis may absorb more than 10 times more iron than normal. This excess iron then accumulates in the body's tissues and organs, such as the liver, pancreas, skin, and brain. Since women lose iron in menstruation, they are less likely to show the full effects of the disease.

Q & A

My doctor tells me that I have hereditary hemochromatosis and that it is a recessive disorder. What does that mean?

The most common form of the disease is caused by a mutation in a gene on the arm of chromosome 6, which is present in about 10 percent of all white people. All genes exist in pairs; most people carrying the gene have only one in the pair with the mutation. A recessive disease shows itself only if both genes in the pair have the mutation. If your parents did not have the disease, they must both have been carriers of the mutation.

Severe symptoms

The early symptoms of hemochromatosis include joint pain, fatigue, and palpitations. The condition may interfere with a woman's menstrual cycle. Men may become impotent. Eventually, the buildup of iron in the body causes organ damage.

Unless there is a family history of the disease, it may become apparent in a patient only in middle age. For example, the skin may become discolored with deposits of melanin. Scarring of the liver, called cirrhosis, may eventually result in liver cancer and total liver failure. A buildup of iron in the pancreas may cause diabetes. In the joints, hemochromatosis can cause a painful condition known as rheumatism. In the heart, the condition can lead to heart muscle failure.

Detection and treatment

The symptoms can be avoided if the condition is identified as soon as possible. The treatment involves removing blood to take excess iron from the body. A unit of blood may be taken once or twice a week until the iron falls to a safe level, then less often.

People with hemochromatosis must avoid iron supplements, but they can still eat foods containing iron. However, it is important also to avoid high doses of vitamin C, because this vitamin increases the body's uptake of iron. It is also important to limit alcohol, which increases the risk of liver damage.

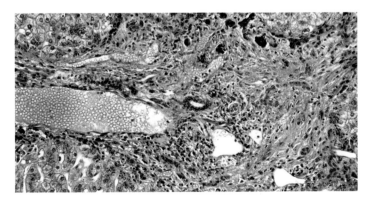

This is a light micrograph of a section through the liver of a patient with hemochromatosis.

SEE ALSO

BLOOD • GENETIC DISEASES AND DISORDERS • LIVER

Hemophilia

Hemophilia is an extremely serious hereditary disease in which the blood does not clot normally because the body does not make enough of a blood-clotting substance called factor VIII and bleeding cannot be halted without medical attention. Hemophilia often used to be fatal, but modern methods of treatment enable hemophiliacs who take care of themselves and receive treatment to live a relatively normal life.

Abnormal gene

Hemophilia is caused by an abnormal gene, which is located on an X chromosome. Females have two X chromosomes, and the chance of their having two such abnormal genes is extremely small. One normal chromosome guarantees that females will produce factor VIII; however, although they remain unaffected themselves, they will pass any abnormal gene to their children. Males have only one X chromosome. Any male who inherits an abnormal hemophilia gene from his mother will have the disease; girls are carriers, because they will inherit a second, normal chromosome from their father. Depending on how much factor VIII is produced, hemophilia can be mild or severe.

Symptoms

The symptoms of hemophilia appear early. Affected babies bruise extremely easily and any cuts or scrapes bleed for a long time. Falls can cause internal bleeding. As children get older, they may begin to bleed into their joints, particularly the knees and ankles. This bleeding is extremely painful and eventually deforms the joint. Any operation causes great problems; even having a tooth pulled can cause severe and prolonged bleeding. A bad cut can cause hemophiliacs to bleed to death if they are not given immediate medical treatment.

Treatment

Hemophiliacs are treated by giving them concentrated factor VIII when bleeding starts. They should carry a card with them in case of an accident and should avoid sports that involve knocks, falls, cuts, or scrapes. Soon after the beginning of the AIDS epidemic, some hemophiliacs became infected by the AIDS virus as a result of contaminated factor VIII transfusions. Donated blood is now screened to avoid such contamination in the future.

Q & A

My brother has hemophilia, but I don't. If I eventually have children, will they be affected?

Since hemophilia is a sex-linked condition, the answer to your question depends on whether you are male or female. If you are male, you cannot have the mutant gene, so your children are safe. However, if you are female, there is a 50–50 chance that you are a carrier of the mutation, in which case some of your sons may be affected by the condition and some of your daughters may be carriers. Before having any children, you should discuss the situation with a doctor or a genetic counselor.

Is it ever possible for a girl to develop hemophilia?

Yes. If a female carrier has children with a male hemophiliac, it is possible that half of their daughters will develop the disease and that the other half will be carriers. Such unions are rare, however. Hemophilia is such a serious disease that few people would wish to risk passing it on to their children. That is why genetic counseling is so important.

> **SEE ALSO**
>
> AIDS AND HIV • BIRTH DEFECTS • BLOOD • BLOOD DISEASES AND DISORDERS • CELLS AND CHROMOSOMES • GENES

Hemorrhoids

Hemorrhoids, or piles, are swollen and twisted veins present in the anal canal, the short tube that connects the last part of the bowel (the rectum) with the outside of the body. Hemorrhoids can be caused by constipation and straining to pass feces. Those that form inside the anus are called internal hemorrhoids; if present nearly at the opening, they are called external hemorrhoids. Sometimes, an internal hemorrhoid prolapses; it bulges out of the anus during a bowel movement or remains outside the body. If the blood in a hemorrhoid clots, it may become painful.

Hemorrhoids are easy to treat; if they are small, they can be injected with a substance that makes them shrivel, or they can be shrunk with a freezing instrument. The blood clot of an external hemorrhoid can be cut away. Another common treatment is to encircle the neck of the hemorrhoid with a very tight rubber band. These treatments are not painful and can be performed on an outpatient basis in a hospital.

Serious hemorrhoids can be removed surgically under a general anesthetic. Hemorrhoids can usually be prevented if constipation is avoided by eating a high-fiber diet.

Does high blood pressure cause hemorrhoids?

No. A person with high blood pressure may be more likely to bleed from hemorrhoids than a person with normal blood pressure, but high blood pressure certainly does not cause hemorrhoids.

Can a person get hemorrhoids from sitting on a hot radiator?

This is an example of an old wives' tale. Sitting on a hot surface does not cause hemorrhoids. However, in a person who already has them, increased local heat could make the hemorrhoids swell and become more pronounced.

I have heard that the types of food you eat can affect whether or not you get hemorrhoids. Is that true?

Any food that tends to cause constipation is likely to aggravate hemorrhoids, and any food with a high roughage content, such as fruits, vegetables, and nuts, is likely to help prevent them.

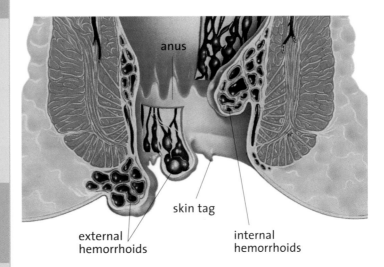

anus

skin tag

external hemorrhoids

internal hemorrhoids

Hemorrhoids may occur internally or externally. They form in areas of the rectum where networks of veins, known as plexuses, are concentrated. Skin tags seldom cause a serious problem and are not true hemorrhoids, but they are often diagnosed and treated as if they were.

SEE ALSO

BLOOD • CIRCULATORY SYSTEM • VEIN DISORDERS

Hepatitis

Hepatitis is an inflammation of the liver. It is an extremely infectious disease caused by viruses. The three main types of hepatitis, caused by different viruses, are known as hepatitis A (infectious hepatitis); hepatitis B (serum hepatitis); and hepatitis C. There are several other less common forms of hepatitis.

Hepatitis A is usually spread by food or water contaminated with the feces of an infected person. Outbreaks happen in overcrowded areas with poor sanitation and in schools and other institutions if standards of hygiene are poor. Hepatitis B is more severe and is usually transmitted by infected blood. People get hepatitis B from using unsterilized hypodermic needles, razor blades, or tattoo needles; from a transfusion of infected blood or plasma; or from sexual contact. Many heroin addicts are carriers of the hepatitis B virus. Hospital workers are particularly at risk of infection. Hepatitis C is transmitted in the same way.

Many hepatitis infections are mild. The patients may not notice them, but blood tests show they have had the illness. A severe attack inflames the liver so much that bile cannot drain from it. The patient becomes jaundiced; the skin and the whites of the eyes become yellow, because bile pigments are building up in the blood. The feces are pale because the liver cannot secrete bile into the intestine, and it is bile that normally colors the feces. Patients feel ill for some time before the jaundice appears. They have little appetite, pain high on the right side of the abdomen and in the joints, and sometimes a rash. Attacks usually clear up after six weeks, but in a few cases, the liver becomes chronically inflamed and cirrhosis of the liver develops. In the worst cases, liver failure causes coma and death.

Q & A

My mother is being treated for infectious hepatitis at home. Should we take special precautions to avoid being infected as well?

During the infectious stage, you should cook her food in separate pots and use different utensils; you should also take extra care with personal hygiene. However, your mother will stop being infectious soon after the jaundice begins to disappear.

I read that you can't be a blood donor if you've had hepatitis. Is this true? If so, why?

Yes, it is true. The organisms that cause this disease can go on living in your blood long after you have recovered. If this blood were given to others, they could be infected with the disease.

My sister had glandular fever and has now developed jaundice. Why would that happen?

People with glandular fever sometimes develop jaundice that is due to hepatitis. That also happens in other viral diseases; numerous viruses can cause liver inflammation.

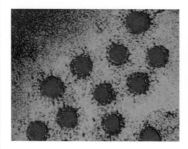 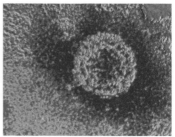

Under a microscope, doctors can identify several hepatitis A viruses (left) and the hepatitis B virus (right) in a patient's liver tissue.

SEE ALSO

BLOOD • INFECTIOUS DISEASES • JAUNDICE • LIVER • SEXUALLY TRANSMITTED DISEASES • VIRUSES

Hernia

A hernia is a bulge of soft tissue that forces its way through an opening or weak place in the surrounding muscles and fibrous connective tissues. If it is an external hernia, the bulge of tissue is covered with a layer of fat and skin. The bulge usually contains either a loop of small intestine or part of the fatty membrane that covers the intestines. Hernias most often appear in the abdomen. A hiatal hernia, for example, is formed when part of the stomach pushes up into the chest through a weak place in the diaphragm. Other hernias may occur in the groin (inguinal or femoral hernia) and near the navel (umbilical hernia). Hernias may be caused by straining the muscles while doing heavy work or by allowing muscles to become weak through lack of exercise.

Symptoms and treatment

Some hernias produce no symptoms, but those near the surface of the abdomen may cause a tender lump, which disappears temporarily when pressed. A hiatal hernia may allow food and acid to move from the stomach back into the gullet. That causes a burning pain behind the breastbone. Sometimes, the blood supply to the hernia may be totally cut off. When this happens, the tissues within the bulge swell, die, and decay. This condition is known as a strangulated or incarcerated hernia. It is extremely painful and needs an immediate operation.

Most hernias need to be treated by surgery. The bulging tissue is pushed back into place and the defect repaired. This is usually a fairly simple surgical procedure carried out in a hospital. The symptoms of a hiatal hernia can be eased by losing excess weight, taking antacids, and eating small, frequent meals.

Q & A

Don't hernias hurt? My uncle has a hernia, but he says he's not in pain.

Hernias do not usually hurt, except when they first occur—for example, during heavy lifting. Afterward, they may be a bit uncomfortable, but they are usually not painful. If a hernia does hurt, it may be strangulating because its blood supply is cut off; medical advice should be sought.

Can a tendency toward hernias run in families?

Yes, but there is no definite hereditary link. Members of some families tend to do the same types of jobs—for example, those involving heavy labor, which are more likely to cause a hernia.

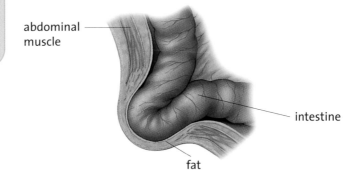

abdominal muscle

intestine

fat

Groin or inguinal hernias are extremely common. They occur more often in men than in women. The soft lump bulges when the patient coughs but disappears when he lies down. This type of hernia can be treated by wearing a truss or by a simple surgical operation.

SEE ALSO

DIGESTIVE SYSTEM • DIGESTIVE SYSTEM DISEASES AND DISORDERS • MUSCLE

Herpes

Q & A

My grandmother has shingles, and my mother wants to keep me away from her so I won't catch it. My aunt says it's nonsense to say I can catch shingles. Who is right?

They are both right, in part. You cannot catch shingles from your grandmother, but you could catch chicken pox, if you have not already had it; the same virus that causes chicken pox causes shingles. Doctors think that shingles is contagious only during an outbreak of active lesions. Chicken pox is a mild illness, and a person is usually immune after one attack.

The term *herpes* refers to infections caused by the seven herpes viruses that infect humans. These are herpes simplex virus type 1 (HSV-1), which causes cold sores, mainly around the mouth or nostrils; herpes simplex virus type 2 (HSV-2), which causes genital herpes; the varicella-zoster virus (VZV), which causes chicken pox and shingles; the cytomegalovirus (CMV), which infects people with AIDS; the Epstein-Barr virus (EBV), which causes glandular fever (infectious mononucleosis); human herpes virus type 6 (HHV-6), which causes the mild childhood disease roseola infantum; and human herpes virus type 7 (HHV-7), which does not appear to cause any disease. Usually, the term *herpes* refers to HSV-2, which appears to be incurable. Genital herpes is acquired during sexual intercourse with an infected person; it is most contagious when symptoms are present.

Symptoms and treatment

The first symptoms of genital herpes appear within a week of exposure. There is pain in the genital area and a red rash on the genitals and often on the thighs and buttocks. The more widespread the rash, the more severe the pain. The red patches become covered with small blisters known as vesicles, which occur in successive crops. These vesicles contain a fluid teeming with millions of herpes viruses; when they are present, the affected person is highly infectious to sexual partners. The vesicles then break down to form shallow ulcers, which tend to join together so that quite large areas of skin are ulcerated.

These raw areas are extremely painful. At this stage, the lymph nodes in the groin become enlarged and tender, and there may be a slight fever. Around two weeks after the beginning of the attack, the pain and discomfort subside, and a week later the ulcers crust over and begin to heal. However, there is usually a recurrence after four months that may start with tingling and sensitivity in the areas about to be affected. Such recurrences are not as severe as the first attack and are usually of shorter duration. When there are blisters or a rash, the person is highly infectious, and further recurrences are likely.

No treatment eradicates herpes, but the drug acyclovir (Zovirax), taken orally, reduces the severity of attacks and shortens their duration. It is the most effective and safest treatment that has been developed to date.

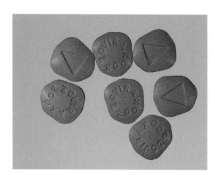

Zovirax, a brand name for a drug called acyclovir, is an oral antiviral that is used to treat herpes infections.

SEE ALSO

AIDS AND HIV • CHICKEN POX • SEXUALLY TRANSMITTED DISEASES • SHINGLES • SKIN • ULCERS • VIRUSES

Hormones and Hormonal Disorders

Hormones act as chemical messengers, stimulating the body to carry out specific functions. They are responsible for the smooth running of important processes such as growth, metabolism, and reproduction. Most hormones are produced by ductless, or endocrine, glands; they discharge their products directly into the bloodstream, rather than through the ducts.

The main endocrine glands are the pituitary, thyroid, parathyroid, ovaries, testes, pancreas, and adrenal glands. Together, these hormone-producing glands make up the endocrine system. The hormones are carried through the bloodstream to other body cells, known as target cells. Each hormone has to find a target with the correctly shaped receptor site to which it can attach itself. Most hormones control or influence the chemistry of the target cells; they might trigger these cells to produce milk, hair, or some other substance, or they might set the rate at which the cells utilize food. For example, the hormone secretin is made in the duodenum and travels to the pancreas, stimulating it to release a flood of watery juices containing enzymes that are essential for digestion.

Hormones play an essential part in the complicated regulation of the body and are also responsible for a number of illnesses. For example, too much or too little of a particular hormone can stunt growth, impair function, or cause serious emotional problems. In addition, hormone production can be upset by a tumor growing in a gland. Such a tumor can be removed surgically or destroyed by freezing or radiation.

Doctors are now skilled in treating hormone-related disorders. They can stop a gland from producing too much of a hormone or stimulate it to produce more. If necessary, they are often able to give patients a synthetic hormone to replace one that the body cannot produce.

OXYTOCIN: triggers release of milk when newborn baby suckles

brain

posterior pituitary gland releases oxytocin

duodenum produces secretin when food is present

pancreas

ACETYLCHOLINE: substance produced at nerve endings that instructs muscle cells to contract

SECRETIN: makes pancreas produce digestive enzymes

Hormones are the body's chemical messengers. They may act locally (for example, acetylcholine and secretin) or at some distance from where they are made (for example, oxytocin).

HORMONE-RELATED DISORDERS AND THEIR TREATMENTS

Hormone (gland)	Disorder	Symptoms	Treatments
Growth hormone (pituitary)	Too little	Failure of growth; may be linked with failure of sexual maturity	Growth hormone given
Growth hormone (pituitary)	Too much (usually owing to a tumor)	Gigantism in childhood; in adults, bones thicken, organs and other structures enlarge, skin thickens, and voice deepens (acromegaly)	Treatment of gland by radiotherapy or removal of part of the gland; drugs to control hormone production
Prolactin (pituitary)	Too much	Periods stop, breasts may produce milk and be tender; infertility	Tablet treatment to reduce production
Antidiuretic hormone (pituitary)	Too little	Production of large quantities of very dilute urine (diabetes insipidus)	Synthetically produced hormone, usually given as nasal drops
Thyroxine (thyroid)	Too much	Body processes speed up (weight loss, palpitations, trembling, anxiety, excess body heat); swelling in the neck (goiter); popping eyes (Graves' disease)	Surgery to remove part of the gland; radioactive iodine by mouth to destroy part of the gland; antithyroid drugs
Thyroxine (thyroid)	Too little	Body processes slow down (weight gain, slow heartbeat, lassitude, thinning hair, thickening skin, sensitivity to cold); cretinism in infants (failure of physical and mental development)	Replacement hormones needed for life
Hormones of adrenal cortex (steroids)	Too much	Muscle wasting and weakness; thin limbs; obese trunk; fragile bones and blood vessels; purple marks on skin; high blood pressure, diabetes, Cushing's syndrome	Drugs to block hormone production; if single gland involved, it is removed. Usually, both glands are involved as a result of a tumor (in the pituitary or elsewhere), which is removed.
Hormones of adrenal cortex (steroids)	Too little	Faintness, nausea, vomiting, loss of weight, low blood sugar, and increased pigmentation of skin (Addison's disease)	Replacement hormone pills for life
Adrenaline (adrenal medulla)	Too much (usually owing to a tumor)	Palpitations, raised blood pressure, faintness, paleness, and sweating	Removal of adrenaline-secreting tumor (usually in adrenal medulla)
Insulin (pancreas)	Too little	High blood sugar, large quantities of urine, thirst, weight loss, tiredness; can lead to diabetes mellitus	Carefully controlled low-sugar diet, regular insulin injections; in mild cases, pills to lower blood sugar
Male sex hormones	Too little	Failure of growth and sexual development; impotence (in adults)	Regular replacement of hormones
Female sex hormones	Too little	Failure of growth and sexual development; early menopause	Regular replacement of hormones

SEE ALSO

BODY SYSTEMS • CANCER • DIABETES • GLANDS • HAIR AND SCALP DISORDERS • METABOLIC DISORDERS

HPV

HPV stands for human papillomavirus. There are about 30 types of human papillomaviruses. They are passed from one person to another during sexual intercourse. Doctors estimate that 20 million Americans have an HPV infection. By the time a woman reaches the age of 50, there is an 80 percent chance that she has been infected with HPV at some point in her life.

Symptoms

Most people infected with HPV do not have any symptoms, and their immune system deals with the infection. However, some types of HPV cause small growths, called warts, on the genitals (sex organs). These warts are not dangerous, but a few HPVs are more dangerous. They have been linked to cancers in the sex organs. Genital warts are soft, flesh-colored swellings. They are sometimes cauliflower-shaped. They grow on their own or in groups and in a wide range of sizes. Genital warts grow on or inside the sex organs and sometimes spread to the thighs. It normally takes several weeks after infection by an HPV virus for warts to appear. People might decide to ignore genital warts and wait for them to disappear on their own. However, while they wait, these people may transfer the disease to other people.

Transmission

HPVs are transmitted between people whose genitals touch each other, usually during sexual intercourse. There is no effective way of stopping this from happening other than avoiding sex with an infected person. However, this is difficult because most infected people do not have any symptoms of HPV. The only way to avoid picking up an HPV is to not have sex with anyone—or to have a sexual relationship with just one, uninfected person. In a few, extremely rare occassions, a pregnant woman might transmit the virus to her unborn baby. Infected babies might develop warts in the throat.

Looking for HPV

Doctors who see patients with genital warts do not need to test for the presence of HPV. The warts are treated directly with creams or gels. However, because the warts are often in sensitive areas, regular wart treatments would be too painful and might cause other injuries and scars. Instead, doctors have developed milder treatments especially for use in the genital area.

In some cases, HPV can cause cancers. Cancers caused by HPV in the male genitals or anus are very rare. The most common cancers caused by HPV grow in the cervix, which is the opening of the uterus (womb). The cancer-causing viruses do not produce

Q & A

My doctor is recommending that I get the HPV vaccine, but I am not sexually active. Why should I get it?

In June 2006, the Food and Drug Administration (FDA) approved a vaccine that protects girls from getting some of the more dangerous strains of HPV. Even though you are not sexually active, your doctor wants you to get the vaccine as a preventive measure for the future.

What type of illnesses can HPV cause?

Human papillomavirus (HPV) can cause genital warts, one of the most common sexually transmitted diseases. The virus can also cause cervical cancer.

I've heard that the HPV vaccine can make me sick. Is that true?

No. The vaccine is made by genetic engineering. Genes are used to make large quantities of the viral protein. That protein is then used to make the vaccine. Since the vaccine contains only a protein and not the entire virus, the vaccine cannot cause the HPV infection.

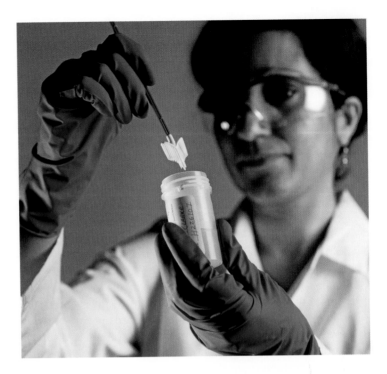

A clinician transfers cells from a cervical smear test from a scraper to a vial of preservative solution. These cells will be tested for the presence of HPVs.

any other symptoms before the cancer appears. By that time, the problem might be too large to cure. As a result, women are tested regularly for high-risk HPVs using a cervical smear (formerly called a Pap test). The wall of the vagina and cervix is gently scraped so a small amount of the lining comes away. The cells in this lining are put on a slide and stained so they can be seen through a microscope. A technician checks the cells from the test. He or she is looking for cancer cells or for cells that have changed in ways that might later become cancer.

If the cervical smear shows a problem caused by HPV, the lining of the cervix and vagina is removed using a simple procedure. A new, HPV-free lining grows back. This action is usually enough to remove the danger of cancers. Regular smear tests, every two years or so, ensure that many cervical cancers are prevented or detected early. Of the 10 million American women with HPV at any time, about 10,000 will develop cervical cancer, and just under 4,000 of them will die from it.

SEE ALSO

CANCER • INFECTIOUS DISEASES • SEXUALLY TRANSMITTED DISEASES • VIRUSES

Huntington's Disease

Q & A

My great-grandfather is mentally active and enjoys playing chess, but he sometimes makes involuntary twitching movements. Could he have Huntington's disease?

Probably not. Although the onset of Huntington's disease is gradual, it usually begins between ages 35 and 50. Also, one of the features that his family would soon notice is mental deterioration, and it sounds as if your great-grandfather is in excellent mental health.

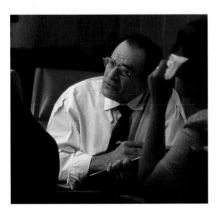

If there is a history of Huntington's disease in the family, couples wanting to have children should see a genetic counselor. They can discuss the chances that their children will be affected.

This rare disease, also called Huntington's chorea or progressive hereditary chorea, was first described by the American physician George Huntington (1850–1916). It is caused by an abnormal dominant gene on chromosome 4. To develop the disease, a person must inherit the abnormal gene from either parent. Someone who develops the disease has a 50 percent chance of passing it on to his or her children. Chromosomes exist in pairs, which are separated during the formation of sperm in males and eggs in females. Thus, chromosome 4, which enters the sperm or the egg, has a 1 in 2 chance of being the one that is carrying the mutation. Since the symptoms do not appear until later in life, parents may pass on an abnormal gene before they are aware that they are carrying the disease. However, a genetic test to reveal whether or not someone has inherited the gene from his or her parents can be carried out at any age. It is important that affected families have genetic counseling. The gene can be detected at an early stage in pregnancy.

Symptoms and outlook

People who carry the gene for Huntington's disease are usually symptom-free until about the age of 35 to 50 years. The onset of the disease is gradual and insidious, and the earliest features are often psychiatric. These features may be mild problems (such as irritability or apathy) or serious psychotic disorders, which may have symptoms similar to those of schizophrenia or bipolar disorder. This stage is followed by motor (movement) disorders, which are the most striking features of Huntington's disease. Facial grimacing, flicking movements of the hands or feet, involuntary twisting of the body, a jerky gait, staggering, and abnormally relaxed muscles are common. Affected people may find it impossible to put out their tongue for more than a second or so at a time. These movement disorders are accompanied by a progressive deterioration of the intellect.

The disease is degenerative and there is no complete cure or treatment. Eventually, there is an inadequate production of neurotransmitting substances, and brain changes occur. Although there is no cure, drugs can control some of the symptoms, such as facial jerks. The disease progresses to disability and dementia. In the final stages, institutional care is necessary, but by then the affected person has little awareness of what has happened.

SEE ALSO

BRAIN • GENES • GENETIC DISEASES AND DISORDERS

Hypertension

Hypertension is the medical term for higher-than-normal blood pressure. If there is no known physical cause, the condition is called essential hypertension. A less common problem is organic hypertension, caused by diseases of the heart and arteries, kidney disorders, or hormonal disturbances. Essential hypertension is believed to be caused by stress. It damages the arteries of the brain, the heart, and the kidneys and can cause a stroke or heart attack, but it has few symptoms until it becomes serious. Then, the patient may have swollen ankles, shortness of breath, headache, visual disturbances, dizziness, and nosebleeds. Some types of hypertension can be treated with drugs. People with the condition should reduce stress levels, stop smoking, reduce their weight, and exercise regularly.

Q & A

My father's doctor described his high blood pressure as "essential." What does this mean?

In medical terms, "essential" means that, although the doctor can identify and treat your father's symptoms, the problem seems to have started of its own accord for some unknown reason.

I've heard that it's possible for stress to cause hypertension. Is that true?

Doctors no longer believe that all stress is necessarily bad or that it is always a cause of raised blood pressure. A certain amount of stress improves performance in some sports, for example; excessive stress, however, can cause tiredness, headaches, and muscle pain, which may lead to raised blood pressure. It is reasonable for a doctor to ask a patient to look at the stresses in his or her life, because identifying them might go a long way toward reducing their effect. Techniques such as yoga, which teach people how to relax, may be of benefit to them.

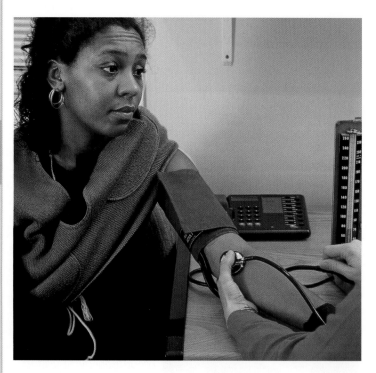

This woman is having her blood pressure taken. Everyone should have his or her blood pressure checked regularly, because hypertension, unless very severe, has few symptoms. Hypertension can be avoided by keeping the weight down, exercising, avoiding undue stress, and not smoking.

SEE ALSO

ARTERY DISEASES AND DISORDERS • HEART • HEART ATTACK • KIDNEY • KIDNEY DISEASES AND DISORDERS • STROKE

Hypoglycemia

The main fuel of the body is a sugar called glucose. This substance is present in the blood and is required by every cell in the body. Glucose is especially important for the brain, because alternative emergency fuels such as fatty acids cannot pass from the small blood vessels in the brain to reach the brain cells. A shortage of glucose, therefore, always causes serious (and sometimes dangerous) effects on the brain. As a result, control of the minimum required level of glucose in the blood is essential to maintain health. A drop below the minimum blood level of glucose is called hypoglycemia. The term comes from three Greek roots: *hypo*, "under" or "less than"; *glyco*, "sugar"; and *haem*, "blood." Hypoglycemia most commonly occurs in people with diabetes.

Causes

The most common cause of hypoglycemia is an overdose of insulin in people with diabetes. A normal dose of insulin can cause hypoglycemia if the person is using up blood glucose faster than normal, as might be the case with unusual physical exertion. Diabetic people who wish to engage in sports and other strenuous activities must therefore adjust their insulin dosage accordingly. Taking certain drugs normally used to treat type 2 diabetes—diabetes that ususally develops during adulthood—can cause hypoglycemia. Hypoglycemia can also be caused by prolonged starvation. Rarely, hypoglycemia occurs because of some other serious medical condition such as disease of the liver or a pancreatic tumor. Hypoglycemia is also a feature of a rare condition called Addison's disease, in which the adrenal glands produce insufficient cortisone.

Symptoms and treatments

Hypoglycemia causes faintness, sweating, trembling, mental confusion, slurred speech, headache, double vision, and seizures. An affected person may give the impression of drunkenness, with irrational and disorderly behavior. Unless treated with glucose or another sugar by mouth or injection, hypoglycemia can lead to coma and death. Diabetic people should always carry some candy to eat whenever they feel a hypoglycemic attack coming on, and they should wear a warning bracelet or necklace informing people of their condition.

Sources of blood glucose

The most immediate source of glucose is the carbohydrates present in food. Some carbohydrates, such as sucrose (cane sugar), lactose (milk sugar), and maltose (malt sugar), consist

Q & A

My mother is on a sugar-free diet. Will being on this diet reduce her blood sugar to a dangerously low level?

No. Serious malnutrition can cause hypoglycemia because of a lack of calories but not because the diet is specifically short of sugar. In a well-nourished person, a diet low in sugar is probably beneficial, because the body is designed to synthesize glucose from a whole range of foods, and it should be allowed to do so naturally.

When my best friend is under a lot of pressure, she sometimes becomes dizzy and even faints. Could this problem be related to hypoglycemia?

For many years, popular medical literature attributed a range of symptoms to hypoglycemia, including dizziness, fainting, lethargy, depression, fatigue, and loss of libido. Informed medical opinion is that most of these symptoms are not caused by hypoglycemia. Also, not all doctors agree that emotional upset can cause hypoglycemia.

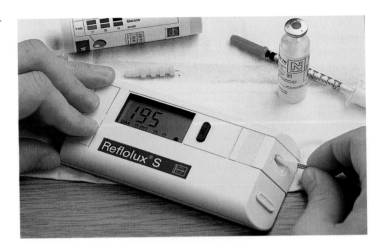

Diabetic patients can easily monitor their blood sugar levels at home by using a glucose meter. A drop of blood is placed on a test strip and the strip is then inserted into the meter, which registers the blood sugar reading.

of two sugars linked together to form molecules called disaccharides. Other carbohydrates, such as starches, are more complex molecules called polysaccharides, which consist of many small sugar molecules, such as glucose and fructose, linked together. In the intestine, these carbohydrate molecules are acted on by various enzymes that break them down to their constituent sugars, releasing glucose into the body. Maltose, for example, consists of two linked glucose molecules, and sucrose is a linked fructose and glucose molecule.

Glucose is so important to the functioning of the body that other foods, such as fats and proteins, can also be converted to glucose. In the liver, which is the largest organ in the body, glucose molecules are linked to form a polysaccharide called glycogen that releases glucose molecules whenever the body needs more glucose.

Control of blood glucose

Control of blood glucose occurs in several ways. If levels fall normally, glucose is released from glycogen stores in the liver. Once these stores are exhausted, body fat stores are converted to glucose. In extreme situations, such as starvation, even the protein of the muscles is converted to glucose. Extremely high levels of blood glucose are controlled by the release of the hormone insulin from the pancreas.

SEE ALSO

BLOOD • BODY SYSTEMS • BRAIN • CANCER • CIRCULATORY SYSTEM • DIABETES • LIVER • MALNUTRITION

Immune System

The body's defense against illness is known as the immune system. This system protects the body from attack and infection by bacteria and viruses. The lymphatic system runs alongside the blood circulation, and together they form part of the body's immune system. The lymphatic system filters out foreign particles and cancer cells, while white blood cells in the blood protect the body against infection, toxins, cancers, and viruses.

T lymphocytes, B lymphocytes, and phagocytes

A virus is an infectious particle that is capable of reproducing only inside a living cell of another organism, such as that of a human. A virus invades the healthy host cell and uses the host cell's reproductive machinery to replicate itself. The first line of

Q & A

Can a baby get prenatal immunity to some diseases from its mother?

Yes. There are some antibodies that cross the placenta and give the baby some protection for the first six weeks to three months of life while his or her immune system is still immature. An example of this is protection of the baby from infection by the measles virus. However, if the mother has not suffered from measles, she will not be able to pass on the antibody created to fight this infection.

After having an illness once, is there any chance that I can get it again?

Yes, this may well happen. If your immune system is working well and you are healthy, you should be able to make antibodies to many infecting agents. However, these antibodies will not always prevent you from having the same illness more than once. Antibodies do not stop you from getting an illness again; they simply fight the infection faster if you do get it.

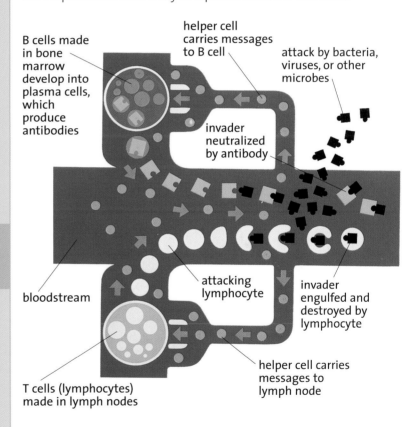

B cells made in bone marrow develop into plasma cells, which produce antibodies

helper cell carries messages to B cell

attack by bacteria, viruses, or other microbes

invader neutralized by antibody

bloodstream

attacking lymphocyte

invader engulfed and destroyed by lymphocyte

T cells (lymphocytes) made in lymph nodes

helper cell carries messages to lymph node

In the immune system, the antibody-producing cells are the B lymphocytes (or B cells, made in the bone marrow) and the T lymphocytes (or T cells, made in the lymph nodes). Both types of cells are alerted by helper cells to attack foreign tissues and viruses. These helper cells send messages to the cell-producing parts of the body, which begin to work at once, producing antibodies customized to kill the invaders.

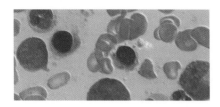

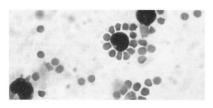

The body's immune system depends on the ability of the B cells (top) and the T cells (bottom) to recognize an invading bacteria or virus. Then these cells go into action against the invader.

defense a virus meets is formed by white blood cells known as T lymphocytes, or T cells. The T cells identify the intruder and immediately organize the right kind of help by activating the spleen and lymph nodes, which begin making other cells to fight the danger. When the T cells recognize the foreign protein (antigen) of the virus, they multiply and fight a battle with the infected cells by enveloping them. The body cells are then activated to rapidly produce a new group of killer T cells should the same virus attack on a later occasion. These cells contain toxic proteins and memory T cells, which are stored to protect the body against that virus. Some of the memory cells remain in the bloodstream for years after the initial attack.

More help against infection is provided by B lymphocytes, or B cells. When bacteria enter the body, some of them are engulfed by phagocytes, which are immune cells that bring the invading bacterial antigens into contact with B cells that match some of the bacteria. The phagocytes can also destroy other microorganisms and other foreign matter. The matching B cells produce two types of cells: memory B cells (which are stored in the body in case of future invasion) and plasma cells (which produce antibodies that destroy the bacteria). The B cells engulf the antigen of the bacterium, and then the antibodies released by the plasma cells lock onto the bacterial antigens and inactivate them. Finally, more phagocytes rush to the area and destroy the inactivated bacteria.

The stages of dealing with an infection

The battle against infection occurs in four stages. The enemy is identified; the necessary cells are produced to fight it; the body's cells move into the attack and kill off the invaders; and finally, another group of the body's lymphocytes, called suppressor T cells, come into action to call off the attack. The body can quickly produce large numbers of the appropriate antibodies to destroy a virus. Then it is said that the body has become immune, or partly immune, to a particular disease. Some viruses, such as those causing the common cold, change to prevent recognition, and the body has no defense against them. The AIDS virus is particularly deadly, because it can invade and kill T cells, thereby sabotaging the body's immune system.

> **SEE ALSO**
>
> **AIDS AND HIV • ANTIBODY AND ANTIGEN • BACTERIA • BACTERIAL DISEASES • IMMUNODEFICIENCY • INFECTIOUS DISEASES • LYMPHATIC SYSTEM • VIRUSES**

Immuno-deficiency

The body's immune system is its means of defense against invading organisms and agents. Sometimes, a fault develops in this system, and the body can no longer rely on its normal immune responses to fight disease.

There are two kinds of immunodeficiency disorders. In some cases, a person's body does not produce sufficient antibodies after an infection or in response to immunization. As a result, the person does not have the usual protection against an attack of this infection. This disorder is caused by a B-cell defect and may affect the body's production of one particular antibody or of several different ones. In another type of defect, the body does not produce enough of the white blood cells called T lymphocytes, with which it destroys invading organisms. As a result, the body cannot fight off some infections and foreign substances.

Immunodeficiencies can be caused by several rare inherited diseases. If the thymus gland is missing at birth, for example, the lymph glands that manufacture the lymphocytes do not work properly. The baby usually dies in a few months from a viral infection against which its body has no defenses. However, immunodeficiencies are more often the result of an illness. The best-known is AIDS, which is caused by a virus that destroys some of the white blood cells. Some cancers (including leukemia), diabetes, measles, infectious mononucleosis, chronic hepatitis, malnutrition, and aging can also cause immunodeficiency. Drugs, such as steroids, and radiotherapy can cause temporary immunodeficiency. People who do not produce enough antibodies can sometimes be helped by antibodies from other people, usually given in the form of monthly injections.

Q & A

I don't get sick as often as I did when I was younger. Why?

When a germ invades your body, lymphocytes make antibodies that clear the germ from your body. If the same germ is presented to the immune system again, the antibodies are already there to fight it. Therefore, you are sick less often because your immune system "remembers" and fights the germs that made you ill when you were younger. However, if any part of this system does not work properly, an immunodeficiency may result and your body will be less able to defend against illness.

RESISTANCE TO DISEASE

When a population is exposed to infection over a long period, it may develop resistance to a particular disease. Although people may still have the disease, it will be in a milder form. In Europeans, for example, measles is an unpleasant, but seldom deadly, illness. When it first spread into other areas such as the South Pacific, where the population had never come into contact with the illness, measles caused many deaths.

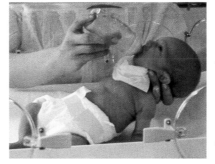

A premature baby lacks immunity to disease, a protection usually passed on from the mother in the last months of pregnancy. For this reason, the baby is kept in a germ-free incubator. That lessens the risk of infection for which the baby has, as yet, no defense system.

SEE ALSO

AIDS AND HIV • ANTIBODY AND ANTIGEN • CANCER • DIABETES • HEPATITIS • IMMUNE SYSTEM • INFECTIOUS MONONUCLEOSIS • LEUKEMIA • LYMPHATIC SYSTEM • MEASLES

Infectious Diseases

Infectious diseases were once often fatal. Now, improved hygiene, sanitation, immunization, and antibiotics have dramatically reduced the spread of infections and infectious diseases. An infection is an invasion of the body by microorganisms such as bacteria and by infective agents such as viruses. Inside the body, the pathogen (disease-causing agent) grows and reproduces itself. It may interfere with the working of the body's cells, destroy it, or produce poisonous substances called toxins (in the case of bacteria). Infections may affect only a small area (such as an abscess), one of the body's systems (as when pneumonia affects the lungs), or much of the body (as in bacteremia and septicemia). Infectious diseases may cause minor ailments (such as a cold or influenza) or fatal illnesses (such as rabies).

How infections enter the body

If an illness is infectious, it is possible to catch the illness from another person. The medical term for this is *communicable*. Some infectious diseases are caught directly by contact with another person (or with objects he or she has handled) or by breathing in infected droplets that have been coughed, sneezed, or breathed out. Some infections, such as herpes, can be sexually transmitted. These infections are known as contagious diseases.

Other communicable diseases can be spread indirectly through infected food or water, or transmitted through bites by carrier animals such as mosquitoes, fleas, or other insects. Some infections enter the body via wounds and scrapes.

Causes of infections

Microorganisms that cause infections include bacteria (such as chlamydia), fungi, and protozoa. Viruses are infective agents rather than microorganisms. The most significant infections are caused by bacteria and viruses. Some of these agents attack only one of the body's organs. The hepatitis virus, for example, lodges only in the liver. Other organisms, such as *Staphylococcus* bacteria, may produce disease in any part of the body. Carried around in the bloodstream, these microorganisms may settle far away from the point at which they entered the body. There, they can multiply and may cause an abscess. The tetanus bacterium produces a toxin that affects only the nervous system; the cholera organism produces toxins that cause severe diarrhea.

How the body defends itself

Microorganisms enter the body in various ways. Some even live in the body, where they usually do no harm. They are a problem only if the body's resistance to infection is lowered. Then they multiply

Q & A

Are childhood diseases more severe in adults?

Generally, yes, although this does not apply to all childhood illnesses. It is especially true of mumps and chicken pox.

Is it possible to have a disease without knowing it?

Yes. Some people may be exposed to an infection and gain immunity to it without developing the full-blown symptoms of the disease. This is a subclinical infection. It seems to occur in young children with mumps and in many people with rubella (German measles).

I seem to catch one infection after another. Could there be something wrong with the way my body copes with infection?

People vary in their ability to fight off infections, but if you have had one, your resistance is lowered and you are more likely to catch another. Therefore, even if you do seem to have nasty runs of infections, you are probably quite normal in the way you respond to them.

and spread. The immune system then defends the body, with specialized white cells neutralizing or engulfing foreign material. Some of the symptoms of an infection are caused by the fight between attacking organisms and the body's defenses. Redness and swelling result because extra blood is carrying white cells to the battleground; dead cells and organisms collect to form pus.

Incubation and quarantine

When the invading organisms of an infection enter the body, they spend some time growing and multiplying before any symptoms appear. This time is known as the incubation period. Depending on the organism, this period can last from one day to several years. Some diseases are infectious before any symptoms appear, and the patient may have been in contact with many other people. For this reason, people who have been in contact with certain infectious diseases are kept in quarantine, that is, out of contact with other people for a time, until there is no chance that they could be infectious.

Preventing disease

Infectious diseases used to kill millions of people. Epidemics of diseases such as smallpox and bubonic plague would sweep through whole communities, killing as many as one in four people. Other less serious infectious diseases were so common that almost everyone had them. Some were known as the infectious diseases of childhood. They included chicken pox, measles, mumps, and rubella (which are all caused by viruses), as well as whooping cough, scarlet fever, and diphtheria (which are all caused by bacteria). In many cases, after one attack of the infection a person remained immune in later life.

Things are very different now. As people learn more about the organisms and agents causing infectious diseases and how the body fights them, people have learned to prevent their spread, treat them, and protect against them. The spread of diseases such as cholera and typhus has been prevented by making sure that people live in clean conditions with a supply of pure water and by controlling carriers such as insects and rats. Doctors have also learned how to use immunization for giving the body built-in protection against some diseases.

Immunization against infection

Once the body's defense system has come across certain invading organisms or agents, it primes special cells to attack them if they ever appear again. Therefore, people very seldom have diseases such as measles twice. Immunization works by

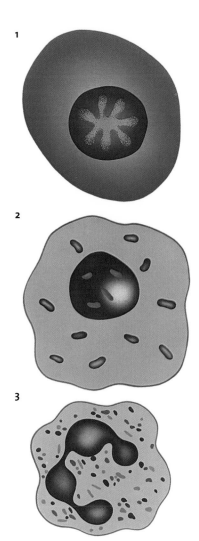

1

2

3

How white blood cells fight infection: When a viral or bacterial infection attacks the body, the number of white blood cells in the bloodstream increases. By studying the type of white cell that predominates in the blood, doctors can determine whether a viral infection (1) or a bacterial infection (2 and 3) is being fought.

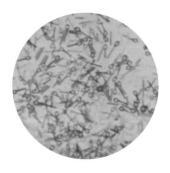

The tetanus bacterium enters via a skin wound. It produces a toxin that causes lockjaw and other spasms that affect the nervous system.

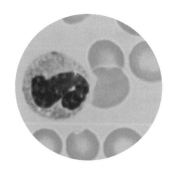

Malaria is contracted from a bite by an infected mosquito. The protozoal agent multiplies in the blood and causes a fever.

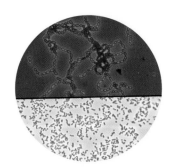

The throat infection bacterium and the pneumonia bacterium are transmitted by droplet infection and cause inflammation.

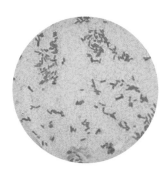

The typhoid bacterium enters the intestines via infected water or food, causing fever, headache, and diarrhea.

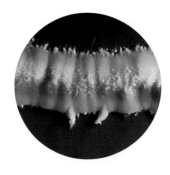

The candida fungus causes the disease thrush. This fungus can be caught from infected towels.

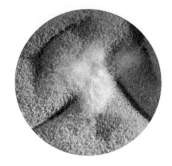

The athlete's foot fungus is picked up from infected ground or from towels. It causes itchy, peeling skin.

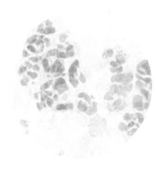

The rickettsial organisms, which cause typhus, are transmitted by louse, tick, and flea bites.

giving the body a tiny amount of a substance (usually dead or harmless versions of bacteria or viruses), which makes the immune system ready to attack the disease in the future but which does not give the person any symptoms of the disease, except perhaps a slight fever. Some immunizations last for life, but others need to be repeated every few years.

It is now possible to immunize people against many of the most serious diseases. In developed countries, most children are immunized against measles, mumps, rubella, diphtheria, tetanus, whooping cough, and poliomyelitis in the first two years of life. Much research has gone into the production of vaccines against AIDS, but to date, no satisfactory vaccine has been developed.

Other immunizations are available, but they are given only when someone is likely to come into contact with a disease (for example, when traveling to a country where it is common).

SOME INFECTIOUS DISEASES AND THEIR TREATMENTS

Disease	Cause	Source of infection	Immunization available	Symptoms	Medical treatment
Chicken pox	Virus	Person to person	Not widely	Rash, light fever	None
Common cold	Virus (many types)	Person to person	No	Runny nose, sore throat, cough	None
Diphtheria	Bacterium producing toxin	Person to person	Yes	Fever, headache, sore throat	Antibiotics and antitoxin
Hepatitis	Virus (at least three types)	Personal (often sexual) contact; infected blood, food, and water	Yes, for virus A; preventive injections for virus B	Jaundice, influenza symptoms	None
Influenza	Virus (many types)	Person to person	Yes, but not widely effective	Cold symptoms, chills, fever, aches	None
Legionnaires' disease	Bacterium	Air-conditioning or water systems	No	Influenza symptoms, pneumonia, diarrhea, vomiting, kidney and respiratory failure	Antibiotics
Malaria	Protozoa (three types)	Mosquito bite	No	Bouts of chills; then fever, recurring every few days	Antimalarial drugs, also given to prevent infection
Measles	Virus	Person to person	Yes	Runny nose and eyes, fever, cough, rash	None
Meningitis	Virus or bacterium	Person to person	Yes, for meningitis A and C	Fever, headache, nausea, neck pain, pain caused by light, drowsiness	Nursing care (viral type); antibiotics (bacterial meningitis)
Mumps	Virus	Person to person	Yes	Salivary glands swell; may spread to testes and ovaries; fever	Anti-inflammatory drugs for severe swelling
Pneumonia	Bronchopneumonia (bacterial or viral)	Person to person	No	Cough, breathing difficulties, fever	Antibiotics
	Lobar pneumonia (bacterial)	Person to person	Yes, for patients at risk	Cough, chest pain, high fever	Antibiotics
Ringworm	Fungus	Infected person or animal	No	Rash	Antifungal drugs applied to skin
Scarlet fever	Bacterium	Person to person	No	Sore throat, high fever, rash	Antibiotics
Tetanus	Bacterial toxin	Infected soil; bacteria enter wound	Yes	Lockjaw and other spasms	Antibiotics, antitoxin, muscle-relaxants, respirator support
Tuberculosis	Bacterium	Person to person, usually by droplet infection	Yes	Tiredness, weight loss, slight fever, persistent cough with blood	Antibiotics
Typhoid	Bacterium	Infected food or water, person to person	Yes	Influenza symptoms accompanied by high fever, headache, diarrhea, rash on abdomen	Antibiotics

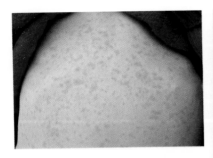

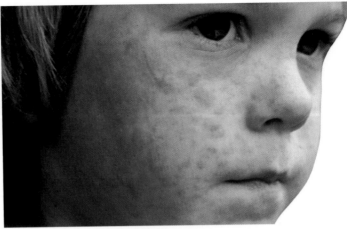

Measles is a highly infectious disease. It is characterized by a rash on the face (right), as well as on the abdomen (above) and other parts of the body.

Precautions against infections

People can avoid many infections by taking a few simple precautions; for example, regular hand-washing prevents the spread of the cold and influenza viruses. Infections can also be spread through dirty towels, bedsheets, and washcloths, so these items should be laundered regularly in hot water.

Precautions should also be taken during a vacation, especially in developing countries. Infected food or water is extremely common in areas where there is poor hygiene. All drinking water should be boiled, or bottled drinks or mineral water should be drunk. Hepatitis and dysentery are two common infections often contracted when these simple health rules are ignored.

Treating infectious diseases

The development of antibiotic drugs has made it possible to clear up many infections and infectious diseases very quickly. They kill the bacteria but do not harm human cells. Antibiotics also kill chlamydia and rickettsial diseases. However, it is important to take antibiotics only when necessary; otherwise, there is a chance of developing drug-resistant bacteria. Other drugs have been developed to kill protozoa and to combat fungal infections, but as yet, no drugs can kill viruses.

GLOBAL KILLERS

Some deadly diseases are making a comeback because of poverty, poor hygiene, and the fact that people travel more widely. Bubonic plague, spread by rats, killed millions in Europe in the Middle Ages. It has recently been reported in Africa, Asia, South America, and even in the United States. Tuberculosis is also on the increase. About 100 million people are infected with tuberculosis each year. It is estimated that about one-third of the world's population is infected with the tubercle bacillus. Malnutrition, poor health, and the spread of AIDS are blamed for the rapid increase of this disease.

SEE ALSO

BACTERIAL DISEASES • CHICKEN POX • COLD • COMMUNICABLE DISEASES • DIPHTHERIA • DYSENTERY • FUNGAL INFECTIONS • HEPATITIS • HERPES • INFLUENZA • MALARIA • MEASLES • MUMPS • POLIOMYELITIS • RUBELLA • SEXUALLY TRANSMITTED DISEASES • TETANUS • TROPICAL DISEASES

Infectious Mononucleosis

Q & A

I have infectious mononucleosis and feel uncomfortable and very unhappy. Why is this?

Among the side effects of your condition are malaise and depression; many patients feel low and lack energy and drive, often for several weeks. It is important that your family and friends understand this. You will soon return to normal.

One of my friends from school has infectious mononucleosis. What can I do to absolutely guarantee that I don't catch it?

The virus is transmitted only by close personal contact, so staying away from this friend for a while might help. However, there are no really effective preventive measures, because the virus is carried long after the illness is over; some people even seem to carry the virus without any symptoms at all. It is just one of those illnesses that young people may or may not get.

Infectious mononucleosis is also known as "mono" or glandular fever. The infection is caused by the Epstein-Barr virus (EBV) and is found mainly in young people. The virus causes the lymphocytes (white blood cells) to enlarge and multiply. As a result, the lymph glands swell and become tender. The virus is passed from one person to another through tiny droplets in the breath and commonly via saliva during kissing. This is why the infection is sometimes known as the "kissing disease."

About four weeks after the initial infection, the patient will begin to feel tired and listless. Then, other symptoms develop, including headache and chills, fever, sore throat, and swollen glands in the neck and possibly in the armpits and groin. Some patients also have a slight rash. These symptoms may be accompanied by a poor appetite and resulting weight loss.

Many people have the illness so mildly that they do not realize what is wrong with them. In severe cases, the symptoms are more obvious. Infectious mononucleosis is usually diagnosed from the swollen lymph nodes, fever, and sore throat. Sometimes, a blood test may also be taken to identify antibodies in the blood that will confirm the original diagnosis.

Most symptoms disappear within two to three weeks, although it may take six to eight weeks to recover completely. Some patients take as long as six months. In the early stages, they should rest in bed, taking painkillers for a headache and gargling for a sore throat. Some people have recurring mild bouts of mono for a year or so after the first attack.

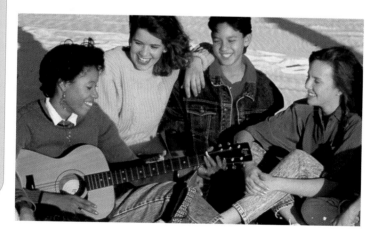

Young people are those most likely to be affected by mononucleosis. It is passed from person to person by close contact. However, not all people who come into contact with it develop the illness.

SEE ALSO

BLOOD • GLANDS • IMMUNE SYSTEM • INFECTIOUS DISEASES • LYMPHATIC SYSTEM • VIRUSES

Influenza

Influenza (flu) is one of the most common and most infectious illnesses in the world. It is caused by several strains (types) of viruses. These viruses are always changing, and that is how they defeat the body's defense system. People do not suffer from the same type of influenza twice, because the body becomes immune to the infecting strain of virus. However, the body will have no immunity to a new strain. Therefore, people who have had influenza once can still have many other attacks.

Epidemics of influenza occur fairly often in winter and usually affect many people in a community. The infection is passed around by an infected person through coughing, sneezing, and body contact. Tiny droplets containing the virus are sprayed into the air and breathed in by other people or are carried from hand to nose or mouth. The affected person will start to have the symptoms from about one to three days later.

Q & A

Should I get an influenza injection, and will it have harmful side effects?

An injection will not do you any harm, and the only side effects that may occur are a sore arm and a raised temperature for about 24 hours. The injection offers 60 percent protection against influenza in the winter of the year when you have the injection; and if you do get influenza, the infection may be milder than it would otherwise have been.

My brother, who is 12, has influenza. He shares a room with our younger brother. Should they be separated?

People who are ill usually sleep badly, and your brother who has influenza may need attention during the night. Therefore, it would be better to move your younger brother out of the bedroom. However, it is probably too late to prevent the younger boy from catching the influenza, which is infectious for one or two days before the symptoms occur. It is almost impossible to keep influenza from spreading.

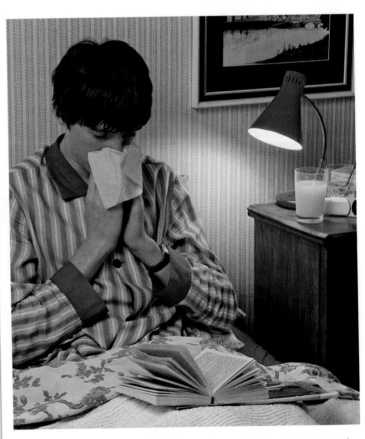

It is best to go to bed when the first symptoms of influenza appear, and to drink plenty of fluids. A person with influenza should be careful to cough and sneeze into a tissue; that limits the spread of infection.

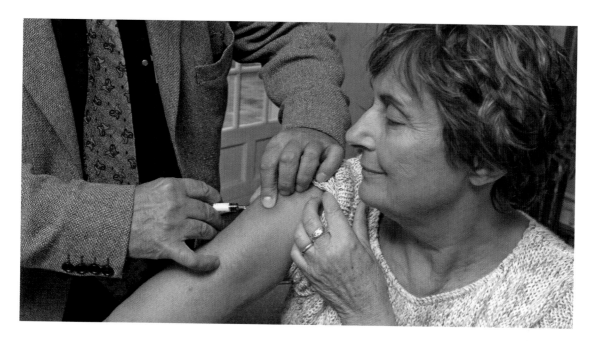

A woman receives an injection against influenza. This form of immunization will offer some protection against a particular strain of influenza.

Influenza symptoms come on suddenly. The patient feels shivery and has aches in the arms, legs, and back. Other symptoms include a headache, aching eyes, a sore or dry throat, and sometimes a cough and a runny nose, diarrhea, and abdominal pain. The temperature is usually between 101° and 102°F (38.3° to 38.8°C), although it may be a degree or so higher. The symptoms and the fever continue for two to five days, and the patient feels tired and weak. It is quite usual to feel tiredness and depression for several weeks after having influenza.

Dangerous complications

There is no cure for influenza. The patient should rest in bed, drinking as much fluids as possible and, if necessary, taking drugs to lower the temperature. Elderly people in particular may have complications with an attack of influenza. These complications include chest infections, caused by bacteria, which affect the body because its resistance is lowered. The doctor may prescribe an antibiotic to prevent these secondary infections. Some symptoms of influenza are similar to those of a cold, but the responsible viruses are quite different.

H1N1 INFLUENZA

First detected in the United States in April 2009, the 2009 H1N1 virus is a new type A influenza virus. Because the H1N1 virus includes genes that were similar to genes found in influenza viruses that normally affect pigs (swine), the disease quickly became known as swine flu. However, H1N1 also includes bird (avian) and human genes, so it has now become more common to refer to the disease as H1N1 influenza.

SEE ALSO

AVIAN INFLUENZA • COLD • EPIDEMIC • IMMUNE SYSTEM • INFECTIOUS DISEASES • VIRUSES

Irritable Bowel Syndrome

Irritable bowel syndrome is a common disorder that features abdominal symptoms for which no organic cause can be found. In the past it was given other various names, such as nervous diarrhea, spastic colon, or idiopathic diarrhea. The term *idiopathic* simply means that the cause is unknown. In the United States, about half the patients seeking medical attention for bowel upset are suffering from irritable bowel syndrome.

Symptoms

The condition usually develops between the ages of 20 and 30 and is twice as common in females as in males, but people of any age and of both sexes can suffer from it. Symptoms are varied and tend to be intermittent. Some pain in the abdomen is usual. Recurrent episodes of pain are commonly localized in one of the four corners of the abdomen and may be relieved by emptying the bowel. The pain may start soon after eating, and many sufferers are convinced that it is brought on by a meal. Eating also often induces an urgent need to use the toilet.

Diarrhea is common and often alternates with constipation, but the condition may involve unduly frequent, but otherwise normal, bowel motions. There may be a constant sense of abdominal fullness and an awareness that something is happening in the intestines. The sufferer is conscious of abdominal noises (borborygmi) and excessive gas production (flatus), and there may be nausea and headache. Sometimes, there is a feeling that there is incomplete emptying of the bowel. Sufferers often notice that the stools are small and rounded or occasionally ribbonlike. Stools may also contain visible mucus. A common feature of the syndrome is anxiety about intestinal function and other health matters.

Normal movement of the bowel contents is brought about by a process known as peristalsis. This is a continuous process organized by a network of nerves in the wall of the intestine, which involves automatic tightening and relaxation of short segments so there is a progressive shifting of the contents in the direction of the rectum. Healthy people are rarely aware of peristalsis, but people suffering from irritable bowel syndrome are acutely conscious of it. This is partly because peristaltic contractions are stronger and more frequent than normal and partly because there is undue awareness of body function.

Causes

People with irritable bowel syndrome are often convinced that they are allergic to certain kinds of food, and that this is the cause of the problem. Food allergy, however, is far less common

Q & A

My sister always has diarrhea and stomach pains before exams. Does she have irritable bowel syndrome, or is this just her nerves acting up because of the exams?

Many people have this kind of reaction before exams. The whole nervous system is affected, and this causes the intestine to become overactive. An irritable intestine causes a similar kind of spasm, but it lasts much longer and may arise without obvious stress.

My doctor thinks I may have irritable bowel syndrome, and he wants me to go to the hospital to have some tests done. I don't like medical tests. Are they really necessary?

There are no symptoms that positively distinguish irritable bowel syndrome from other types of bowel disorders. Diagnosis has to be made by excluding other possible reasons for your symptoms. This can be done only by hospital tests. It does not mean that your doctor is expecting to find anything serious, but having the tests done will provide reassurance.

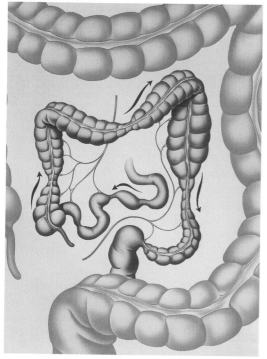

The larger blue structure shows a normal colon; the red one depicts the distension and constriction that is common in irritable bowel syndrome. Muscle movement in the red colon is shown in yellow, and arrows show the direction of the flow of feces.

than is generally supposed, and most doctors do not accept this theory. The syndrome invariably has either a psychological basis or a strong psychological element. It is notoriously common in women of high intelligence and driving ambition, especially those with a tendency to tension and anxiety about professional, financial, and family matters. The syndrome often starts after a life crisis or a period of emotional stress. Many sufferers have developed irritable bowel syndrome after a divorce or a bereavement. In some cases, there is a strong, but not always realized, fear of cancer.

Diagnosis and treatment

Doctors recognize that it can be a serious error to make a premature diagnosis of irritable bowel syndrome without full investigation. Before concluding that a person's symptoms are due entirely to irritable bowel syndrome, it is necessary to exclude a number of other possibilities by carrying out some tests. One of the most important of these is a barium meal X-ray. Barium is an element that X-rays cannot pass through, so it is used to outline internal organs. In irritable bowel syndrome, a barium meal X-ray shows no structural abnormality, but it may indicate an unusual degree of contraction of the circular muscle fibers of the bowel. This suggests that the colon is in a state of abnormally high activity.

Some people with irritable bowel syndrome may require drug treatment to relieve their underlying anxiety. Careful examination to exclude an organic cause, followed by strong reassurance, is often enough to provide a cure. A diet high in vegetable fiber is also helpful in regulating bowel activity. A number of drugs have a specific sedative effect on peristalsis. These calm down excessive contractions in the intestine and relieve abdominal pain. If patients have psychological symptoms, such as anxiety, the doctor may refer them to a therapist, who can give advice on how to alleviate stress. Some people learn to use mind and body relaxation techniques to help reduce their stress and so improve their bowel symptoms.

SEE ALSO

ALLERGIES • CANCER • DIARRHEA • DIGESTIVE SYSTEM • DIGESTIVE SYSTEM DISEASES AND DISORDERS

Jaundice

Sometimes, the whites of people's eyes and their skin take on a yellow tinge because they are suffering from jaundice. This is not a disease in itself, but it is a symptom of a number of diseases and disorders, some of which are serious.

The yellow color of jaundice is caused by a substance called bilirubin. It is produced when worn-out red blood cells are broken down by the spleen. Normally, bilirubin is processed in the liver and then excreted in the bile. If the liver becomes diseased, or the bile ducts are blocked, preventing excretion of bilirubin, the level of bilirubin in the blood will rise. The yellow color shows in the whites of the eyes and then in the skin. Sometimes, so many blood cells are being broken down that the bilirubin in the blood rises even though the liver is working properly. Some diseases, including malaria, cause this to happen. Any disorder of the liver can upset the normal processing of bilirubin.

Causes of jaundice

There are many different causes of jaundice. The viral diseases of the liver, called hepatitis, are a common cause. So is drinking too much alcohol, which damages the liver, often beyond repair. Any obstruction that prevents the bile from passing through the bile ducts and gallbladder to the intestines also causes jaundice. In these cases, the dammed-up bilirubin leaks back into the blood. It passes through the kidneys and into the urine, turning it a dark yellowish brown, whereas the feces are pale.

Jaundice in newborns is common; it develops if the baby's liver is not yet able to cope with the normal breakdown of red blood cells. In severe cases of jaundice, a complete change of blood is necessary in the first days of the baby's life.

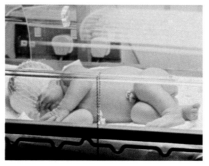

It is very important to find out the cause of jaundice so that the disorder may be treated. Often, bed rest and a low-fat diet are necessary, and alcohol must be avoided. Obstructions of the gallbladder and bile ducts need to be corrected by surgery.

Q & A

My baby brother developed jaundice a few days after he was born, and he was given treatment under a powerful light. Why?

Ultraviolet light increases the breakdown of bilirubin, the substance released by used red blood cells and excreted by the liver. Jaundice is common in young babies before the liver is functioning properly. High levels of bilirubin can be dangerous. Treatment with ultraviolet light tides the baby over until his or her liver matures.

My skin looks sallow and yellow when I'm tired. Is this jaundice?

You may have a slightly higher level of bilirubin in your blood than normal. There is a common congenital disorder called Gilbert's syndrome that may cause long-term, low-grade jaundice. This condition may be worsened by fasting or infection but is usually harmless.

This newborn baby has jaundice and is being treated by exposure to a powerful light that helps break down bilirubin. The baby's eyes are bandaged to protect them from the light.

SEE ALSO

BLOOD • GALLBLADDER AND GALLSTONES • HEPATITIS • LIVER • LIVER DISEASES AND DISORDERS • MALARIA

Joint Disorders

The joints undergo a great deal of wear and tear, so it is not surprising that they suffer from a number of disorders. Some disorders are easily cured with treatment and time, but others may need surgery. Sprains and strains caused by awkward or accidental movements and falls are the most common injuries to joints. They cause swelling and may be extremely painful. These injuries are treated with bandaging and rest of the affected limb.

Knee joint disorders

The knee joint is often injured in sports when it is accidentally twisted and wrenched. It contains two floating pieces of cartilage, which may be torn or crushed. Such an injury causes severe pain and sometimes stops the knee from bending. If this happens too often, the cartilage may have to be removed. In time, the muscles of the knee grow strong enough to take the place of the cartilage.

Sometimes, the whole knee swells after an injury, a condition called water on the knee. Like many other knee problems, it clears up with rest. Too much kneeling on a hard surface or a blow to the knee may cause one of its soft lubricating pads, or bursae, to become inflamed. In this disorder, known as bursitis, or housemaid's knee, a painful, fluid-filled swelling develops in front of the kneecap. Other joints where bursitis may develop include the elbow, the heel, and the base of the big toe.

Dislocations

Accidents may also lead to dislocation, when one bone of a joint is wrenched out of its socket. This displacement prevents normal movement of the joint and is usually extremely painful. The muscles, nerves, and blood vessels around the joint are damaged and the tissues swell. Skilled treatment is needed to reposition the bone as quickly as possible. The shoulder, jaw, and hip are particularly likely to be dislocated.

Spinal joint injuries

The joints of the spine are often injured. The spinal bones (vertebrae) are joined by fibrous tissue. Small disks of pulpy material surrounded by rings of fibrous tissue act as shock absorbers between vertebrae. When the vertebrae are crushed together, as in heavy lifting, the pulp may be forced through the fibrous tissue and press against the spinal cord or a nerve root. This condition is known as a slipped, or prolapsed, disk and can be very painful. Symptoms may come on suddenly or over a period of time. Treatment includes bed rest (lying on a firm mattress for support) and taking painkillers.

Q & A

I dislocated my right shoulder a few months ago. Now it dislocates easily, and I have had to give up playing football. Is there anything I can do to strengthen the joint?

It is possible to have an operation, known as the Putti-Platt operation, to increase the strength of the joint if a shoulder repeatedly dislocates. This procedure builds up the bone at the front of the shoulder to increase the depth of the socket, making it more difficult for the bone to slip out. Healing takes about two months.

I am double-jointed. Am I more likely to develop rheumatism when I get older?

People who are said to be double-jointed do not, in fact, have double joints. They do have greater than normal flexibility and can move their bodies and limbs through a wider range of movement than most people. As a result, their joints are subjected to unusual stresses and strains through overuse. "Double-jointed" people may be more prone to aches and pains in their joints later in life.

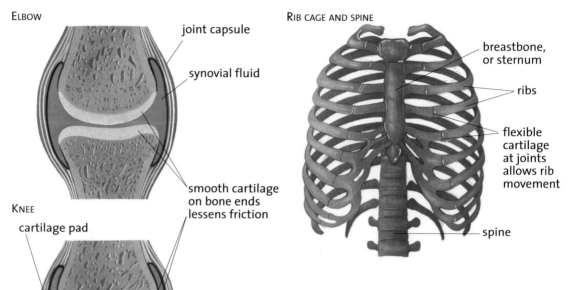

ELBOW

joint capsule

synovial fluid

smooth cartilage
on bone ends
lessens friction

KNEE

cartilage pad

RIB CAGE AND SPINE

breastbone,
or sternum

ribs

flexible
cartilage
at joints
allows rib
movement

spine

*Highly mobile joints, which include the
elbow (top left) and the knee (bottom
left) are particularly susceptible to injury.
These joints are enclosed within fibrous
tissue, known as the joint capsule, and
contain synovial fluid, which acts as a
lubricant. The knee joint also contains
shock-absorbing cartilage pads. Certain
joints on each of the ribs (top right),
however, are formed from bone and
cartilage. These cartilaginous joints allow
movement without the need for fluid-
filled synovial membranes, as in the
elbow and knee.*

Other joint disorders

Inflammation of the synovial membrane that lines a joint can be
caused by an injury or by rheumatoid arthritis. Sometimes, it can
lead to ankylosis, or permanent fixation of the joint. This most
often affects the area around the spine and the pelvis. The joints
may also be affected by osteoarthritis, which causes the cartilage
around them to wear away gradually.

People whose joints are badly worn away, creating pain and
limiting movement, can now be fitted with new joints made of
metal, plastic, or ceramic. These artificial joints help relieve the
pain, and, with exercise and practice, the patient may, in time,
regain full movement of the joint.

Rheumatism

Rheumatism is a term used to describe a range of aches and
pains. It is not a disease in itself; it is more a collection of
symptoms. The aches and pains, including swelling, tenderness,
and stiffness, affect the joints and other surrounding structures,
such as muscles, tendons, and ligaments.

> **SEE ALSO**
>
> ARTHRITIS • BONE • BONE DISEASES AND DISORDERS •
> FRACTURES AND DISLOCATIONS • GOUT • HEMOPHILIA •
> IMMUNE SYSTEM • MUSCLE • OSTEOARTHRITIS • SKELETAL
> SYSTEM • SLIPPED DISK • SPINAL COLUMN • SPORTS INJURIES
> • SPRAINS AND STRAINS

Kidney

The kidneys are two bean-shaped organs that act as the filtering units of the body. They remove waste products from the blood and maintain the correct balance of water and salts in the body. The kidneys also produce hormones that play a part in the production of red blood cells and help regulate blood pressure.

Located at the back of the abdomen on each side of the spine, the kidneys are approximately 4 inches (10 cm) long and are protected by the lower ribs. Each kidney consists of an outer layer called the cortex and an inner layer called the medulla. A long narrow tube known as the ureter runs from the inside of each kidney to the bladder.

Structure of the kidney

Each kidney contains between one million and two million filtering units called nephrons. The end of each nephron expands into a knot-shaped structure called the glomerulus, which is located in the cortex. Within each glomerulus is a cluster of minute blood capillaries where the majority of blood filtration takes place. The remainder of the nephron consists of a long, coiled tubule, which includes Henle's loop.

Filtering out water and waste

Blood enters the kidneys through the renal artery at an astonishing rate: 15 gallons (75 l) per hour. Blood containing waste products enters the glomeruli, where water and waste products are filtered out and substances needed by the body, such as glucose, are reabsorbed into the bloodstream. The blood then flows through the network of capillaries. There, certain essential substances such as water and some salts are reabsorbed into the blood. This purified blood returns to the main circulation via the renal vein. The remaining waste products and excess water, which make up urine, pass from the kidneys through the ureters and into the bladder, ready to be expelled from the body.

Overleaf: This enlarged and simplified view of a kidney shows its different parts and how they work. The renal artery carries blood to the kidney; it splits into smaller blood vessels (A), forming millions of nephrons, each of which ends in a glomerulus (B), inside a Bowman's capsule. Materials carried in the blood, such as water, salts, and hormones, filter through the wall of the glomerulus into the renal tubule. Useful materials pass back across the tubule wall into the blood (C), while waste products are carried away in the urine. The filtered and purified blood then flows back into the body's main circulatory system through the renal vein, along Henle's loop.

Q & A

If one kidney fails, can the other one cope on its own?

Yes. In fact, humans have so many nephrons (filtering units) in each kidney that we can easily do without not just one, but almost half of the other kidney as well. For this reason, it is perfectly reasonable to remove a kidney from a healthy person and donate it to someone else. The donor can live with one healthy kidney for the rest of his or her life.

Does drinking cranberry juice help the kidneys to function better?

Yes, a number of studies have concluded that cranberries are beneficial to the kidneys and the urinary tract. One study reported that out of 60 patients with urinary tract infections who were given two cups (473 ml) of cranberry juice per day for three weeks, 70 percent showed moderate to excellent improvement. There is some evidence that cranberry juice prevents bacteria from adhering to the bladder lining. Cranberry taken in tablet form is also thought to be beneficial.

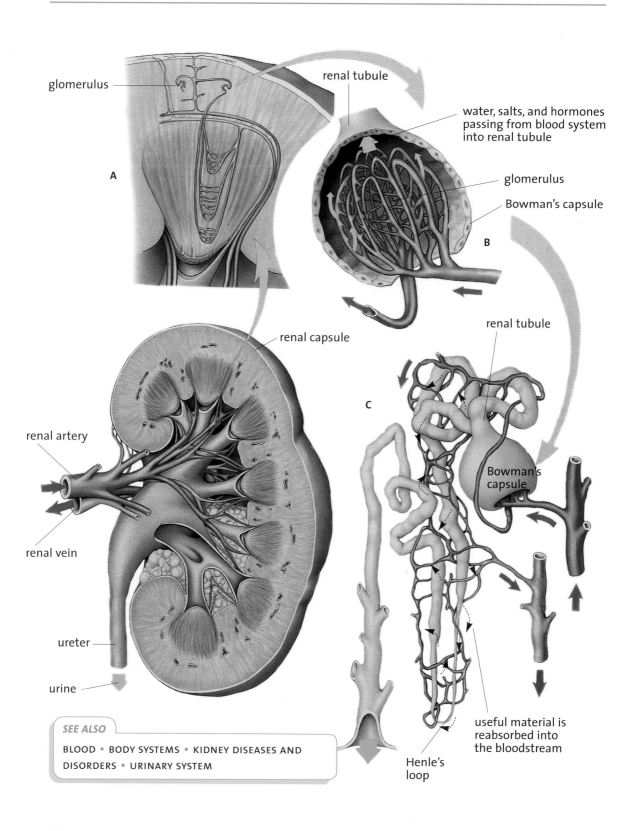

glomerulus

renal tubule

A

water, salts, and hormones passing from blood system into renal tubule

glomerulus

Bowman's capsule

B

renal tubule

C

Bowman's capsule

renal capsule

renal artery

renal vein

ureter

urine

useful material is reabsorbed into the bloodstream

Henle's loop

SEE ALSO

BLOOD • BODY SYSTEMS • KIDNEY DISEASES AND DISORDERS • URINARY SYSTEM

Kidney Diseases and Disorders

Q & A

My uncle has high blood pressure. Will this harm his kidneys?

High blood pressure causes the small blood vessels to thicken. This causes damage to the kidneys' filtering units (called nephrons), and as these are lost, so is the kidneys' ability to remove waste products. This may result in kidney failure unless the condition is treated.

I have diabetes mellitus. Is it likely to damage my kidneys?

Four out of 10 people who have had diabetes mellitus for more than 15 years develop diabetic kidney disease. However, most people with diabetes mellitus are monitored to detect kidney damage at an early stage.

My father has kidney stones, and his doctor has suggested that he be treated by lithotripsy. What does this involve?

Lithotripsy is a technique that uses a machine called a lithotripter to send high-energy ultrasonic shock waves onto the stones to break them up. The fragments pass out in the urine.

Inflammation of the kidney is called nephritis. It has several causes, which result in different degrees of illness. Some types of nephritis are easily treated; others may lead to kidney failure. When the kidneys are not working properly, the waste products and water usually processed and eliminated by them build up in the body's tissues. The tissues become waterlogged and swollen, particularly around the ankles. The affected person may urinate more frequently and feel increasingly tired. This sort of chronic kidney failure is often the result of repeated infections, which may have started in childhood and gone unnoticed, or of a single infection that causes an abnormal immune reaction in the kidneys. These infections are usually caused by microorganisms, such as bacteria, which reach the kidneys by traveling up the ureter from an infected bladder, or along the bloodstream.

Some acute kidney infections develop rapidly. The patient may feel cold and nauseated and experience severe lower back pain and a fever as high as 104°F (40°C). The urine may be cloudy or pinkish, and urinating may be difficult. Kidney infections usually clear up quickly with antibiotics. The patient should rest in bed, eat lightly, and drink water to flush through the kidneys.

The kidneys secrete a hormone that controls blood pressure. When the blood supply to a kidney is abnormally reduced, more of this hormone is produced; the result may be dangerously high blood pressure (hypertension). Some of the drugs used to treat hypertension block the action of this hormone.

Acute kidney failure

If the kidneys suddenly stop working—a condition known as acute kidney failure—the patient produces less and less urine, loses his or her appetite, and feels nauseated, drowsy, and confused. Eventually, the patient may go into a coma and may even die because of the accumulation of waste products. Acute kidney failure can be caused by some poisons or infections, by a reaction to some drugs, or by a sudden drop in blood pressure, which cuts off the blood supply to the kidneys.

Knocks and stones

The kidneys are well protected by the ribs, but they can be bruised by a direct blow or a kick, or crushed in an accident. Damage to the kidneys causes severe pain in the back and possibly blood in the urine. A doctor will X-ray the patient's kidneys and probably recommend that the patient spend a week or more in bed to give the kidney time to repair itself.

Sometimes, stones form in a kidney. These stones are collections of solid material, usually including the mineral

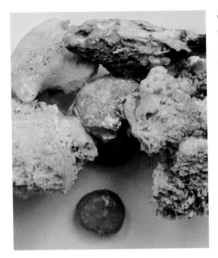

These objects are kidney stones—collections of solid material that have built up in the kidneys over a period of several years. Small stones may not cause any problems, but large ones can block the ureter and can be extremely painful.

calcium, that build up gradually over a number of years. Some stones travel out of the kidney, move along the ureter to the bladder, and pass out in the urine. Tiny stones cause no trouble, but larger ones can be extremely painful as they travel along the ureter. Other stones remain in the kidneys and grow too large to pass out. They may grow to 1 inch (2.5 cm) or more in diameter. Stones in the kidneys may not cause any problems unless they block the ureter, damming up the urine. Then they need to be removed by surgery. This is now usually done by a machine called a lithotripter focused on the stones from outside the body. This device uses powerful shock waves to smash the stones to fine gravel so that they can be passed out naturally with the urine via the ureter and bladder.

Kidney dialysis

Usually, the kidneys work so efficiently that the body can function quite normally with only one kidney. However, if neither kidney works properly, the patient may need dialysis, which is sometimes called hemodialysis. A dialysis machine takes over the principal functions of a real kidney, filtering the blood outside the body, removing impurities, and returning the "clean" blood to the body. While in the filtering system, the blood flows through tubes made of a membrane that allows the waste products (which are much smaller than blood cells) to pass out through it. The waste products pass through the membrane into a dialysis solution (dialysate) and then out of the machine. The clean blood is carried on through and returned safely to the body. This happens over and over again throughout the dialysis

SYMPTOMS OF KIDNEY DISORDERS

A doctor's advice should always be sought if
- the urine is cloudy or discolored, particularly if it is red
- there is pain passing urine and the pain lasts for more than two days
- urine is passed frequently for more than three or four days
- the ankles are swollen

To test for nephritis, a measurement is made of the level of protein in the urine. A dipstick is put in a urine sample and the color is checked against a chart.

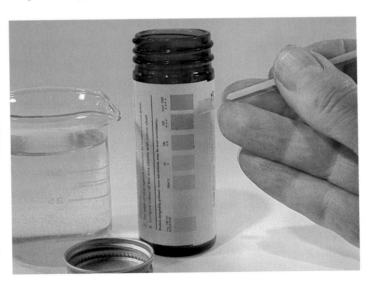

This man's kidneys are functioning so poorly that he needs regular dialysis— a treatment in which an artificial kidney filters his blood. Tubes carry blood from his body to a filtering machine beside the bed and bring purified blood back again through a vein in the arm. Some patients need dialysis several times each week.

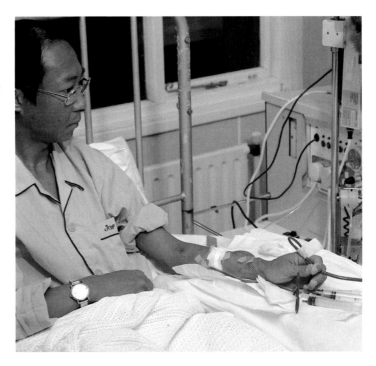

session. Each time the clean blood is returned to the body, it picks up more waste products from the cells it circulates through and brings these newly collected toxins back to the dialysis machine to be removed. Fresh dialysate is passed through continuously, to make the rate of the cleaning process as fast as possible.

Some patients can have dialysis at home, but most have it done in the hospital. They may need two to three periods of dialysis each week, with each treatment lasting up to five hours.

Kidney transplant

The most satisfactory solution to kidney failure is a kidney transplant operation, which is usually successful. The donated kidney is positioned in the pelvis, while the damaged kidneys are normally left in place. The transplanted kidney starts to function immediately. Many people who have had a kidney transplant are able to have a normal lifestyle, although they may need to take drugs to prevent rejection of the new kidney. The main constraint is the lack of donated kidneys for transplantation.

NEPHRECTOMY

In most cases, the removal of a kidney—a nephrectomy—is not dangerous and has no ill effects on a person. However, the operation is carried out only when all other treatments have failed or are not possible. The other, healthy kidney will take over the work of the first. There are various reasons for a nephrectomy. Some people are born with a congenital abnormality of the kidney; it has not formed properly and does not function. The presence of a kidney tumor or serious damage to a kidney as the result of an accident will also result in the removal of the kidney.

SEE ALSO

BLOOD • HYPERTENSION • KIDNEY • URINARY SYSTEM

Legionnaires' Disease

Legionnaires' disease is a serious chest infection caused by a bacterium that lives in mud, in soil, and, particularly, in water. If it contaminates the water used in an air-conditioning system, the bacteria from the water are taken up into the air and can spread throughout the system. Most reported cases have been spread through the air-conditioning systems of large buildings, such as hotels and hospitals.

The incubation period for this illness is between three and five days. The patient then develops influenza-like symptoms, including headache, aching muscles, and a general feeling of illness. A day or two later, the patient may have a high fever, often accompanied by uncontrollable fits of shivering and a dry cough. Other symptoms can include diarrhea, vomiting, abdominal pain, sleepiness, and confusion. Some patients have only the symptoms of a mild chest infection. Others develop severe pneumonia, which affects their kidneys, digestive system, and nervous system. This condition can prove fatal. Less severe symptoms can be treated with antibiotics.

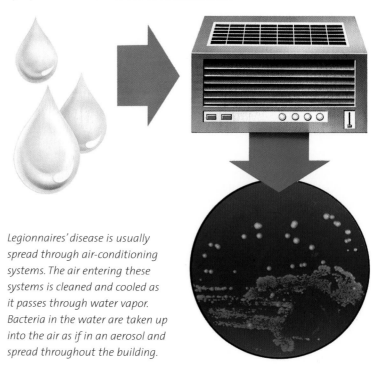

Legionnaires' disease is usually spread through air-conditioning systems. The air entering these systems is cleaned and cooled as it passes through water vapor. Bacteria in the water are taken up into the air as if in an aerosol and spread throughout the building.

Q & A

Are there certain people who are more likely than others to get Legionnaires' disease?

Yes. Legionnaires' disease is more common in patients whose immune systems are suppressed, either by disease or by treatment such as that given to prevent rejection of kidney transplants. Men are three times more likely to get the disease than women, and mostly it affects people in their mid-fifties.

Is it possible to get Legionnaires' disease in any country?

There have been outbreaks in countries outside the United States, especially in hospitals that have air conditioners. It does seem to be more common in warmer climates, but this may be because air conditioners are used more often in such regions.

Can you disinfect water to prevent Legionnaires' disease?

Yes. The bacterium that causes the disease is sensitive to disinfectants, which are commonly used to prevent the disease from growing in air-conditioning systems.

SEE ALSO

COLD • DIARRHEA • INFECTIOUS DISEASES • PNEUMONIA

Leukemia

Leukemia is a form of cancer that affects the white blood cells. It is an extremely serious illness, but because of modern treatments many people with this once fatal disease now survive.

White blood cells are made in the bone marrow and in the lymph nodes. Their job is to fight infections. Normally, they die after a few days or weeks and are replaced by new cells. In leukemia, abnormal white cells that cannot fight infection are produced. The cells also live longer than normal. As a result, they clog up the bone marrow, which cannot produce the normal amounts of red blood cells and platelets. The abnormal cells spread and prevent the body's organs from working properly.

The symptoms of leukemia include fatigue and anemia, because the marrow is not producing enough red cells. Patients may bleed from the gums and nose. They bruise easily, because the blood has insufficient platelets to enable clotting to take

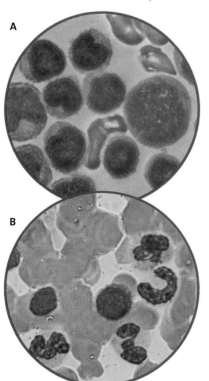

A

B

place. The liver and spleen become swollen. The patient has little resistance to infections and may lose weight and develop a fever.

Leukemia can be acute (with serious symptoms developing rapidly) or chronic (with milder symptoms appearing gradually). A blood test shows the abnormal cells. Treatment consists of chemotherapy or radiotherapy to destroy the abnormal cells. The body then produces normal cells again, at least for a time. Further treatment may be needed later. Blood transfusions are often given to boost normal cell levels.

Q & A

Can leukemia run in families? My uncle recently died of leukemia, and my father is very worried.

There are a few unusual hereditary diseases that are associated with an increased incidence of leukemia. They are mainly immunodeficiency diseases and those associated with an abnormal fragility of chromosomes. Both of these conditions are rare.

I have heard that X-rays can cause leukemia. Is it true?

Yes, this is true, but even if you have undergone X-rays on many occasions, it is very unlikely that you will be at an increased risk. People who spend their lives taking X-rays have only a slightly increased risk of developing any form of leukemia. In contrast, those who have been heavily exposed to radiation, such as the survivors of the atomic bomb dropped on Hiroshima in 1945, have a greatly increased risk.

In these two samples of blood cells, the white cells have been stained purple. In leukemia (A), the white cells are greatly increased in number and are immature compared with normal blood cells (B).

SEE ALSO

ANEMIA • BLOOD • BLOOD DISEASES AND DISORDERS • CANCER • IMMUNE SYSTEM • LIVER • LYMPHATIC SYSTEM

Liver

The liver is the largest organ in the body. It weighs between 3 and 4 pounds (1.36 and 1.80 kg). It lies in the right side of the abdomen and is protected by the lower part of the rib cage. The liver is a mass of tissue. It contains millions of cells that are richly supplied with blood vessels, and it is the body's chemical processing plant. A body cannot survive without a liver.

All the blood from the intestines passes through the liver on its way to the heart, entering the liver through the portal vein. The hepatic artery brings oxygenated blood to fuel the liver cells. Blood from the intestines is full of freshly digested nutrients—protein, carbohydrates, and fats. The liver either stores these nutrients or converts them into a form that the body can use immediately. Proteins are broken down into simple amino acids and rebuilt into the proteins needed to form tissues such as skin, bone, hair, and nails. The liver breaks down carbohydrates and converts fats into forms that renew fatty tissue. The liver makes glucose (which provides instant energy) and glycogen (which is stored for future energy use). The liver also stores certain vitamins and minerals, particularly iron. It removes waste products and poisons from the blood and breaks down excess red blood cells. Waste products are converted by the liver into bile. The bile drains through the common bile duct for storage in the gallbladder and is used to break down fats.

The liver is unusual; almost all of its structural units are exactly alike. If part of the liver is destroyed, more liver cells grow to replace it.

Nutrients enter the liver from the intestines through the portal vein. Processed blood collects in the hepatic vein to return to the heart. The enlarged section of this liver reveals the blood vessels, veins, and special cells that process nutrients and waste.

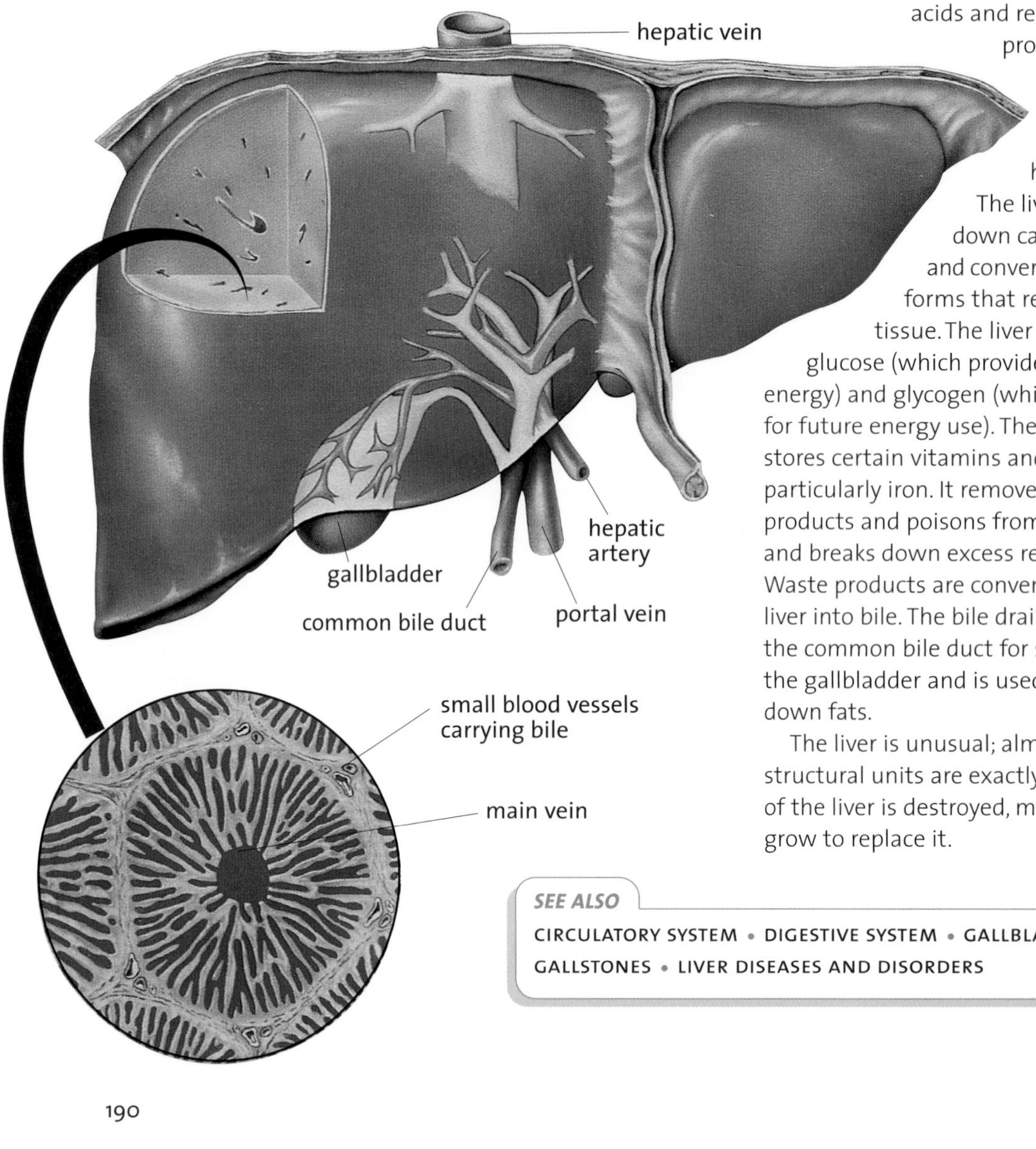

hepatic vein

hepatic artery

gallbladder

common bile duct

portal vein

small blood vessels carrying bile

main vein

SEE ALSO

CIRCULATORY SYSTEM • DIGESTIVE SYSTEM • GALLBLADDER AND GALLSTONES • LIVER DISEASES AND DISORDERS

Liver Diseases and Disorders

The liver is exceptionally good at renewing itself. Even if a whole lobe is removed during an operation, it will regrow in only a few weeks. Sometimes, however, the liver cells are destroyed faster than they can be replaced. When this happens, it can lead to acute (immediate) liver failure.

Causes of liver disorders

The most common cause of liver disorders is infection by viruses (as in viral hepatitis, yellow fever, and rubella) or by bacteria (as in amebic dysentery, leptospirosis, or streptococcal infections). The liver can also be poisoned by harmful substances, such as arsenic, chloroform, carbon tetrachloride, poisonous mushrooms, and too much alcohol or an overdose of acetaminophen. Liver problems are also caused by inborn defects, such as the failure of the enzymes in the liver to remove excess bile. This condition is most common in premature babies. Also, the enzymes that make and store glucose may not be working normally. That causes rapid falls in the blood sugar level.

A great deal of blood passes through the liver. Therefore, cancerous cells from another part of the body can be spread to the liver through the blood and cause a secondary tumor there. Primary liver cancers (cancers that appear in the liver first) are quite rare in the Western world.

Cirrhosis

Infections or poisoning of the liver can cause its cells to be destroyed more quickly than they can be replaced. Such destruction leads to

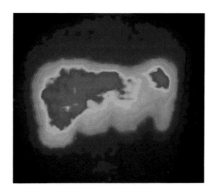

Cirrhosis of the liver is a serious disorder, generally caused by heavy drinking. The liver cells are destroyed and replaced with fibrous tissue. Both of these pictures show affected liver tissue; in the top image, a radioactive tracer shows the damage.

Q & A

Are liver transplant operations performed often?

Yes. Liver transplants are common. However, although 90 percent of kidney transplant patients survive their first year, only 80 percent of liver transplant patients—who are usually much sicker—do. Improvements in the drugs used to control the body's tendency to reject the new organ may increase the operation's success in the future.

I've heard that eating shellfish sometimes causes hepatitis. Why is this?

Shellfish, such as oysters and mussels, commonly grow near sewage outlets, because of the rich supply of food they provide. Sewage usually contains a virus that causes hepatitis; if this is absorbed by the shellfish, it may affect humans, especially if the shellfish are eaten raw. If you go to collect mussels, check whether it is the right season. Leave them in freshwater for 12 hours before cooking. Mussels constantly pass fluid through their bodies, and the freshwater helps clean them.

LIVER DISEASES AND THEIR TREATMENTS		
DISEASES AND CAUSES	SIGNS AND SYMPTOMS	TREATMENTS
Acute liver failure, brought on by hepatitis virus, alcohol, acetaminophen poisoning	Coma and jaundice	Liver transplant, low-protein diet, vitamin K, blood transfusion, antibiotics, intravenous fructose
Cirrhosis—alcohol and viral hepatitis are the best-known culprits, but there are several unknown causes	May be none until quite late in the disease, when signs associated with hepatitis and finally liver failure develop	Liver transplant; stop drinking; special diet with vitamin supplements
Hepatitis, caused by hepatitis virus A and B, glandular fever, and other viruses	Influenza-like symptoms, abdominal pain, nausea, loss of appetite, jaundice	Bed rest; low-fat diet; abstinence from alcohol for at least six months after the jaundice has disappeared
Kernicterus, caused by jaundice in newborn babies	Yellowing of eyes and skin—if allowed to persist, brain damage may result	Jaundice is common in babies, but if severe should be treated by complete replacement of the blood, known as exchange transfusion

scarring. If the damage is bad, cirrhosis of the liver may follow. The liver hardens and shrinks and becomes less and less able to function, until eventually it fails completely.

Symptoms of liver disorders

The first sign of a liver disorder is often jaundice. Since the liver is not processing and excreting waste products efficiently, they accumulate in the blood, and the patient's skin and eyeballs become yellowish. The liver may become enlarged and tender. The patient loses his or her appetite and feels nauseated, and blood sugar levels fall. The brain cannot function properly, and the patient becomes confused.

The liver cannot produce the proteins that cause the blood to clot, and therefore the patient will bleed and bruise easily. Fluid may collect in the ankles and the abdomen. Liver failure eventually causes death.

Patients with liver disorders must give the liver a chance to recover. They need to rest in bed for a time, eat sensibly, and avoid all alcohol for some months after the illness. Hepatitis and other infections usually clear up after a few weeks. Liver tumors can be treated by surgery and radiotherapy. The progress of cirrhosis can be slowed by avoiding all alcohol.

SEE ALSO

BACTERIA • CANCER • DYSENTERY • HEPATITIS • JAUNDICE • LIVER • RUBELLA • VIRUSES • YELLOW FEVER

Lung

Living organisms must breathe to survive. In humans, the lungs are responsible for this function. They bring life-maintaining oxygen into the body and expel waste carbon dioxide from it.

Humans have two lungs that are suspended in the chest cavity, one on each side of the body. Each lung consists of soft, spongy tissue made up of millions of tiny air sacs called alveoli. Each alveolus is surrounded by a network of tiny blood vessels. The heart is tucked between the lungs, and all three organs are protected by the rib cage. The trachea (windpipe) runs down from the throat to the lungs, where it divides into two branches, or bronchi, one leading to each lung.

Inside the lungs, each bronchus subdivides many times into smaller branches, which carry air to the alveoli. The oxygen breathed in passes through the thin walls of the alveoli into the blood and is carried around the body. At the same time, carbon dioxide is collected from cells all over the body. It travels from the blood into the alveoli, to be expelled in breathing out.

The lungs work automatically. Together, the downward movement of the diaphragm and the outward movement of the ribs increase the internal volume of the chest, so that air is sucked into the lungs, which expand passively. Breathing out occurs when the diaphragm rises and the chest falls.

Q & A

I get short of breath when I run. What is wrong with my lungs?

You are probably just not particularly fit. When you have been running for a while, you may notice that you bring up phlegm. This is quite normal, and if you continue to exercise it will gradually get better and your performance will improve.

Does it hurt to have the inside of your lungs examined?

No. The instrument used is a bronchoscope: a flexible tube containing a bundle of glass fibers that is passed down the windpipe and into the lung.

I've heard that just one cigarette can damage the delicate tissues of the lungs. Is this true?

It is doubtful, but smoking is now recognized to be the single most dangerous avoidable health hazard. It is especially likely to damage the lungs.

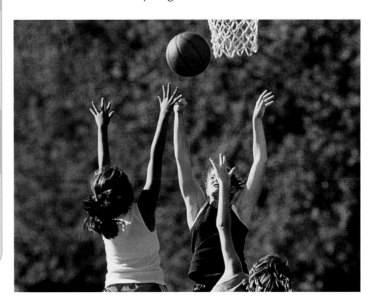

Activities such as basketball exercise the lungs as well as the limbs; people breathe faster and more deeply to draw in the extra oxygen the body needs when it is working hard.

SEE ALSO

HEART • LUNG DISEASES AND DISORDERS • RESPIRATORY SYSTEM

Lung Diseases and Disorders

Q & A

Can measles cause serious lung disease?

Yes, but this effect is extremely rare. Although the measles virus may infect the lungs, it may also reduce the patient's resistance to other infections, and it is usually these other infections that cause the trouble. If a child develops a persistent cough after a measles infection, he or she should see a doctor.

I've read that some dusts are more dangerous to inhale than others. Why?

Although it is not desirable to have any foreign particles enter the lungs, some dusts are more harmful than others. A person who inhales marble dust has practically no chance of getting lung disease. However, with sandstone dust, the risk of lung disease and death caused by inhaling the dust would be high. The reason for these differences is not fully understood. Many types of dusts, such as asbestos (once widely used in the building industry), are a special danger and can cause cancer of the lung and the pleura (linings of the lung).

The air people breathe contains millions of tiny particles, including dust and pollen, chemicals, tobacco smoke, viruses, and bacteria. All these particles can damage the lungs.

The most common disorder of the lungs in Western countries is bronchitis, or inflammation of the bronchi (the lung's main air passages). The principal cause of bronchitis is smoking, but other atmospheric pollutants and infections may contribute. Everyone has occasional attacks of bronchitis, which usually clear up in a few days. Some people develop chronic (long-lasting) bronchitis. Another common lung complaint is emphysema, in which the tiny air sacs of the lungs become damaged and the patient becomes breathless. Another condition that causes shortness of breath and wheezing is asthma. It can be triggered by an allergic response or by a stress-related disorder.

Pneumonia, pleurisy, and tuberculosis

Inflammations of the deepest parts of the lungs are called pneumonia. There are several causes of pneumonia. One of the most common causes is a bacterial infection. Pneumonia can also be caused by viral and fungal infections, and one rare type of pneumonia is caused by inhaling vomit. The different types vary in their severity from mild to extremely serious.

The symptoms of pneumonia also vary in speed of onset and severity. Bacterial pneumonia can develop within a matter of hours. Symptoms include a severe cough that may contain bloody sputum, a chest pain, fever or confusion, and shortness of breath when at rest. Other types of pneumonia may develop more slowly, over a matter of days. Symptoms include a general feeling of ill health, loss of appetite, and fever. Healthy young people may recover within a few weeks, but pneumonia can cause death in very young or very old people, or those who already have some other illness.

Pneumonia sometimes leads to pleurisy, which is an inflammation of the membranes that surround the lungs. When this happens, the membranes, which normally glide smoothly over each other, grate together, causing a sharp pain in the chest. Occasionally, pneumonia results in a lung abscess.

Breathing in dust particles irritates and scars the lungs. This sort of illness is still common in miners and stoneworkers. Tuberculosis (TB) of the lung is caused by the bacterium *Mycobacterium tuberculosis*. This disease greatly declined in developed countries in the twentieth century owing to improvements in health care. However, cases of TB have increased in recent years owing to the development of antibiotic-resistant strains of the bacteria.

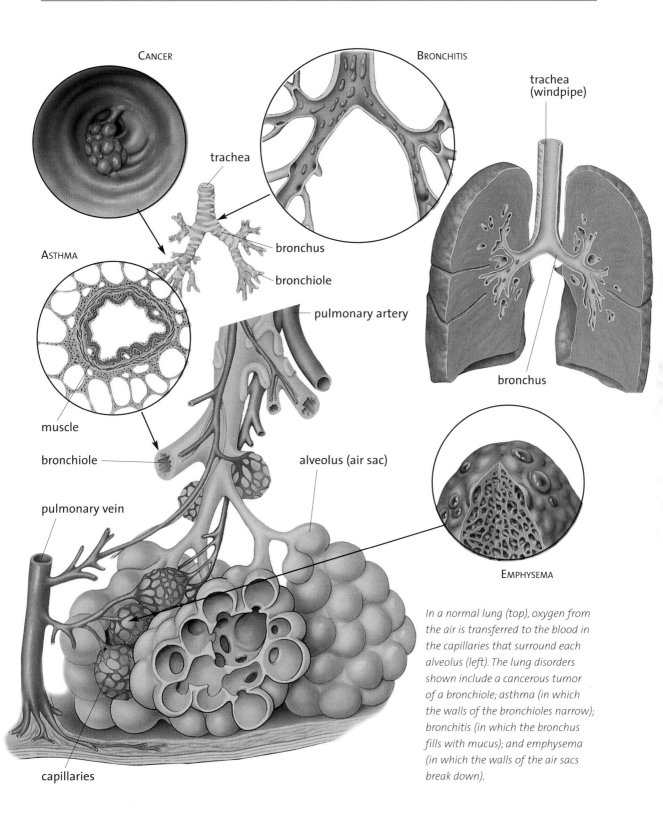

CANCER

BRONCHITIS

trachea
(windpipe)

trachea

ASTHMA

bronchus

bronchiole

bronchus

pulmonary artery

muscle

bronchiole

alveolus (air sac)

pulmonary vein

EMPHYSEMA

In a normal lung (top), oxygen from the air is transferred to the blood in the capillaries that surround each alveolus (left). The lung disorders shown include a cancerous tumor of a bronchiole; asthma (in which the walls of the bronchioles narrow); bronchitis (in which the bronchus fills with mucus); and emphysema (in which the walls of the air sacs break down).

capillaries

COMMON LUNG DISORDERS

Condition	Signs and symptoms	Causes	Treatments
Asthma	Breathlessness and wheezing	Allergies—commonly to dust mites or pollens, household pets, irritants, and some foods; some types aggravated by stress	Identification and avoidance of allergen, drugs to prevent attacks, and bronchodilators; hospital treatment for severe attacks may include muscle relaxants and connection to a respirator
Chronic bronchitis	Persistent cough with phlegm for more than three months of the year for two years in succession; breathlessness and wheezing	Smoking and industrial air pollution	Stopping smoking; wearing an approved face mask for dust protection in industry; antibiotic protection may be needed in winter; avoid cold and damp if possible
Emphysema	Breathlessness and enlargement of the chest	Smoking, air pollution, long-standing chronic bronchitis, and inherited susceptibility	Stopping smoking; breathing exercises
Lung cancer	Weight loss, persistent cough (sometimes with bloodstained phlegm), chest pains, breathlessness, wheezing, and hoarseness of the voice	Smoking, exposure to asbestos dust, exposure to silica dusts (as in mining), and industrial pollution	Surgical removal or radiotherapy and anticancer drugs; painkillers
Pneumonia	Cough, dry or with green or yellow phlegm, occasionally streaked with blood; fever, sweating, chest pains, and breathlessness	Bacteria and viruses; smoking makes adults more susceptible	Antibiotics (ampicillin or tetracycline); stopping smoking

Cancer of the lung

Lung disorders are made worse by smoking, which can also cause serious and fatal lung cancer. There are various types of lung cancers, all of which arise in the bronchi. All but a very few types are caused by smoking. There may be no obvious symptoms until the disease has spread within the body. Weight loss, persistent cough (sometimes with bloodstained phlegm), chest pains, wheezing, breathlessness, and hoarseness of the voice are common signs and symptoms. Surgical removal of a cancerous lung tumor is possible in only a few cases. Chemotherapy and radiotherapy help treat the disease.

SEE ALSO

ASTHMA • BRONCHITIS • CANCER • EMPHYSEMA • LUNG • PNEUMONIA • RESPIRATORY SYSTEM • RESPIRATORY SYSTEM DISEASES AND DISORDERS • TUBERCULOSIS

Lupus Erythematosus

Q & A

My aunt suffers from lupus, and I'm afraid I'll inherit it. Recently, my fingers and wrists have been aching. Is this a symptom of lupus?

There is a small chance of inheriting lupus, but you will not necessarily do so. The ache in your hands could be a symptom of rheumatoid arthritis or tenosynovitis (swelling in the membranes around the tendon caused by overuse—for example, from using a computer keyboard). If you are worried, you should see your doctor.

Lupus erythematosus is a disease that can produce a variety of symptoms. The one common symptom is a rash on each side of the nose, often forming a butterfly shape. People used to think this made the face look wolflike, hence the name *lupus*, which is the Latin word for "wolf."

In the mild form of lupus, called discoid lupus erythematosus (DLE), the rash may develop scaly patches and spread to the lips, hands, and forearms. The rash is extremely sensitive to sunlight, and those who have it should keep the face shaded. The more serious form of the disease, systemic lupus erythematosus (SLE), can affect various organs. Symptoms include a rash and possibly a fever, pains in the joints, inflammation of the lungs, and heart or kidney problems. All kinds of strange and seemingly disconnected symptoms may appear.

The cause of lupus is not fully known, but it seems to be connected with abnormalities of the body's immune (defense) system, which attack the body's own tissues. Steroids can be used to control it, and steroid cream is prescribed for discoid lupus. As the drug may have to be taken over a long period of time, doctors prefer not to use it for systemic lupus; instead, they use newer immunosuppressive drugs.

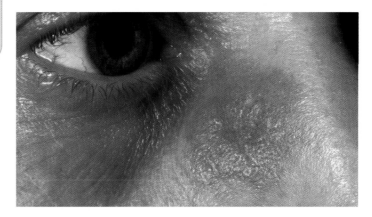

In the condition lupus erythematosus, a rash develops on either side of the nose and may spread to some other parts of the body. This may be the only symptom of discoid lupus, which is the mild form of lupus erythematosus.

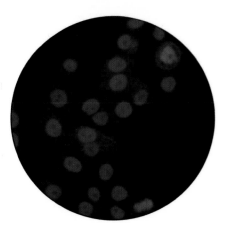

Green-stained antibodies in the blood of a person with the more serious form of lupus called systemic lupus erythematosus (SLE).

SEE ALSO

HEART • IMMUNE SYSTEM • IMMUNODEFICIENCY • KIDNEY • KIDNEY DISEASES AND DISORDERS • LUNG • SKIN • SKIN DISEASES AND DISORDERS

Lyme Disease

Lyme disease is named after Old Lyme, the town in Connecticut where it was first recognized in 1975. The cause was found to be an infection from the bites of tiny ticks that usually live on deer in the wooded areas nearby. The bacterium that causes Lyme disease is *Borrelia burgdorferi*; it enters the bloodstream through the tick bite and then spreads throughout the body.

Since it was first discovered, Lyme disease has been reported in many other states (particularly those on the northeastern coast and in California and Oregon) and in other parts of the world.

The first sign is a red spot that appears at the site of the bite and then develops into a spreading circular rash that lasts for a few weeks. Patients may feel chills and fever, with a headache and stiff neck. Later, they may develop symptoms that affect the heart, joints, and nervous system and that can lead to a form of meningitis and arthritis.

Antibiotic treatment is helpful early in the illness. If people are walking in long grass where ticks are common, the arms, legs, and feet should be covered, particularly in summer and early fall.

Any ticks on the skin should be removed as soon as possible. The tick must generally be attached to the host for 48 hours before enough of the bacteria can be transmitted to establish an infection. Not all ticks carry Lyme disease. It is relatively rare to contract Lyme disease from a single tick bite.

Q & A

Does Lyme disease have permanent effects, or does early treatment guarantee a complete cure?

Early treatment makes a cure more likely but does not guarantee it. If the joints are damaged permanently, the condition is similar to a mild case of rheumatoid arthritis. In a few cases of Lyme disease, the heart is also affected, as is the nervous system, where meningitis can develop.

Are some people more likely to get Lyme disease than others?

The disease is carried by a tick and is sometimes transferred to dogs, so it is more likely to affect people who live in or visit the countryside.

Is there any way I can avoid getting Lyme disease?

The best way is to cut down on the chances of getting tick bites. Cover as much of your body and head surface as possible when out walking, use insect repellent, and check yourself thoroughly when you return home.

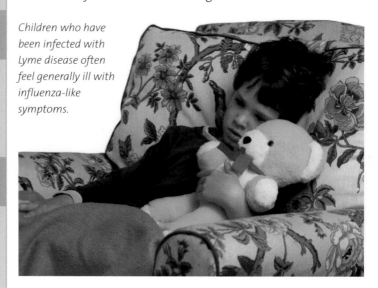

Children who have been infected with Lyme disease often feel generally ill with influenza-like symptoms.

SEE ALSO

ARTHRITIS • BACTERIA • BLOOD • HEART • JOINT DISORDERS • MENINGITIS • NERVOUS SYSTEM

Lymphatic System

Q & A

My sister has repeated attacks of tonsillitis, accompanied by swelling in her neck. Why does this happen?

The tonsils and adenoids are small patches of lymphoid tissue in the upper part of the throat. Both structures can become infected by the bacteria and viruses that are inhaled, causing inflammation. The infection then spreads along the lymphatic channel to other lymph nodes lower in the neck, so that the neck appears to swell. If the situation persists and there are no other alternatives, your sister may need to have her tonsils removed.

When my older brother became ill at college, the doctor said he had infectious mononucleosis. What is this?

Infectious mononucleosis is a disease caused by the Epstein-Barr virus. The infection invades all the lymphatic tissues and may cause lymph node enlargement in the groin, the armpits, and the neck, as well as enlargement of the spleen and liver. The mainstay of treatment is general rest.

The lymphatic system is part of the body's transport and defense system. It consists of a complicated network of very fine tubes or vessels. These vessels, or lymphatics, run through every part of the body except the central nervous system. They collect surplus fluid called lymph from the blood vessels and body tissues and return it to the bloodstream via two veins in the base of the neck.

At certain points in the body, such as the groin, armpits, and neck, the lymphatic vessels join to form lymph nodes, which are commonly called lymph glands. These glands play a vital role in the body's immune system. They manufacture white blood cells called lymphocytes, which produce antibodies to fight specific diseases. Lymph nodes also filter harmful bacteria and viruses. They can also trap cancer cells that have entered the lymph from the blood and body tissues.

Lymph nodes frequently become swollen and inflamed. This is usually a sign that they are fighting an infection. If the swelling persists, a doctor should be consulted. Among the most common disorders of the lymphatic system are tonsillitis and infectious mononucleosis. Lymphoma, or cancer of the lymph nodes, is comparatively rare; Hodgkin's disease, the best known form of lymphoma, can now be treated successfully if diagnosed early.

The thymus gland forms part of the body's immune system. Located in the upper chest under the breastbone, the thymus

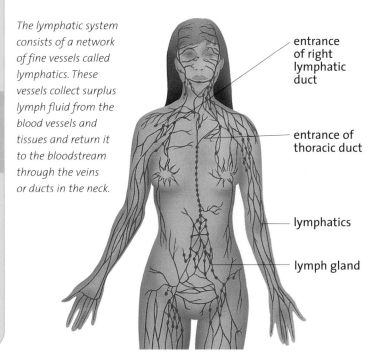

The lymphatic system consists of a network of fine vessels called lymphatics. These vessels collect surplus lymph fluid from the blood vessels and tissues and return it to the bloodstream through the veins or ducts in the neck.

entrance of right lymphatic duct

entrance of thoracic duct

lymphatics

lymph gland

DISEASES AFFECTING THE LYMPHATIC SYSTEM

Disease	Causes	Symptoms	Treatments
Elephantiasis	Blockage of lymph channel in limb, in tropical countries caused by worm infestation	Swelling of affected limb, thickened and discolored skin, and difficulty in passing urine	Ethyl-carbamazine drug to kill worms; elevation of affected leg; compression stocking on limb
Infectious mononucleosis (glandular fever)	Virus infection, spread by close contact	Listlessness, fatigue, headache, chills, high fever, and sore throat; swollen lymph nodes in the neck, armpits, and elsewhere	Each symptom is treated separately: gargles, painkillers, bed rest, and hot-water bottle to relieve swollen glands; convalescent period of six to eight weeks
Lymphangitis	Bacterial infection from a cut or abscess that has spread to the nearest lymph nodes	Chills, fever, and swelling of the lymph nodes; red lines spread up the arm or leg as the channel becomes inflamed	Antibiotics; elevation of affected part; application of hot, wet, or dry compress
Lymphedema	Blockage of lymph vessels can be congenital, or following childbirth or surgery for breast cancer	Swelling of affected area	Usually disappears in time, or with treatment for cause
Lymphomas, lymphosarcomas (including Hodgkin's disease)	Tumors of the lymphatic system; no cause known	Fatigue and loss of energy, appetite, and weight; affected glands harden and swell; fever and night sweats; itchiness of skin; pain in glands	Radiotherapy in early stages of disease; surgical removal of affected glands; radiotherapy and chemotherapy in later stages
Tonsillitis	Bacterial or viral infection of lymphoid tissue of tonsils	Chills, high fever, headache, and sore throat; difficulty in swallowing; sometimes, painful swollen glands under the jaw	Antibiotics; if persistent, removal of tonsils may be necessary

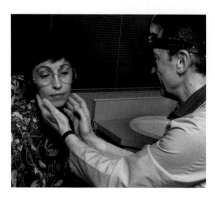

Tonsillitis causes swollen lymph glands in the neck.

is responsible for processing a class of white cells, called lymphocytes, that are present in the blood, the bone marrow, the lymph nodes, and the spleen. These lymphocytes are called T lymphocytes, or T cells. They help protect the body against cancers and viral infections and produce antibodies that fight disease. The thymus gland is at its largest in children. It appears to program how the immune system works and ensure that the system does not work against the body's own tissues.

SEE ALSO

ANTIBODY AND ANTIGEN • BACTERIA • BODY SYSTEMS • GLANDS • IMMUNE SYSTEM • INFECTIOUS MONONUCLEOSIS • LYMPHOMA • NERVOUS SYSTEM • VIRUSES

Lymphoma

Lymphoma is cancer of the lymph nodes and tissues of the lymphatic system, the complex network of lymphoid organs, nodes, ducts, tissues, capillaries, and vessels that produce lymph fluid and transport it from tissues to the circulatory system. The lymphatic system is a major component of the immune system. In a person with lymphoma, the immune cells become cancerous and multiply rapidly in the lymph nodes.

There are two major forms of lymphoma: Hodgkin's disease (in which the cancer stays mostly within the lymph nodes) and non-Hodgkin's lymphoma (in which the cancer spreads to other organs). In the early stages of a lymphoma there may be no symptoms, but as the illness progresses, the most common signs are tiredness, loss of energy, loss of appetite, loss of weight, and long-term fevers that rise in the evening. The patient may also have enlarged lymph nodes in the neck. Enlarged nodes caused by a lymphoma feel rubbery and painless. In advanced stages, blood abnormalities, such as anemia, can develop.

If lymphoma is suspected, doctors do tests, including blood tests or computed tomography (CT) scans. Biopsy (taking a small piece of a lymph node) is used to differentiate Hodgkin's disease from non-Hodgkin's lymphomas. The earlier treatment starts, the better the chance of a cure. The treatment for Hodgkin's and non-Hodgkin's is similar. In the early stages, radiotherapy can cure a person. In the later stages, or if the cancer has spread to other organs, chemotherapy is used. Depending on the stage when it is discovered, Hodgkin's disease is curable. However, the cure rate for non-Hodgkin's lymphomas is not as promising.

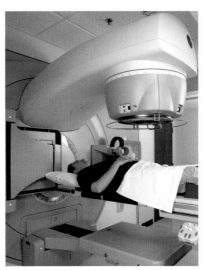

A patient with lymphoma receives radiotherapy.

SEE ALSO

ANEMIA • BLOOD • BODY SYSTEMS • CANCER • CELLS AND CHROMOSOMES • CIRCULATORY SYSTEM • LIVER • LYMPHATIC SYSTEM

Q & A

My sister had a swollen neck after a sore throat. Could she have a lymphoma?

It is unlikely. Swelling of the lymph nodes, particularly in the neck, is common after an upper respiratory tract infection. If the nodes are tender, lymphoma is even less likely.

My grandmother's doctor says that she has a lymphoma. Could it be malignant?

Unfortunately, yes. A malignant disease is one that spreads to other areas of the body, distant from its place of origin. Since the lymphatic system circulates throughout the body, lymphomas are particularly dangerous. However, there are degrees of malignancy; some cancers spread slowly and others spread quickly. Lymphomas are fairly slow-growing and can be cured if they are diagnosed early enough.

Is it true that you will know if you have a lymphoma because the affected area swells up?

No. The swelling can be seen only if the nodes affected are near the skin surface.

Malaria

Malaria is an infectious disease that is caused by parasites called plasmodia. The disease used to be found in many parts of the world but is now present mainly in tropical areas. Malaria can be transmitted to humans only by a bite from an infected female anopheles mosquito. If an insect without the disease feeds on the blood of an infected person, it becomes infected itself and passes on malaria when it bites someone else. The malarial parasites enter the human bloodstream and go to the liver. They multiply during an incubation period of one to four weeks and then return to the bloodstream, where they penetrate red blood cells. These cells eventually rupture and release parasites that infect other red blood cells. Malaria parasites may stay dormant in the liver. They can cause outbreaks of the disease long after the original infection if left untreated. The main symptom of malaria is a high fever. Other symptoms include headache, nausea, and possibly vomiting and diarrhea.

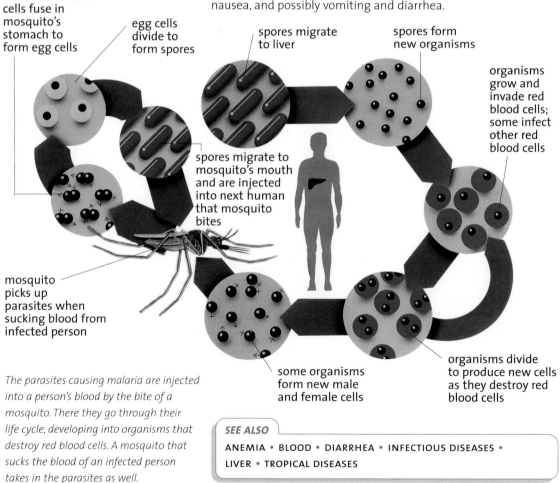

male and female cells fuse in mosquito's stomach to form egg cells

egg cells divide to form spores

spores migrate to liver

spores form new organisms

organisms grow and invade red blood cells; some infect other red blood cells

spores migrate to mosquito's mouth and are injected into next human that mosquito bites

mosquito picks up parasites when sucking blood from infected person

some organisms form new male and female cells

organisms divide to produce new cells as they destroy red blood cells

The parasites causing malaria are injected into a person's blood by the bite of a mosquito. There they go through their life cycle, developing into organisms that destroy red blood cells. A mosquito that sucks the blood of an infected person takes in the parasites as well.

SEE ALSO

ANEMIA • BLOOD • DIARRHEA • INFECTIOUS DISEASES •
LIVER • TROPICAL DISEASES

Malnutrition

Q & A

My great-grandmother says she lost all her teeth because of malnutrition during World War II (1939–1945) in England. Is this likely?

No. It seems more probable that she just had poor teeth prone to decay. As a result of government action, the standard of nutrition in Britain during the war was better than before. There was no junk food; there were plenty of vegetables; free milk, cod liver oil, and orange juice were provided for children; and common foods, such as margarine, were supplemented with vitamins.

Could an old man who cannot afford meat have malnutrition?

If he eats other protein, such as nuts and cheese, his diet should be adequate. However, the elderly can easily become malnourished, especially in the winter.

Are vitamin supplements really necessary?

If people eat a balanced diet containing all the proteins, fats, carbohydrates, vitamins, and minerals they need, there should be no need for supplements.

Malnutrition is any form of poor health caused by not eating enough food or by eating the wrong kind of food in the wrong amount. People should eat appropriate quantities of quality food, and it should contain all the vitamins, proteins, carbohydrates, fats, and minerals needed to keep the body healthy. In developed countries, obesity due to a poor diet with high levels of fat and lots of junk food is a type of malnutrition. Elderly people and hospital patients may also suffer from malnutrition, because they may not be able to look after themselves properly and may be too weak or ill to eat properly.

The most obvious malnutrition, however, is the starvation that occurs in some countries in the developing world. Their food generally lacks protein, and there may be far less food than people need. In many countries, half the children die before they reach the age of five. Conditions are made worse by famine, drought, and war. These countries cannot afford to import food. Moreover, it often proves difficult to distribute donated food to those who most need it. As a result, people suffer from varying degrees of starvation and do not get enough nutritious food to maintain health.

Lack of protein

The most common cause of malnutrition is lack of protein, which occurs in some African countries. Kwashiorkor and marasmus are two diseases that afflict young children. Weight loss; retarded growth; wasted muscles; dry, inelastic, cold skin; and sparse hair are typical symptoms of these diseases. Antibodies are made of proteins, and a severe shortage of protein therefore results in a failure to make antibodies. That causes severe immune deficiency and probable death from infection. If treated early with a diet based on milk and high-calorie food supplements, protein-deficiency diseases can be cured.

Voluntary starvation

Few people endure starvation out of choice. Some, however, fast for dietary or religious reasons, and such fasting can cause severe malnutrition if practiced regularly. Anorexia nervosa is a starvation disease that is common in young girls who begin dieting to lose weight. Soon, losing weight becomes a compulsion, and the sufferer may take appetite suppressants and laxatives. If untreated, anorexia nervosa can result in death.

The elderly

As people grow older they generally become more frail and experience loss of strength and balance. It is therefore

When a child suffers from malnutrition, the limbs may become wasted while the belly is distended. The child becomes more and more lethargic, and the face becomes pinched and gray, with sunken eyes. This condition is known as marasmus. The most common cause is starvation, although marasmus can also be a symptom of certain illnesses that stop the child from taking in nourishment from his or her food.

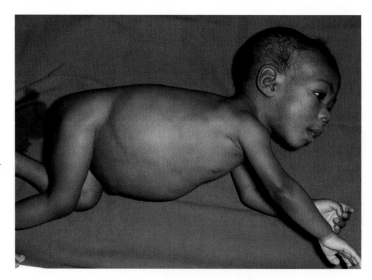

particularly important that the elderly eat sufficient amounts of suitable food, including protein, selected vitamins, and dietary supplements to help overcome these effects of aging.

Studies have shown that a lack of specific nutrients—including protein; vitamins A, D, and C; and the B vitamin folate—increases the risk of becoming frail. As people age, their ability to absorb nutrients from food also decreases. In addition, many elderly people may have a fixed income, which affects the quality and quantity of the food eaten. However, frailty may be easily prevented and even reversed: meat, beans, and nuts are excellent sources of protein and folate, and fruits and vegetables are good sources of vitamins A, C, and D.

Treatment

Malnutrition is treated, whenever possible, by gradually giving the patient a full, balanced diet (a sudden change in eating patterns could be too much for a malnourished body to cope with). Sometimes, vitamin and mineral supplements may be necessary for a while, and any medical problems need to be treated. Normally, however, there is no need to take extra vitamins or minerals, and they can even be harmful. Eating properly should provide all the nourishment needed.

> **SEE ALSO**
>
> ANOREXIA AND BULIMIA • ANTIBODY AND ANTIGEN •
> IMMUNE SYSTEM • NUTRITIONAL DISEASES • OBESITY •
> SCURVY

Marfan Syndrome

Q & A

What is Marfan syndrome?

Marfan syndrome is a genetic disorder that affects the body's connective tissue. Connective tissue is present everywhere in the body. It is the "glue" that helps support the organs, blood vessels, bones, joints, and muscles. The defect causes this connective tissue to be weaker than normal.

The doctor says my friend should not play basketball because he has Marfan syndrome. Why?

Weakened connective tissue can lead to problems in many parts of the body, especially the heart, eyes, and joints. The most serious complication of Marfan syndrome involves the heart. Over time, the aorta can dilate and tear. A large, sudden rupture can be fatal. In addition, heart valve problems can occur, causing blood to leak backward through the heart. This condition may result in shortness of breath, fatigue, and palpitations.

People with Marfan syndrome have extremely long limbs and fingers (left) compared with other people (right). They are also tall, thin, and loose-jointed.

Marfan syndrome is a genetic disorder of connective tissue that has potentially fatal effects. Connective tissue is one of the most abundant and diverse of the basic types of tissues of the body. It connects parts of the body; supports, strengthens, and insulates organs; transports nutrients, gases, and wastes through the body; and marshals the immune response. Connective tissues include bone, blood, lymph, cartilage, fat, ligaments, tendons, and muscle.

Connective tissue is made of cells embedded within a matrix that gives the tissue its special properties. The matrix includes fibers (collagen, elastic, and reticular) that provide strength and support (all three fibers), flexibility (collagen only), or the ability to stretch and return to its original shape (elastic only). In Marfan syndrome, an inherited mutation weakens the elastic fibers and may adversely affect the skeleton or blood vessels.

People with Marfan syndrome are typically tall, thin, and loose-jointed. Their arms, legs, fingers, and toes may be disproportionately long. Many people with Marfan syndrome have impaired vision, caused by a weakening of a ligament that holds the lens of the eye in place. The curvature of the spine may be affected, leading to disorders such as scoliosis.

In the case of large arteries, such as the aorta, the walls may be weakened, leading to the development of bulges in the walls called aneurysms. Aneurysms may suddenly burst, leading to massive internal bleeding and death. Several noted athletes, such as Flo Hyman (captain of the 1984 U.S. Olympic women's volleyball team) and Hank Gathers (Loyola Marymount College

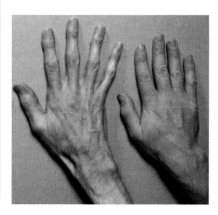

men's basketball player) died without warning as a result of burst aneurysms. They were young and seemed to be at the peak of their athletic prowess and health, but the demands on their circulatory system, combined with the weakness of their blood vessels, proved too much.

SEE ALSO

ARTERY • ARTERY DISEASES AND DISORDERS • BLOOD • BONE • EYE DISEASES AND DISORDERS • IMMUNE SYSTEM • LYMPHATIC SYSTEM • MUSCLE • SKELETAL SYSTEM

Measles

Measles is arguably the most serious of the preventable infectious diseases commonly caught by children. Although it is often mild itself, it has a high rate of complications, including pneumonia and encephalitis. It is now common to immunize children against measles. In many parts of the United States, students must be vaccinated before starting school. Children are usually vaccinated at one year of age. Once someone has had an attack of measles, he or she should not get the disease again.

Symptoms and treatments

Measles is a contagious disease, caused by a virus that is passed from one person to another on the tiny droplets of moisture people constantly breathe in and out. Measles is so infectious that epidemics quickly spread through schools and communities. For the first seven to 14 days after the virus has entered someone's system, it incubates or multiplies in the cells of the throat and the passages leading to the lungs. Then comes the first, catarrhal stage of measles. The patient develops a bad cold with a husky cough. The nose runs, and the eyes are red, watery, and swollen. There may be a fine red rash that lasts for only a few hours. Most children have a slight fever, lose their appetite, perhaps feel nauseated, and have diarrhea.

On about the third day, tiny white spots like grains of salt appear on the inside of the mouth. The temperature rises to about 103°F (39.4°C). A dusky red rash appears on the forehead and behind the ears and spreads over the face and trunk. This stage takes about 36 hours. The rash may itch. The cough gets worse, and light may hurt the eyes. At this stage, the patient may feel very ill. However, the rash begins to fade after a couple of days, and the patient soon begins to feel better.

Mild measles requires no treatment other than careful home nursing, although the doctor should be informed of any suspected case. The patient should be kept in bed until the fever and rash have gone. Mild drugs can be given to reduce the fever. Calamine lotion helps ease the itching spots. The patient should be given plenty of fluids to drink, and the curtains should be drawn if light hurts the eyes. Measles is extremely contagious. Until the rash has disappeared, patients should be kept away from anyone who has not had the disease.

Q & A

How do you identify measles for sure when so many childhood illnesses produce a rash?

The only way to be sure is to look for what are called Koplik's spots, named after the man who first identified them. They appear in the mouth (on the inner lining of the cheeks) on the third day after the initial symptoms (a fever and runny nose) appear. They look like grains of salt surrounded by a rosy, slightly inflamed area.

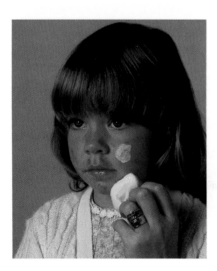

The most obvious symptom of measles is an itchy rash, which may spread over the whole body. It may be soothed by dabbing the rash with calamine lotion.

SEE ALSO

COLD • DIARRHEA • ENCEPHALITIS • EPIDEMIC • INFECTIOUS DISEASES • PNEUMONIA • VIRUSES

Meningitis

Q & A

Can meningitis be inherited?

No, there is no chance of inheriting meningitis. You can catch it only from someone who has the germ.

My neighbor's child has meningitis. Am I at any risk?

If you were in contact with the sick child, your parents should tell your doctor, who can find out from the hospital if you need protective antibiotics. If your parents saw the sick child, they may need antibiotics, too.

My 70-year-old grandfather, who lives with us, has TB of the lung. Can I catch meningitis from TB?

Yes, tuberculosis (TB) is a rare cause of meningitis. Public health officials should visit you to see if any of you have caught TB meningitis.

If meningitis is caused by a virus (1), the illness is quite mild. Meningitis caused by meningococcus bacteria (2) is very dangerous, and the patient can die within 12 hours. Small children are now routinely vaccinated against a type of influenza called Haemophilus influenzae *type B, which is a common cause of meningitis.*

Meningitis is inflammation of the meninges, the thin layers of tissue covering the brain and the spinal cord. Between these layers is the cerebrospinal fluid (CSF). There are several causes of meningitis. Sometimes, a germ enters the CSF from the bloodstream, from an ear infection, or from a head wound. It irritates the meninges, which then become inflamed. The most common form of meningitis is caused by a virus and may be a mild, influenza-like illness. More serious but less common cases are bacterial meningitis, which is sometimes life-threatening and requires urgent medical treatment in the hospital.

The symptoms of meningitis may develop very quickly or quite slowly. The patient develops a bad headache, finds bright light painful, has a stiff neck, feels nauseated, and vomits. Bending and straightening the legs may be painful. In some cases of bacterial meningitis, a purpura rash, which looks like bruising, may develop on the body. This red or purple rash does not fade when pressed. It can be identified by pressing a glass against the skin; if the rash does not disappear underneath the glass, then this may be a sign of meningitis. The patient also feels feverish and ill and may become confused and drowsy. In a baby, the main symptoms of meningitis are fever, vomiting, convulsions, and poor feeding. Its neck may be stiff, and its body may be floppy. The soft part of a baby's skull, called the fontanelle, may bulge.

Anyone who has the symptoms of meningitis should be seen by a doctor at once. Viral meningitis can be nursed at home and often clears up within two weeks. A patient with bacterial meningitis is treated in a hospital with large doses of antibiotics. Some types of meningitis are very infectious; occasionally, cases occur in clusters, for example, in a school or college. Most people recover completely within a few weeks, but some people die from meningitis. Others may be left with a serious handicap such as deafness, epilepsy, cerebral palsy, or mental retardation.

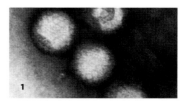
1

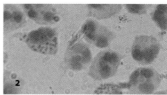
2

SEE ALSO

BACTERIAL DISEASES • BRAIN • BRAIN DAMAGE AND DISORDERS • CEREBRAL PALSY • INFECTIOUS DISEASES • VIRUSES

Menstrual Disorders

Q & A

I become constipated just before my period. Why does this happen?

High levels of progesterone in the blood tend to make the intestine less mobile at this time, causing constipation. You should make sure you eat fruit and drink plenty of fluids. If this fails, talk to your doctor.

My 15-year-old sister becomes impossible to live with immediately before her period. She's very grumpy and argumentative. What can I do to help her?

She may be suffering from premenstrual syndrome (PMS). Start by discussing what you have noticed and see if she has noticed a pattern of negative feelings that immediately precede her periods. If she has, her doctor may be able to help. Avoid getting into arguments with her; they will only make both of you feel angry and depressed. She may find it useful to read a book about premenstrual syndrome so that she can understand what is happening to her; this may make it easier for her to cope with it.

Many women feel little or no pain or discomfort at all when they menstruate. Others, however, experience problems, including irregular or very heavy periods and painful cramps; some women experience both.

One of the most common problems associated with the monthly period is premenstrual syndrome (PMS), which is thought to be caused by the hormonal changes that occur around this time. PMS usually occurs in the week before a period and then disappears when the period begins. Some women, however, may experience PMS as early as two weeks before the start of their period. Symptoms include tenderness and swelling in some parts of the body, weight gain, and skin problems. Some women may feel depressed or anxious and increasingly irritable.

Menstrual cramps (dysmenorrhea) are particularly common in the first few years of menstruating. They may be caused by spasms in the muscles of the uterus (womb). A substance called prostaglandin, released by the cells lining the uterus, may be another cause. A woman may also experience bad backache, nausea, and even vomiting. A mild painkiller can often help relieve the pain. Holding a heating pad or a hot water bottle next to the abdomen is soothing, and gentle exercise can often help bring relief. Tablets such as aspirin, which block prostaglandin production, may be prescribed. For some women, taking a contraceptive pill can also help lessen these cramps. Often, dysmenorrhea stops after a woman has her first child.

Unusually heavy periods (menorrhagia) are inconvenient but not usually serious. However, a physician should be consulted if a woman has heavy periods regularly, because they could cause anemia. Hormonal tablets can be prescribed. Sometimes, fibroids (harmless growths in the uterus) cause heavy periods.

Missing a period can be worrying. Occasionally, a woman's periods never start, a condition called primary amenorrhea. A girl whose periods have not begun by the time she is 16 should talk to her doctor in case something is wrong with her reproductive system or her hormonal system. When someone who usually menstruates misses a period, the most obvious reason is pregnancy. Emotional upsets, stress, hormone deficiency, anemia, prolonged athletic activity, and anorexia nervosa can also cause a missed period.

> **SEE ALSO**
>
> ANEMIA • ANOREXIA AND BULIMIA • BLOOD • BODY SYSTEMS • ENDOMETRIOSIS • FIBROIDS • HORMONES AND HORMONAL DISORDERS • PREMENSTRUAL SYNDROME

Metabolic Disorders

Metabolic disorders are illnesses caused by disorders in the body's chemistry that prevent it from functioning properly. For example, some babies are born lacking the ability to make certain enzymes. As a result, poisons can build up in the body. Many metabolic disorders are caused by gene mutations.

Genetic diseases

In the disorder phenylketonuria (PKU), the body lacks the enzyme necessary to break down certain waste products. If these build up, the nervous system may be damaged. In developed countries, babies are tested for PKU when they are about six days old. Those babies with the disorder are given a formula or milk substitute to enable them to develop normally.

Babies with the rare, inherited condition galactosemia lack the enzyme to break down milk sugar and may become mentally retarded and develop cataracts unless milk is removed from their diet. In Wilson's disease, the body absorbs harmful amounts of copper. Foods high in copper are avoided and drugs are taken to prevent the absorption of the mineral. These diseases are classed as inborn errors of metabolism.

Hormonal disturbances

Other metabolic disorders are caused by disturbances in the production of certain hormones. For example, diabetes is caused by the body's failure to produce enough of the hormone insulin. As a result, the body cannot absorb and break down glucose, which accumulates in the blood.

Diabetes can be treated with insulin injections. The condition is believed to be caused by environmental factors, such as viral infections operating on a genetically predisposed person to damage the insulin-producing cells of the pancreas. In rare cases, obesity can also result from disturbances in the production of hormones.

Early treatment

Many metabolic disorders are now treated early in a baby's life and do no lasting harm. People with a disorder in their family can have genetic counseling before they have children, so that they know the risks of passing on the disorder.

Q & A

My new baby sister has phenylketonuria and has to be given a special formula diet. Why is that?

Human milk contains phenylalanine, an amino acid that the baby's body cannot handle. The high levels of this amino acid that occur in the first few months or years of life lead to intellectual and developmental impairment. The brain is at its most sensitive at this time in a child's life.

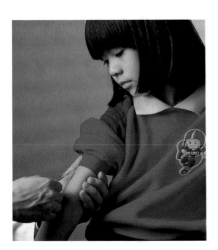

This little girl has diabetes. She will need to take insulin for the rest of her life. However, because of newly developed techniques, people with diabetes may no longer have to inject themselves daily.

SEE ALSO

BODY SYSTEMS • DIABETES • GENES • GENETIC DISEASES AND DISORDERS • HORMONES AND HORMONAL DISORDERS • NERVOUS SYSTEM • PHENYLKETONURIA

Migraine

The term *migraine* is a modification of two Latin words: *hemi*, meaning "one side," and *cranial*, meaning "of the head." In a true migraine, pain is felt on one side of the head only. People with a migraine have a violent headache, may feel nauseated, and may vomit. They may not be able to see, hear, or feel properly. Sometimes, they even find it hard to speak. These usually severe headaches may last for some time. People who suffer from them often have difficulty in leading a normal life.

Migraines affect mainly young and middle-aged women, although anyone can suffer from one occasionally. Tens of millions of people in the United States suffer from regular migraine attacks.

Modern scanning techniques such as magnetic resonance imaging (MRI) have shown that migraine headaches seem to result when the blood vessels in the head narrow and then expand again, upsetting the flow of blood to the brain and therefore triggering the disturbances in perception and producing a painful headache. Doctors do not yet understand just what causes this effect. For some people, eating foods such as chocolate and cheese or drinking alcohol can trigger a migraine. The tendency to suffer from migraines often runs in families.

Prevention and treatment

Susceptible people should avoid substances and activities that set off migraines. While having a migraine, they should lie quietly in a dark room and get plenty of rest. Doctors can prescribe drugs to help the symptoms, but these drugs must be taken carefully, because they can cause unpleasant side effects. Some of the common treatments for migraines can also interact with each other to cause undue narrowing of arteries. Some migraines require treatment by a doctor.

Simple painkillers, such as soluble aspirin, acetaminophen, or codeine, are suggested for pain relief. However, as the stomach becomes inactive early in an attack, drugs may not be well absorbed and may be vomited, so antivomiting drugs may have to be taken first. For most people, the headache is the most painful part of a migraine attack and is often unaffected by simple painkillers. Therefore, vasoconstrictive drugs called ergotamines (which constrict the swollen blood vessels in the head) are often prescribed. Sumatriptan is also an established treatment.

Q & A

I've tried all the pharmaceutical drugs available for migraines, and none of them helped. Are there any alternative treatments I could try?

Yes. You could try homeopathic medicine or acupuncture, in which fine needles are inserted at different points in the body. Bioenergetic therapy, on the other hand, treats physical symptoms such as migraines by exploring emotional tension and repressed feelings. Research is also being done on an herb called feverfew, which has been claimed to relieve migraines if taken over a few months. It can be obtained from many health food stores.

During my migraine attacks I often feel sad and want to cry. Is this a normal reaction?

Emotional tension, especially holding in strong feelings, can be a factor in causing migraines. It is perfectly normal to cry if you wish to, and you may find that this brings some relief. Symptoms can become worse while you are crying, but the attack may pass more quickly than usual.

SEE ALSO

BRAIN • BRAIN DAMAGE AND DISORDERS • EYE AND SIGHT

Motor Neuron Disease

Q & A

What exactly is a motor neuron?

A neuron is a nerve cell. It has a small, spiky body and a long nerve fiber called an axon. Sensory neurons carry nerve information to the brain, and motor neurons carry activating signals from the brain to the muscles and glands.

Are the sensory nerves affected in motor neuron disease?

No; only the motor nerves are affected. There is no reduction in sensation, and there is no disturbance of mental functioning.

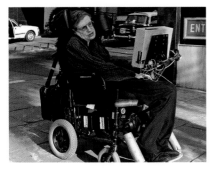

The distinguished British physicist Stephen Hawking (b. 1942) has suffered from amyotrophic lateral sclerosis for nearly 40 years. He still writes books and gives lectures with the help of a speech synthesizer and computer.

Motor neuron disease (amyotrophic lateral sclerosis) is often called Lou Gehrig's disease after the U.S. baseball player Lou Gehrig (1903–1941), who died from it. The cause of this form of motor neuron disease is usually unknown, but in a small minority of people there is a genetic cause. The term *motor neuron disease*, however, covers several similar conditions, of which amyotrophic lateral sclerosis is the most serious.

There are two groups of motor neurons or nerves: the upper motor neurons and the lower motor neurons. The upper motor neurons run downward from the surface of the brain, through the brain and the brain stem and down the spinal cord to end in a series of junctions positioned at the front of the cord from top to bottom. The lower motor neurons emerge from these junctions to run to and activate the muscles. Motor neuron disease may affect either the upper or the lower neurons, or both.

Amyotrophic lateral sclerosis is a combined upper and lower motor neuron disease. It is more common in men and seldom appears before the age of 50. The motor neurons degenerate until their function is destroyed. When the upper part of the spine is involved, there is difficulty in swallowing and speaking, with weakness of the tongue, throat, and voice box. Food may enter the lungs and cause infection, the vocal cords are paralyzed, and the person cannot cough. The muscles of respiration gradually weaken so that unassisted breathing becomes impossible.

The pure lower motor neuron types of the disease are much less severe than amyotrophic lateral sclerosis. They include conditions formerly known as spinal muscular atrophy and progressive muscular atrophy, and they vary in terms of the age of onset. They usually start with wasting and weakness of the muscles of one limb, affecting the hand or foot and progressing until the affected limb becomes useless.

Amyotrophic lateral sclerosis is usually fatal. Death often results, within two years, from an inability to breathe, choking, or pneumonia owing to the inhalation of food. Death may also be due to malnutrition, because of difficulties swallowing.

The outlook in cases of lower motor neuron disease varies with the different forms. The recessive genetic adult form starts at any age from 15 to 60 but usually begins in the forties. Limb weakness and serious difficulty with walking seldom occur until the sixties or seventies.

SEE ALSO

BRAIN • MUSCLE • MUSCLE DISEASES AND DISORDERS • NERVOUS SYSTEM DISORDERS • PARALYSIS • SPINAL COLUMN

Mouth

The human mouth is a cavelike facial opening that contains the teeth and tongue. The mouth is surrounded on the outside by the lips (the most sensitive area of the body), which give the mouth its expression. The lips also allow people to suck and close the mouth, and they play a vital role in speech. At the back, the mouth links up with the digestive system and the lungs. The mouth helps people to eat, digest food, speak, and breathe.

A mucous membrane lines the inside of the mouth. The membrane contains small glands, which produce a sticky fluid called mucus. With the saliva, this mucus keeps the inside of the mouth clean and constantly moist. The roof of the mouth consists of the hard and soft palate. The hard palate lies toward the front. It is formed by the bottom of the upper jawbone (maxilla) and provides a firm surface against which the tongue can press when chewing. Thus, food can be mixed and softened. Toward the back of the mouth is the soft palate, which moves upward as food is swallowed and prevents food from being forced up into the nose. A piece of soft tissue called the uvula, or third tonsil, hangs down from the center of the soft palate. Its function is unknown, but one theory is that it prevents choking when food is swallowed.

The mouth is the entrance to the digestive system. Food passes over the lips and into the mouth, where it is chewed by the teeth and moved about by the tongue. Mucus, along with saliva from three pairs of salivary glands, moistens the food

Q & A

Why do babies always put things in their mouths?

Because babies depend on their mouths for feeding—and therefore for their survival—they find that their mouths can provide them with the most accurate picture of the world around them and, at the same time, satisfy their basic need to suck. That is why babies always put things in their mouths. Parents need to make sure there is no chance of a baby's swallowing or choking on a small object or picking up an infection from dirty objects. Most babies outgrow this behavior by the age of two.

My sister wants to learn to play the trumpet. Will all the blowing stretch her mouth and cheeks?

No, this will not happen. The tissues of the cheeks are packed with muscle cells and other fibrous cells that are elastic enough to cope with the kind of wear and tear your sister's trumpet playing will give them. These elastic tissues begin to lose their springiness only from middle age on.

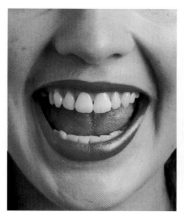 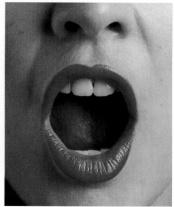

The mouth is involved in many functions, including speech. Each sound is made by a slightly different movement of the lips, tongue, and teeth. The letter "A" (left) is made with the mouth wide open and the tongue on the bottom teeth. The sound "ah" (right) is made with the lips wide open and drawn away from the teeth.

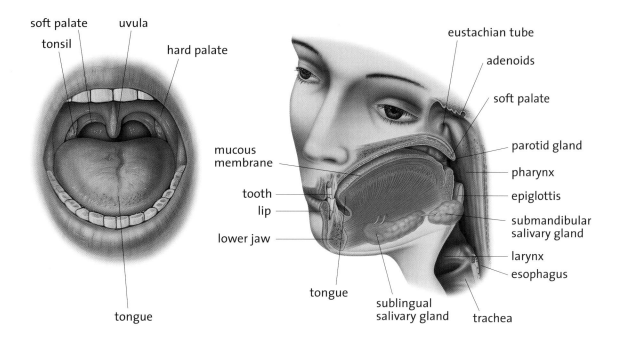

soft palate
uvula
tonsil
hard palate
eustachian tube
adenoids
soft palate
mucous membrane
parotid gland
pharynx
tooth
epiglottis
lip
submandibular salivary gland
lower jaw
larynx
esophagus
tongue
tongue
sublingual salivary gland
trachea
tongue

These diagrams show the structure of the mouth. Hanging down from the center of the soft palate is the uvula. Its function is a mystery, but experts believe it seals the air passages when food is swallowed, thus preventing the possibility of choking.

so it can be chewed and swallowed easily. After the food has been chewed, the tongue pushes it to the back of the mouth into a cavity called the pharynx. A little flap of tissue, the epiglottis, closes the larynx (voice box) off from the pharynx as a person swallows, so that the food is not allowed to pass into the trachea (windpipe).

Breathing and speech

The mouth is involved in speech. It shapes the sounds from the larynx in the throat to make words. It also provides an airway and is involved in breathing. The mouth is not as efficient as the nose, however. Air entering the mouth is not warmed, and harmful particles in the air are not trapped. Ulcers, cold sores, thrush, gum diseases, and tooth decay are among the most common mouth disorders. All of them, however, can be treated.

A serious mouth disorder is cleft palate, a birth defect in which the two halves of the mouth are not properly sealed. This problem can be corrected by surgery.

SEE ALSO

DIGESTIVE SYSTEM • GUM DISEASES • MOUTH DISEASES AND DISORDERS • RESPIRATORY SYSTEM • THROAT DISEASES AND DISORDERS • ULCERS

Mouth Diseases and Disorders

Most mouth disorders heal quickly. They may feel worse than they are; because the mouth has so many nerve endings, any swelling feels large and any slight injury bleeds a great deal.

Mouth infections are common. Viruses cause cold sores and ulcers; bacteria lead to tooth decay and gum infections; fungi cause the white-spotted ulcers of candida (thrush). Bacteria and viruses live in the mouth but do harm only when resistance is low. They multiply and may cause infections in other parts of the body or in a wound. Sometimes, the salivary glands under the mouth become infected and swollen. This problem may be caused by bacteria or by mumps. Pus from the glands can leak into the mouth, causing a salty taste. Salivary glands may swell when a tiny stone blocks the duct. This stone can be removed by surgery. Tumors can form in the glands; usually, but not always, they are harmless. Very rarely, benign or malignant tumors form in the mouth. Oral cancer can result from smoking. The risk of oral cancer increases with the number of cigarettes smoked and the number of years that the person has been smoking. If mouth ulcers last for a long time, a doctor's advice should be sought.

Q & A

My boyfriend says he caught a canker sore (mouth ulcer) from me. I was offended at first, but then I remembered that I did have one recently. Is it possible that my boyfriend is right and that he caught the canker sore from me?

Mouth ulcers are not contagious. Although many infections and diseases can be spread by kissing, most couples find that after a period of time together they develop an immunity to each other's germs.

Whenever I get anxious, I feel a prickling sensation in my lower lip and a cold sore comes up. Is there any connection between cold sores and stress and anxiety, or is it just a coincidence that they seem to go together?

Stress itself will not create a cold sore unless your body has learned to use such situations as a trigger. Cold sores are more likely to occur when you are run-down. This fact could account for the feeling of not being able to cope that accompanies anxiety in many people.

COMMON MOUTH DISORDERS		
CAUSES	SYMPTOMS	TREATMENTS
Cold sores	Herpes blisters on mouth and lips; may occur with common colds and in hot or cold weather	Consult doctor if cold sores are large and painful; apply acyclovir (Zovirax) cream early
Gingivitis	Bleeding and soreness of the gums, especially when teeth are brushed; bad breath; excess watering of the mouth	Consult dentist without delay
Halitosis (bad breath)	Causes include cigarette smoking, indigestion, appendicitis, and tooth decay	Treat at home; if problem persists (and always in cases of severe pain) consult doctor
Mouth ulcers	White or yellowish patches in mouth, surrounded by red, sore area; breath may be bad	Avoid acidic foods and chocolate; apply ointment containing choline salicylate or similar
Candida (thrush)	Ulcers covered with white spots in mouth	A doctor will prescribe antifungal ointment

SEE ALSO

BACTERIA • BACTERIAL DISEASES • CANCER • FUNGAL INFECTIONS • GLANDS • GUM DISEASES • MOUTH • MUMPS • THROAT DISEASES AND DISORDERS • ULCERS • VIRUSES

Multiple Sclerosis

Q & A

I've heard that multiple sclerosis is contagious. Is that true?

No. It is true that the illness is more common in temperate climates, but no one can explain this environmental factor. It is a fact that northern Europeans born and raised in the tropics are unlikely to get the disease. The place with the highest incidence of multiple sclerosis is the Orkneys in Scotland.

Is it possible to recover from a bad relapse in multiple sclerosis, or will it always leave disability?

Many people have had attacks that have given them temporary paralysis or other major symptoms from which they later recover. It is impossible to predict what is going to happen after an attack; sometimes there may be some residual disability, but in other cases the remission may be complete. Multiple sclerosis seldom affects two people in the same way.

People with multiple sclerosis can never know for certain how long their good periods will last, so they usually take full advantage of them and remain active whenever possible.

Multiple sclerosis (MS) is an illness that affects the central nervous system. It varies a great deal. Some people have it mildly, whereas others become severely disabled. As yet, no one knows what causes it or how to stop its development. Women are more likely than men to get MS, and it usually starts when people are in their twenties or thirties.

In MS, parts of the myelin sheath that protects nerve fibers become inflamed, affecting the nerves inside. The nerves affected are those that control physical sensation, coordination, and movement. People who have the disease feel weak and quickly get tired. They may have episodes, usually lasting for about six weeks, in which the vision in one eye is lost. A common symptom is tingling or numbness in the hands, arms, feet, and legs. As the illness gets worse, patients may lose control over their hands or limbs. They may not be able to walk or stand without help and will need to use a wheelchair. They may lose control of the bladder, and their speech may get slurred. The brain, however, will not be affected. Repeated episodes of visual loss lead to permanent impairment of vision.

Relapsing-remitting MS

Symptoms can last for days or weeks and then clear up for months or even years. An active period is known as a relapse; it is usually followed by remission (a period when the disease is inactive). The nervous system tries to heal itself by forming scar tissue. Patients often recover during remissions, but the level of recovery is likely to be lower after each severe attack. About

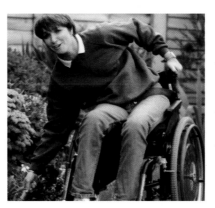

3 in 10 people with MS have chronic-progressive MS, in which the symptoms worsen without any remission. MS may be caused by an abnormal reaction to a common virus. Emotional stress can trigger a relapse. There is no known cure, although scientists hope to discover one.

SEE ALSO

MUSCLE • **NERVOUS SYSTEM** • **NERVOUS SYSTEM DISORDERS** • **PARALYSIS** • **VIRUSES**

Mumps

Mumps is an infectious disease caused by a virus. It is common in childhood, when it is usually quite mild. If an adult catches it, there may be painful complications.

Mumps is spread by droplets exhaled by an infected person. The first symptoms appear two to three weeks after infection. They include a slight fever, a sore throat, and shivering. The next unmistakable sign is a swelling of the parotid gland, the large salivary gland between the upper and lower jaws. Other salivary glands may be affected, and occasionally one side of the face swells and then the other. It may be painful to open the mouth and to eat. The patient may have a fever and the temperature may rise to 103°F (39.4°C). Swelling increases for two or three days and then dies down. The temperature falls, and the patient usually recovers completely within 10 days.

Other complications

Mumps is seldom serious, but the virus can cause complications. It can infect other glands, including the testicles, ovaries, prostate gland, mammary glands, and pancreas. Of these complications, the most usual, and one of the most serious, is inflammation of the testicles in adult males. This is extremely painful and in rare cases can lead to sterility. Mumps very occasionally causes mild meningitis, and even more rarely encephalitis. In a very few cases, these types of complications can lead to disability or even death.

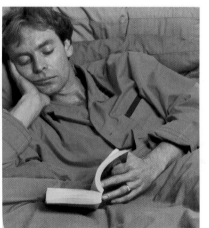

People with mumps should stay in bed and keep warm. They should drink fluids and eat bland food. One attack of mumps gives immunity for life. Many children are now immunized against mumps between the ages of 12 and 15 months.

Only a small percentage of adults catch mumps. Painful swelling in the glands is usually a symptom.

SEE ALSO

COMMUNICABLE DISEASES • ENCEPHALITIS • EPIDEMIC • GLANDS • IMMUNE SYSTEM • INFECTIOUS DISEASES • MENINGITIS • MOUTH • VIRUSES

Q & A

In severe mumps, can the salivary glands be permanently damaged?

No. The mumps virus causes a temporary inflammation of the salivary glands, which clears up completely with no long-lasting effects. In some rare cases, a bacterial inflammation follows mumps, and this can scar some of the saliva-producing cells. However, there are so many of these cells that it has little effect.

When my sister had mumps, she had terrible back pain. Was this a normal symptom?

Your sister may have had mild pancreatitis as a complication of mumps. The pancreas is on the back wall of the abdomen, and it causes back pain if inflamed. This would leave no harmful effects.

I was told mumps had affected only one of my salivary glands. Could I get mumps again?

No. Mumps quite often inflames only one salivary gland and leaves the others unaffected. Because you have had the mumps virus, you now have immunity for life.

Munchausen Syndrome

Q & A

A friend told me that there is a condition called pathomimicry. This must mean that some people pretend to be ill when they are not. Is this possible?

Yes. The condition is commonly known as Munchausen syndrome. People with this syndrome pretend that they are sick and will often even attempt to receive treatment by means of major surgery. The condition is very rare in the United States. It is more common in countries such as England that have a free health service.

Is it true that there is a condition called Munchausen syndrome by proxy? If so, what is it?

This condition is even more horrifying than the basic syndrome. In this variant, the claimed patient is a helpless child who is deliberately abused by his or her parent to produce symptoms that suggest serious illness. The parent aims for the child to receive treatment.

In Munchausen syndrome, doctors are persuaded to carry out routine medical investigations, such as blood tests, to identify some phantom illness.

In this rare disorder, repeated medical treatment is sought for nonexistent illnesses. It was first described in detail in 1951 by the distinguished British doctor and writer Richard Asher (1912–1969), in a paper in the medical journal *The Lancet*. Looking for a name for the syndrome, Asher recalled the set of tall tales attributed to a Hanoverian nobleman, Karl Friedrich Hieronymus, Baron von Münchhausen (1720–1797), reputed to be one of the great liars of all time. Since the publication of Asher's paper, Munchausen syndrome (now the accepted spelling) has become well known, and although it is rare, many cases have been described.

Symptoms and causes

Munchausen syndrome occurs more commonly in men and usually starts before middle age. Its main feature is a recurrent determination to seek unnecessary medical consultation and treatment. To achieve this, affected people pretend to be suffering from a variety of diseases, the more serious and dramatic the better. Their preference is for conditions requiring urgent surgery, and by careful study of medical textbooks, they are able to present a detailed history of the complaint, a convincing set of symptoms, and appropriate physical signs.

Such people deliberately add blood or sugar to a urine sample, inflict injuries on themselves, abrade their skin or use blistering materials to produce symptoms of dermatitis, or swallow foreign bodies. Some people take warfarin, which prevents blood from clotting and so simulates serious blood disorders. Others have bled themselves to the point of causing dangerous anemia.

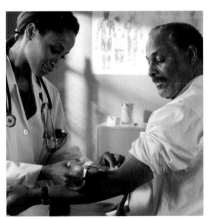

Many people with Munchausen syndrome bear numerous surgical scars. If the deception is discovered, they disappear immediately. People who inflict severe and dangerous injury on themselves to gain medical attention are mentally ill and require psychiatric treatment to deal with the underlying cause of their behavior.

SEE ALSO

ANEMIA • BLOOD DISEASES AND DISORDERS • DERMATITIS

Muscle

All the movements of the body, from the simple twitch of an eyebrow to performing a high jump, are made possible by the muscles. There are three different kinds of muscles: voluntary, involuntary, and cardiac.

Voluntary muscles are under the conscious control of the brain. They are the muscles that are used when a person decides to carry out an action, such as raising an arm, turning the page of a book, smiling, or frowning. This type of muscle is also called striated (striped) muscle, because it looks striped under a microscope. Voluntary muscles are attached to the bones by ligaments and work in pairs to move the bones. Signals from the brain are carried to the muscles by nerves. When a person wants to raise an arm, for example, chemicals are released that make one muscle contract and pull up the arm. The other muscle of the pair relaxes. Voluntary muscles are often subject to injury, but they can self-repair. Sometimes, if one muscle has been damaged, another muscle will grow larger to compensate for the weakened muscle.

Involuntary muscles control all the things that the body does automatically and unconsciously, such as the working of the digestive system and the bladder. They are also called smooth

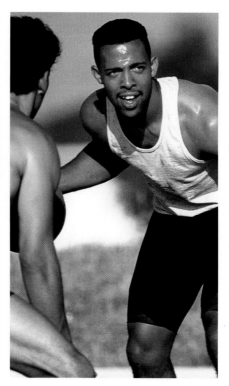

muscles, because they appear unstriped under a microscope. They contract slowly and rhythmically. These muscles may be stimulated by nerves, but some of the chemicals in the body, called hormones, can also control them.

Cardiac muscles make up the main bulk of the heart. Under a

A basketball player uses hundreds of voluntary muscles, unconscious of the hard work being done by his involuntary muscles and heart muscle. Good muscle tone and strength are achieved through regular training.

Q & A

My brother tore a leg muscle playing football, and he's extremely worried about whether or not he will still be able to play. Will this muscle injury trouble him in the future?

The best way to avoid trouble later on is to gradually build up strength in the injured leg, exercising and training carefully for the first two to three weeks after injury until he can do things without pain in the leg muscle. The tendency of recurrent injury to the same muscle is much greater if people rush back to being fully active.

What happens physically to a muscle as it is built up and strengthened?

Adults do not increase the number of fibers in a muscle as they train it; the muscle grows bigger and stronger through an increase in the size of each individual muscle fiber. Whether children can make more muscle fibers by exercise or whether the number of fibers is set by genetic makeup is unclear.

microscope, they look similar to voluntary muscles. They are controlled by a regulating device in the heart itself, and there is no conscious control over this kind of muscle.

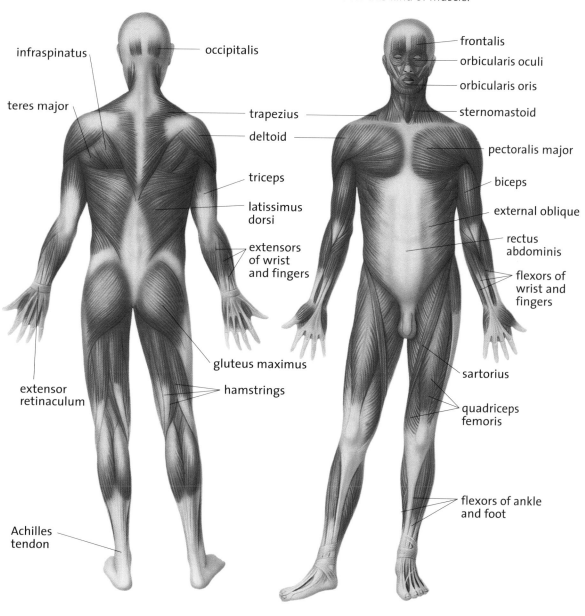

infraspinatus

teres major

occipitalis

frontalis

orbicularis oculi

orbicularis oris

sternomastoid

trapezius

deltoid

triceps

latissimus dorsi

extensors of wrist and fingers

pectoralis major

biceps

external oblique

rectus abdominis

flexors of wrist and fingers

extensor retinaculum

gluteus maximus

hamstrings

sartorius

quadriceps femoris

flexors of ankle and foot

Achilles tendon

These diagrams show front and back views of some of the main voluntary muscles that are located throughout the body.

SEE ALSO

BONE • BRAIN • HEART • MUSCLE DISEASES AND DISORDERS • SPORTS INJURIES • SPRAINS AND STRAINS • WHIPLASH INJURY

Muscle Diseases and Disorders

The most common muscle problems are caused by injuries, which often happen to people who take part in active sports. Pulled, strained, and torn muscles are all the same type of injury.

Muscle injuries

Tearing of the muscle fibers and bleeding inside the muscle cause pain and swelling. This kind of injury usually heals quickly, particularly in young people. Treatment usually consists of resting the muscle as much as possible to give it time to knit together and bandaging it for support. When the pain and swelling have gone down, the muscle can gradually be exercised back into use. If any injury remains swollen and painful for more than a few days, a doctor should be consulted.

Sometimes, the whole muscle is torn, or ruptured. This condition is extremely painful, and the muscle will need to be stitched together again. Occasionally, a torn muscle causes bleeding in the muscle and the formation of a blood clot, which is removed surgically.

Muscle cramps and myositis

A cramp is the painful tightening of a muscle or group of muscles. It occurs most commonly in the leg muscles, particularly in the calf. A cramp can come on suddenly, sometimes when a person is asleep. The muscle fibers contract into a hard knot during the spasm, which can last from a few seconds up to a couple of minutes. A cramp can be caused by poor circulation and by exposure to cold. Heavy sweating due to vigorous exercise in a hot climate can deplete the body of salt, causing a cramp. Young people and others engaging in sports should avoid eating just before physical exertion, because the blood is concentrated around the intestines and away from the muscles during digestion, so a cramp may result. Swimmers are particularly at risk. An attack of cramp can be eased by massaging the affected muscle. Flexing the foot upward or manually lifting the toes helps to relieve leg and foot cramp.

Inflammation of the muscle sheaths is known as myositis. It can be caused by cold, by excess exercise, or by an

Q & A

I strained my thigh muscle last week. The doctor now says I have fibrositis. How did this problem happen?

The strain that affected the muscle has caused inflammation within the muscle, which can be termed fibrositis. More accurately, it might be called fibromyositis—*myositis* implying that the inflammation of fibrous tissue is in the muscle. In time, the injury should heal and the inflammation will die down.

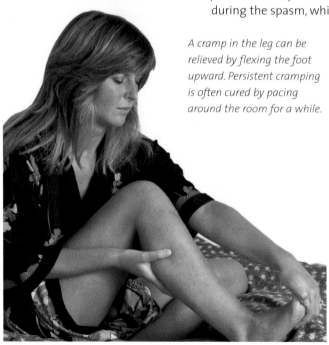

A cramp in the leg can be relieved by flexing the foot upward. Persistent cramping is often cured by pacing around the room for a while.

MUSCLE DISORDERS

Disorder	Causes	Symptoms	Treatments
Pulls, tears, strains, and sprains	Tearing of the muscle fibers, followed by bleeding in and swelling of the affected muscle	Pain, which may become worse during the first few days after original injury; limited movement	Cold (ice packs, water) and pressure with bandages help immediately; later, gentle muscle movement; heat treatment may help
Cramp	Muscle goes into spasm; dehydration may be a cause	Painful tightening of the muscles, often in the calf	Quinine may help; salt and water replacement are vital when dehydration is the cause
Polymyalgia rheumatica	Inflammation of the blood vessels supplying blood to the muscles	Pain, often around the neck and shoulders, and ill-health; affects only the elderly	Anti-inflammatory drugs
Myositis	Painful inflammation of the muscles, often with associated conditions; can be caused by infection	Pain and weakness; blood tests may show that muscle tissue is being broken down	Treatment depends on the cause; rest alone will improve many types, but steroid tablets may help
Muscular dystrophy	Inherited abnormalities in the working of muscle cells	Progressive weakness of muscles affecting different areas according to the form of muscular dystrophy	None, but splints and other aids can be of considerable value
Hypokalemic paralysis	Low level of potassium in blood	Periodic attacks of paralysis	Requires expert medical attention
Hyperkalemic paralysis	High level of potassium in blood	Periodic attacks of paralysis	Requires expert medical attention

PULLED MUSCLES

A muscle can be pulled, strained, or overstretched in an accident or during exercise. The main symptom is pain. The type of injury varies. For example, dropping a heavy load can cause a sudden, sharp movement or moment of acute tension in a particular muscle. Attempting to lift something that is too heavy, or lifting awkwardly or incorrectly, can also cause a pulled muscle. A powerful movement that twists a part of the body into an unnatural position, as often occurs in basketball, may also stretch muscles beyond their natural limit.

infection. Rubbing the area with liniment and taking mild painkillers can ease the pain.

Causes of diseases and disorders

Diseases affecting the muscles are relatively rare. Most muscle weaknesses are caused indirectly: for example, by a problem occurring in the nervous system, which controls the movement of the muscles. Lou Gehrig's disease is this type of disorder or motor neuron disease. Occasionally, a hormonal condition or a lack of vitamin D can result in a weakening of the muscles. Other serious muscle disorders, such as muscular dystrophy, are inherited.

SEE ALSO

MOTOR NEURON DISEASE • MUSCLE • MUSCULAR DYSTROPHY • NERVOUS SYSTEM • PARALYSIS • SPORTS INJURIES • SPRAINS AND STRAINS

Muscular Dystrophy

Q & A

My brother has Duchenne muscular dystrophy, and I'm worried that I might be a carrier. Is that possible?

As a sibling of an affected person, you have a 50 percent chance of being a carrier. You will have to have a blood test for an enzyme called creatine phosphokinase (CPK). This enzyme is released from the muscles into the blood and is present at a raised level in those people who carry Duchenne muscular dystrophy.

My cousin has muscle weakness and was diagnosed as having muscular dystrophy. Our grandmother thinks the diagnosis was wrong and that the weakness will just go away. Is it possible that my grandmother is right?

It is unusual to find muscle weakness in children. When such a problem occurs, muscular dystrophy is a common cause. This, together with positive blood tests, suggests that it is unlikely that the diagnosis is wrong. Your cousin's weakness will not just go away.

Muscular dystrophy is the name given to a group of disorders that produce weakness in the muscles themselves. There are about 20 different types of muscular dystrophies. Three of the disorders are caused by inheriting an abnormal gene. If the affected muscle cells are examined under a microscope, it can be seen that they are being destroyed.

The most severe form, which is also one of the most common, is Duchenne muscular dystrophy. It affects mainly males, and females can be carriers of the disorder; the abnormal gene that causes the disease is carried on the X sex chromosome. Because women have two X chromosomes, the unaffected chromosome cancels out the disorder. However, men have just one X and one Y sex chromosome; thus, they will have the disease if they inherit the abnormal gene.

Symptoms

The first symptoms are a weakness of the thighs and the muscles of the pelvis, which leads to difficulty in standing, walking, and climbing. The weakness usually becomes noticeable between the ages of two and seven, although it can appear even before the child can walk. Later, the condition affects the muscles of the neck, shoulders, and back. The spine may eventually become deformed, and there may be difficulty in breathing. The heart muscle may become involved, too. Most people with Duchenne dystrophy die before the age of 20.

A similar condition, called Becker muscular dystrophy, usually begins after the age of 10 and is much less severe. The other fairly common forms of muscular dystrophy—Landouzy-Dejerine dystrophy and myotonic dystrophy—affect both men and women and can be mild or disabling.

Treatment

There is no known way of stopping the progress of these conditions. Treatment usually consists of exercises to keep the unaffected muscles functioning as well as possible. Anyone with a family history of muscular dystrophy should get advice from a genetic counselor before starting a family. Blood tests show when a woman is a carrier of Duchenne dystrophy; if a carrier has a son, there is a 50 percent chance that he will have the disease.

SEE ALSO

CELLS AND CHROMOSOMES • GENES • GENETIC DISEASES AND DISORDERS • MUSCLE • MUSCLE DISEASES AND DISORDERS

Nervous System

The nervous system is the body's complex communications and control network. It collects information around the body through the senses of sight, hearing, taste, smell, and touch, and then it tells the body what to do in response. The nervous system consists of millions of interconnected nerve cells called neurons; they pick up information and send signals from one part of the system to another. Neurons are easily damaged or destroyed by injury, infection, pressure, chemical disturbance, or lack of oxygen.

The nervous system consists of the peripheral nervous system and the central nervous system. The central nervous system consists of the brain and the spinal cord. Together they receive messages from the body's sense organs, analyze them, and then send out signals to the muscles and glands. Thousands of neurons are involved in the brain during this assessment. The peripheral nervous system consists of all the nerve tissue outside the central nervous system. Nerves branch out from the brain and spinal cord and then divide to supply the body. The peripheral nervous system consists of an outer system (the somatic or body system) and an inner one (the autonomic system).

The somatic system collects information from the body's sense organs and conveys it to the central nervous system along sensory nerve fibers. It carries signals from the central nervous system to the muscles along motor nerve fibers, which are gathered into a bundle called a nerve. Forty-three pairs of nerves emerge from the central nervous system. Twelve pairs come from the brain; the rest of them come from the spinal cord.

The autonomic nervous system controls unconscious functions, such as the heartbeat, the narrowing and widening of blood vessels, breathing, and gland secretion. Autonomic control becomes extremely active in times of sudden physical danger and modifies body function to give the body the best chance of survival.

Each neuron has the same basic structure, but neurons are of various shapes and sizes. Each neuron cell has a number of fine, rootlike fibers, or dendrites, projecting from it. Projecting from the cell is a single, long fiber called an axon. At its far end, the axon either ends in a single tiny knob or divides into a number of branches, ending in a cluster of knobs. Each knob is separated by a minute gap from a dendrite, from another neuron, or from the surface of a muscle cell or a gland cell. Messages are carried across these gaps by substances called neurotransmitters. Every neuron has a thin wall known as the neural membrane, which is vital for the transmission of signals. Many axons have an insulating covering called myelin.

Q & A

A friend said the pain I have in my hands and arms could be caused by a pinched nerve. What is this?

At some point along their length, many nerves have to pass through a restricted space, especially near joints. Any displacement or swelling in this space may squeeze or pinch the nerve, causing pain, muscle weakness, numbness, or a tingling sensation.

Two months ago, my grandfather had a foot amputated. I'm extremely confused because he still feels that the foot is there and even has pain from the missing toes. Why does this happen?

Although his foot has been amputated, the sensory fibers that used to send messages from the foot to the brain are still present in the remaining part of his leg and have their endings in the stump. If these endings are stimulated, the fibers send messages via the spinal cord to the brain, which, from past experience, interprets the message as having come from the foot.

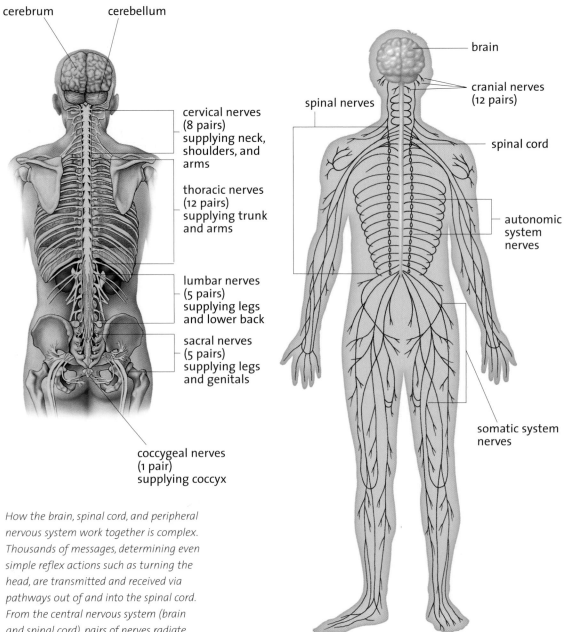

cerebrum

cerebellum

brain

cervical nerves
(8 pairs)
supplying neck,
shoulders, and
arms

thoracic nerves
(12 pairs)
supplying trunk
and arms

lumbar nerves
(5 pairs)
supplying legs
and lower back

sacral nerves
(5 pairs)
supplying legs
and genitals

coccygeal nerves
(1 pair)
supplying coccyx

spinal nerves

cranial nerves
(12 pairs)

spinal cord

autonomic
system
nerves

somatic system
nerves

*How the brain, spinal cord, and peripheral
nervous system work together is complex.
Thousands of messages, determining even
simple reflex actions such as turning the
head, are transmitted and received via
pathways out of and into the spinal cord.
From the central nervous system (brain
and spinal cord), pairs of nerves radiate
all over the body, forming the peripheral
system. This system has two main
subdivisions: the autonomic system
(unconscious control of functions such
as breathing) and the somatic system
(conscious control).*

SEE ALSO

BODY SYSTEMS • BRAIN • CELLS AND CHROMOSOMES • MOTOR
NEURON DISEASE • MULTIPLE SCLEROSIS • MUSCLE • NERVOUS
SYSTEM DISORDERS

Nervous System Disorders

Q & A

My mother suffers from epilepsy. Is it possible that I inherited the condition, too?

Epilepsy does sometimes run in families, but your chances of being affected are only slightly increased—perhaps about five times the national average.

My grandmother had meningitis two years ago. Is it likely to recur?

When she first had the condition, the doctors would have checked carefully for a predisposing cause. If they had found one, they would have told your grandmother and tried to treat it, so she is unlikely to catch it again.

My father sometimes has severe neuralgic pain in his left cheek, but it has recently begun to occur more often. What could be the cause?

It may be that your father is in the early stages of facial neuralgia, or perhaps he has a chronic infection in a tooth or sinus. He should see his doctor so the cause can be established and treatment can be started promptly.

The nervous system is made up of billions of cells called neurons. As the body ages, many neurons wear out, and unlike tissue cells, neurons cannot be replaced. Some of the functions neurons control are therefore affected.

Damage and infection can cause neuritis (inflammation of the neurons) and neuralgia (pain along a nerve path). Symptoms indicating that neurons are not working properly include numbness, loss of physical coordination or balance, dizziness or loss of consciousness, visual problems that cannot be corrected with eyeglasses, inability to find the right words, and acute pain that is unconnected with other symptoms. Anyone who has any of these symptoms should see a doctor.

Stroke

One of the most common disorders of the nervous system is a stroke, when the blood supply to one part of the brain is completely blocked off. Neurons in the brain die quickly, and as a result, some of the functions of the body are affected. Sometimes, other brain cells can take control of these functions. In other cases, nothing can be done.

Injuries and infections

Many nervous system problems are the result of injury. For example, damage to the brain can cause cerebral palsy. Damage to the spinal cord can cause paralysis, the extent of which depends on the injury site. Brain and spinal tumors can press on or invade nerve tissues. Sciatica and spondylosis are caused by pressure or pinching of a nerve. In Ménière's disease, fluid builds up in the ear, pressing on nerve cells. Mild and brief pressure on a nerve can cause pins and needles.

Nervous system infections are not common but they are serious. They can infect the brain, the spinal cord, or the nerves coming from these areas. Infections include meningitis, encephalitis, poliomyelitis, and, less seriously, shingles. Ménière's disease may be caused by infection, but this is not the usual cause (which remains unknown). Some problems are caused by functional disorders. They include epilepsy, migraine, headache, and tics. Other problems, such as Parkinson's disease, dementia, and Lou Gehrig's disease, are the result of neuron degeneration. Multiple sclerosis is caused by inflammation of the myelin sheaths around the nerves.

Long-term heavy drinkers can permanently reduce the ability of the nerve cells to pass signals. Heavy drinking speeds up the rate at which brain nerve cells die, and mental function progressively worsens.

SOME DISEASES OF THE NERVOUS SYSTEM

Disease	Symptoms	Treatments
Brain tumor	Personality change, progressive paralysis	Surgical removal of tumor, radiotherapy
Dementia	Memory loss, inability to concentrate, confusion, loss of interest, untidiness	No cure, except when a specific cause for the condition is known
Epilepsy	Convulsive fits or temporary loss of consciousness	Anticonvulsant drugs
Ménière's disease	Ringing in the ear, giddiness, nausea, vomiting	Antinausea and vasodilator drugs; fluid-drainage drugs
Meningitis	Fever, headaches, neck and back muscle spasms, intolerance of bright lights, convulsions, vomiting, drowsiness	Antibiotic drugs for bacterial meningitis; analgesics and bed rest for viral meningitis
Multiple sclerosis	Weakness in one or more limbs, numbness, pins and needles, visual disturbances, walking difficulties; symptoms vary, may improve for a time and then reappear	No cure; various drugs may cause remission
Neuritis	Numbness, pain, pins and needles, muscle weakness	Underlying cause treated
Parkinson's disease	Tremors, uncoordinated movements, facial rigidity	Anti-Parkinsonian drugs
Poliomyelitis	Headaches, spinal pains, stiff neck, followed by fever, muscle weakness, and paralysis	Prevention through vaccination during childhood
Sciatica	Back and leg pain along course of sciatic nerve	Spinal manipulation, painkilling drugs; surgery when due to slipped disk
Shingles	Fever, pain, skin blistering along the course of affected nerve fibers	Acyclovir (Zovirax) for skin blisters, analgesic drugs for pain and fever
Spastic paralysis	Spasms, partial paralysis, lack of coordination, uncontrolled movements	No cure; special education to make best use of unaffected areas of brain
Stroke	Effects depend on area of brain affected; partial paralysis, speech impairment, severe headaches, visual disturbance, deafness; sometimes fatal	Anticoagulants to help prevent blood clotting; surgery to remove clots or seal any weak blood vessels
Trigeminal neuralgia	Severe pain in the side of face lasting for about a minute; recurs every few hours, days, or weeks	Drugs, surgery to destroy trigeminal nerve or allow more room for nerve
Vestibular neuronitis	Vertigo, vomiting, uncontrolled eye movements	Treatment with drugs

SEE ALSO

CELLS AND CHROMOSOMES • CEREBRAL PALSY • ENCEPHALITIS • EPILEPSY • MENINGITIS • MOTOR NEURON DISEASE • MULTIPLE SCLEROSIS • NERVOUS SYSTEM • PARALYSIS • PARKINSON'S DISEASE • SCIATICA • SHINGLES • STROKE

Nonspecific Urethritis

Q & A

What is the difference between urinary tract infections and urethritis?

Urethritis is an infection specifically of the urethra. A urinary tract infection (UTI) is an infection anywhere in the urinary tract. The main symptom of urethritis is dysuria (painful or difficult urination). Other symptoms include a stinging or burning sensation during urination, itching, redness, and discharge. Symptoms of UTIs depend on the location of the infection. Infections of the kidney (nephritis) include back pain and high fever. Cystitis or bladder infections can cause abdominal pain.

Is nonspecific urethritis caused only by sexual contact?

Any situation in which bacterial germs are introduced to the body can cause illness. Germs responsible for sexually transmitted urethritis include *Neisseria gonorrhoeae* and *Chlamydia trachomatis*. Nonspecific urethritis can be caused by other germs, including *Mycoplasma genitalium*, herpes simplex, and adenovirus.

Urethritis is an inflammation of the urethra, the tube that carries urine from the bladder to be excreted. Bacteriological researchers discovered that the majority of cases of urethritis were caused by *Neisseria gonorrhoeae*, the organism responsible for gonorrhea. However, in a small proportion of cases with similar symptoms, this organism could not be found, and the urethritis was said to be nonspecific, because the cause was unknown. The term *nonspecific urethritis* has been falling into disuse, because it is now known that these cases of urethral inflammation are caused by the bacterium *Chlamydia trachomatis* and by the mycoplasma (primitive microorganism) *Ureaplasma urealyticum*.

Symptoms
Nonspecific urethritis (NSU) is a sexually transmitted disease that shows itself one to four weeks after intercourse. There is discomfort or mild pain on urination, some staining discharge that may be clear or whitish, some redness at the outlet of the urethra, and sometimes a temporary blockage of the external orifice. These symptoms may be much more acute. The symptoms are usually more obvious in men than in women, who may have no initial symptoms. In many cases, however, women have a need for frequent and uncomfortable urination, a changed vaginal discharge, a sore throat, and pain and discomfort during sexual intercourse. Because NSU is often symptomless in women, it has become extremely common, especially among sexually promiscuous young people.

Complications
In women, NSU may eventually spread to other organs, causing more generalized pelvic inflammatory disease (PID), the most common chlamydial infection in the Western world. PID may include inflammation of the fallopian tubes (salpingitis) of such severity as to lead to total blockage and sterility. It may also cause painful inflammation and abscess or cyst formation in the Bartholin glands (mucus-secreting lubricating structures at the mouth of the vagina). In men, NSU can lead to narrowing of the urethra so that urination becomes difficult; inflammation of the epididymis, a structure connected to the testicle; and Reiter's syndrome. This complication of NSU causes arthritis in several joints and a potentially sight-damaging eye inflammation.

SEE ALSO

BACTERIA • GLANDS • GONORRHEA • PELVIC INFLAMMATORY DISEASE • SEXUALLY TRANSMITTED DISEASES

Nosebleed

A nosebleed is caused by the breaking of a small blood vessel inside the nose. It may be the result of direct violence, injury, sneezing, or picking the nose. Some people have a nosebleed when they have an attack of hay fever or have a nasal infection. If the membranes lining the nose become dry and cracked, bleeding may occur. Sometimes, there is no obvious reason for it. Girls who have recently started to menstruate often have nosebleeds with no apparent cause.

A broken nose, one of the most common sports injuries, often results in a nosebleed and requires immediate medical attention. Almost invariably, a broken nose will be out of shape. If it is allowed to heal without being reset by a surgeon, it will lead in most cases to other problems, such as chronic runny nose or sinusitis (inflammation of a sinus).

First aid for a nosebleed

The person with a nosebleed should sit quietly, loosen the clothes around the neck, and lean his or her head slightly forward (not back) to help prevent any blood from being swallowed. He or she should pinch together the nostrils until the bleeding stops, while breathing gently through the mouth. If bleeding continues, a small, clean piece of gauze should be inserted just inside one or both nostrils, which should then be pressed together. It is important not to force anything up the nose. When the bleeding stops, it is important that the patient does not keep touching the nose. If bleeding does not stop, a doctor should be consulted or the patient should be taken to a hospital.

Serious nosebleeds

Sometimes, an artery at the back of the nose is damaged, causing extremely heavy bleeding. That situation needs treatment by a doctor, who will pack the nose. Other nosebleeds also need attention from a doctor: those caused by a blow, those that happen within a week or so of a tonsil or adenoid operation, and those lasting for more than about 20 minutes. Otherwise, home treatment is usually sufficient.

Although nosebleeds can often be alarming, not much blood is lost, even during a heavy nosebleed. Normally, a nosebleed clears up in five to 15 minutes, which is the time it usually takes for blood to clot.

SEE ALSO
ARTERY • BLOOD • CIRCULATORY SYSTEM • SPORTS INJURIES

Q & A

I've heard that a nosebleed is a sign of pressure on the brain. My brother has had several nosebleeds recently. Is this serious?

Nosebleeds are common in children, perhaps because they are so active and thus are likely to have many minor injuries. Some children are more prone to nosebleeds than others. A frequent cause is that blood vessels just inside one or both nostrils have burst, after becoming weakened and enlarged through rubbing and picking, or because of previous nosebleeds. Pressure on the brain is not a cause. However, recurrent bleeding can be a symptom of disease, so your parents should consult your brother's doctor.

My grandmother used to put a cloth soaked in witch hazel across my nose when it bled. Is this an effective cure?

Although some herbs may have properties that help stem the flow of blood, it is more likely that your grandmother's treatment acted as an effective cold compress.

Nutritional Diseases

The body can work properly only if it receives the right materials, including certain vitamins and minerals. Without them, people develop diseases such as scurvy and rickets. In the past, although it was known how to prevent certain diseases, it was not known what the causes were. Experts are now learning more about the substances the body needs. In developed countries, few people suffer from deficiency diseases. However, in some countries in the developing world where people have an inadequate diet, there is a serious problem.

Sometimes, people do not eat properly because they cannot get enough food. Others do not know what to eat or do not eat sensibly. Alcoholics often get deficiency diseases, for example, because they do not eat properly and do not absorb fats and vitamins. Beriberi (degenerative changes of the nerves, digestive system, and the heart) is caused by lack of vitamin B_1 (thiamine). However, most deficiency diseases are easy to cure with a proper diet. The diet may be supplemented with large doses of the substance that has been lacking.

A few people have nutritional diseases even though they are eating properly, because their bodies are unable to take in or use certain substances properly. For example, some people become anemic because their bodies cannot absorb vitamin B_{12}. If people eat sensibly, they should get everything they need from their food. Vitamin and mineral supplements should be taken only if a doctor prescribes them, because too many vitamins can be harmful.

CONDITIONS CAUSED BY NUTRITIONAL DEFICIENCY

VITAMIN OR MINERAL DEFICIENCY	DISEASES AND DISORDERS	DEFICIENCY CORRECTED BY
Vitamin A	Skin diseases, severe conjunctivitis, night blindness	Dairy products, eggs, liver, oily fish, vegetables (especially carrots)
Vitamin B_1 (thiamine)	Beriberi (weakness, swelling), confusion, heart failure	Bran, cereals, pork, liver
Vitamin B (niacin)	Pellagra (a skin disorder), diarrhea, dementia, dermatitis with skin blistering	Liver, kidney, yeast, fish, cereals
Vitamin C	Scurvy, slow wound healing, anemia, hemorrhages from tooth sockets and into joints	Fresh fruits and vegetables
Vitamin D	Disorders of bone formation leading to swelling, softening, and bowing of bones (called osteomalacia in adults and rickets in children)	Milk, egg yolk, cod liver oil, fortified milk and margarine, action of sunlight on skin
Iron	Anemia	Lean meat, liver, spinach, cabbage, legumes, eggs
Sodium	Disturbances of body chemistry	Salt
Iodine	Goiter (swelling of thyroid gland), cretinism	Seafood

SEE ALSO

ANEMIA • ANOREXIA AND BULIMIA • BONE • DIGESTIVE SYSTEM • HEART • MALNUTRITION • RICKETS • SCURVY

Obesity

If the amount of food people eat exceeds the energy used, they will become overweight. If a person's weight is 20 percent or more above normal for his or her height and age, there will be an accumulation of body fat and the person will be obese. Obesity can be prevented by sensible eating and by exercise. It can be cured by dieting and then eating carefully. This is not easy, but it is worth doing. Obesity is a serious condition, because it increases the risk of developing various chronic health problems.

Causes

The amount of food someone's body uses varies a great deal from one person to another, but if a person is gaining weight, he or she is eating more than is needed. The excess food is converted into fat that is stored under the skin, first in cells in the buttocks and around the waist, and later in the thighs, shoulders, and arms.

Very rarely, a medical problem such as an underactive thyroid gland causes obesity by greatly reducing energy expenditure. Medical tests will find out if there is any such cause. Bad eating habits are the most common cause of obesity. Often, all the members of a family are obese, because they have similar habits. Emotional problems can make people overeat for comfort.

Dangers and treatments

Extra weight puts strain on the joints, particularly the knees, hips, and some of the back joints. It causes wear and tear, which may become a painful problem. Someone with a very fat stomach cannot breathe properly, and he or she will have shortness of breath and lung problems. Obesity can cause gallstones; mild

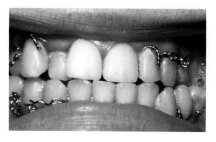

diabetes, in turn causing serious complications in the small blood vessels of the eyes and kidneys; thickening of the arteries, which increases the likelihood of suffering a stroke or heart attack; and high blood pressure.

Q & A

My friend eats the same amount as I do, is about the same height as I am, but is of average weight, whereas I am fat. Why is this?

The way in which people's bodies use food varies widely. People who use their food fuel economically become obese more easily than those who use it extravagantly, because they burn off less energy for the same amount of work. You may also find that you are getting less exercise than your friend, so that you are expending less energy. Finally, you may have acquired an excess of fat as a child, so that even if you eat the same as your friend, you are still not losing your excess stored fat.

Is it true that gland trouble can cause obesity?

People are rarely overweight because of an underactive thyroid gland or overactive adrenal glands, and in these cases, there are other symptoms.

This woman has resorted to desperate measures to help reduce her weight. She has had her teeth wired so that her jaws are clamped together. She can consume liquids only.

SEE ALSO

CIRCULATORY SYSTEM DISEASES AND DISORDERS • DIABETES • GALLBLADDER AND GALLSTONES • HEART DISEASES AND DISORDERS • JOINT DISORDERS • OSTEOARTHRITIS

Obsessive-Compulsive Disorder

Q & A

What is the difference between an obsession and a compulsion?

An obsession is a thought or feeling that keeps recurring over long periods of time. It is an idea that you cannot get out of your mind however much you may try, even though it has little real relevance to your present life. A compulsion is a constant or repeated conviction that you have to do something, often something that you have already done and, rationally, have no need to do over again. Some compulsions, such as repeatedly checking that you have locked a door or washed your hands, are especially common.

An obsessive-compulsive disorder involves carrying out a particular act and then repeating it to the point of obsession. Excessive hand washing, even when the hands are clean, is a common example. Returning home several times to check that all the doors are locked, even when the person knows that they are, may be another example. At the beginning, the thought behind the action may have been a sensible one—to prevent burglars from entering the house. However, the behavior of someone suffering from obsessive-compulsive neurosis begins to interfere with normal daily life.

Obsessive-compulsive disorder tends to run in families, but this is probably not because of a genetic cause. Obsessional mothers may condition their children to similar behavior through social learning; it is known that the children of such mothers are more likely than average to show neurotic symptoms. These disorders often begin during a stressful period, but they are not associated with any particular form of stress.

Complexes and compulsions

In psychology, a complex is a set of strongly linked memories. They are often frightening and have their origin in childhood, when the world is usually a more fearsome place.

If these complexes last into adulthood, they may eventually produce compulsive behavior, which is an attempt to relieve the buildup of anxiety that is the result of the complex. However, compulsions can be removed, and complexes can be treated by psychotherapy.

Treatment

Obsessive-compulsive disorder can be treated. A method that works for some people is systematic desensitization, usually in a clinic. The patient is taught simple exercises that relax the body and the mind and is encouraged to conjure up a relaxing situation, such as lying on a beach in the sun. This approach reduces tension. The person then re-creates the compulsive behavior either in real life or in the imagination and, instead of carrying out the action, summons up the fantasy situation. As a result, anxiety decreases, and the urge to carry out the compulsive pattern disappears.

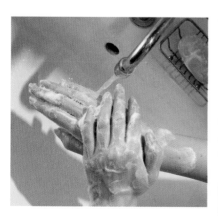

Repeated hand washing is a common example of obsessive-compulsive behavior.

> **SEE ALSO**
>
> BACTERIA • BACTERIAL DISEASES • COMMUNICABLE DISEASES • GENETIC DISEASES AND DISORDERS • INFECTIOUS DISEASES • VIRUSES

Osteoarthritis

The term *osteoarthritis* is misleading. The ending *itis* means inflammation, but this is not essentially an inflammatory disorder, and the basic features of the disease do not include inflammation. Osteoarthritis is the most common form of arthritis and, to a minor extent, affects the weight-bearing joints of nearly everyone over the age of 40. Among people over 45, 10 to 15 percent suffer some pain from osteoarthritis of the knee. In the United States, at least 10 million people have osteoarthritis of one or both knees to a degree that causes pain and disability.

Cause

The cause of osteoarthritis remains uncertain. It was widely believed that osteoarthritis was simply a wearing-out disorder due to weight-bearing damage from constant use. However, although the disease is certainly worse in people who are overweight and is associated with occupations involving joint trauma, there has never been convincing evidence that wear and tear is the principal cause. Recent research has shown that there is a definite genetic element in the causation of osteoarthritis. Studies of identical twins show that if one twin has obvious osteoarthritis, the other is likely to have it to a similar degree. In fraternal twins, the correlation is much less.

Joint trauma certainly has a part to play in osteoarthritis. The condition commonly affects a joint that has had a previous injury and occurs in joints that have been overused. Osteoarthritis is also strongly related to excessive joint pressure as a result of obesity and is known to occur in any condition in which there is a change in the physical relationship of the bone ends forming the joint. This is common in people with congenital bone deformities, bowlegs, or knock-knees. It has been recorded in those who have suffered from rickets, have had a joint infection, or have suffered damage to the nerve supply of the joint. Osteoarthritis is also more likely to occur in people with other joint diseases, such as gout or rheumatoid arthritis.

Symptoms

The first indication is pain, which is usually made worse by bending the joint. Joint stiffness after resting is common, but at first this is relieved by movement. Progression of the condition is slow and gradual, with progressive reduction in the range through which the affected joints can be moved. This may lead to permanent shortening of the muscles that move the joint, so that the affected joint cannot be fully straightened. This is called flexion contracture. At the same time, joint movement will probably cause a grating sensation, and pressure over parts

Q & A

I always thought that exercise was good for you until I read that professional football players often suffer from osteoarthritis. Is football unhealthy?

Aerobic movement that works the large muscle groups (such as the legs) is very good for you; repeated stresses and shocks to your joints are not. So, although exercise is good for you, repeated injuries are not and may cause osteoarthritis. Football players often have a form of arthritis in the middle bones of the foot—probably because of repeated small injuries.

My grandmother says that women are more likely to get osteoarthritis than men are. Is she right?

Osteoarthritis is a disease that particularly affects the elderly. Because women tend to live to a greater age than men, more women appear to suffer from the condition. However, in younger age groups, men and women are almost equally affected—and the condition may even be slightly more common in younger men.

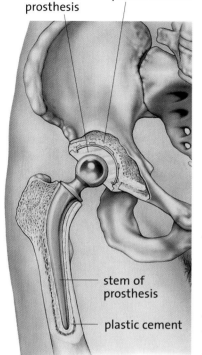

acetabular prosthesis

plastic cement

stem of prosthesis

plastic cement

In severe cases, the hip joint can be replaced with a prosthetic ball and stem.

of the joint may cause some pain. Once the disease is fully developed, affected joints will show enlargement from increased growth of bone, cartilage, ligaments, lining membrane (synovial membrane), and outer capsule. Bone overgrowth is an important feature of the disease and can, in itself, cause problems.

In the later stages of osteoarthritis of hip and knee joints, limitation and pain may be severe. Tendon overgrowth at the knee joint can cause instability and even dislocation. Sometimes, an osteoarthritic knee joint locks, because small pieces of bone or cartilage interfere with movement. In advanced cases, the muscles around the joint often go into painful spasm.

In osteoarthritis of the spine, bone overgrowth (known as osteophyte formation) can press on the spinal cord, causing neurological symptoms, including numbness and weakness. In the neck area, two arteries that provide blood supply to the brain may also be compressed by osteophytes.

In osteoarthritis of the hands, painful, small, bony lumps known as Heberden's nodes may appear on the fingers. The pain soon disappears, but the nodes remain.

Treatment

Treatment of osteoarthritis includes pain control, rehabilitation, a full range of physical activity, maintenance of maximum fitness, and prevention of further deterioration. If the patient is overweight, the first step is weight reduction, which relieves the symptoms. A program of daily exercises designed to improve general health and increase the range of movement of affected joints must be set up. Exercising is alternated with rest to allow for relubrication of the cartilage in the joints. Physical therapy helps maintain good posture, and the patient is taught to sit properly. Someone with osteoarthritis must avoid slumping into a soft armchair and should sleep on a firm mattress. Such a program can halt the progress of the disease and to some extent reverse its severity, especially when the hips and knees are affected. Uncorrected immobilization can speed the progress and worsen the outlook. Osteoarthritis is helped little by drugs, because there is neither inflammation nor infection, but drugs can help relieve pain and relax muscle spasms. In disabling cases, joint replacement surgery can have excellent results.

> **SEE ALSO**
>
> ARTHRITIS • BONE • GENETIC DISEASES AND DISORDERS • GOUT • JOINT DISORDERS • MUSCLE • OBESITY • RICKETS • SKELETAL SYSTEM • SPINAL COLUMN

Osteoporosis

Bones are made of protein, heavily mineralized with calcium and phosphorus salts, which make them strong structural supports for the body. The male and female sex hormones are anabolic (building-up) steroids. While these sex hormones are being produced, protein and minerals are laid down as required, and the bones remain strong, healthy, and robust. Men produce anabolic steroids throughout life and, provided they do not spend most of their time lying in bed or floating weightless in space, need not worry about bone density and strength. It is different for women. From puberty until menopause, a woman's ovaries produce anabolic estrogens that promote body growth and repair and maintain bone strength. However, after menopause, estrogen production stops, and from then on, a woman's bone density begins to decline. In time, the bones may become so reduced in protein and minerals that they become spongelike and brittle.

Symptoms

Most women with osteoporosis are unaware that anything is wrong until a fracture occurs, usually because of minor trauma. This may be no more than a slight stumble, a heavy footfall from miscalculating a step, or even a minor bump on the rib cage. Many of the events brought on by osteoporosis are unnoticed. Elderly women may not realize that they have lost several inches in height from undetected crush fractures of vertebrae or compression from softening of the bone of the vertebral bodies. Marked curvature of the spine may also occur, and spinal pain is common. A high proportion of women over the age of 70 suffer a spontaneous fracture from osteoporosis, often at the neck of the thighbone (femur).

Menopause and hormone replacement therapy

Some doctors believe that women should have the continued protection of estrogens after menopause by way of hormone replacement therapy (HRT). In conjunction with oral calcium and disodium etidronate, HRT helps prevent the development of osteoporosis and protects against heart attacks and strokes in addition to treating menopausal symptoms. The current guidelines recommend using the lowest possible dose of HRT and for the shortest duration of time.

Q & A

My grandmother has a humpback. It seems to have occurred gradually since her seventieth birthday. She calls it her dowager's hump and says that it's not worth worrying about because it doesn't hurt. Is she right?

A dowager's hump is the result of osteoporosis, in which the bones become smaller, lighter, and less robust than normal. Over the years, some of the vertebrae (small bones) in your grandmother's spine have become squashed and others have collapsed into a wedge shape, so that the spine has bent into a hump. Your grandmother is right not to worry about it; a dowager's hump is not life-threatening, it often causes no pain, and severe cases are rare.

Can I avoid osteoporosis if I drink plenty of milk?

Some of the constituents of milk are essential for bone growth, but milk cannot prevent osteoporosis, which is a condition of old age and its accompanying changes in the balance of the body's hormones.

> **SEE ALSO**
> BONE • CANCER • FRACTURES AND DISLOCATIONS • HEART ATTACK • HORMONES AND HORMONAL DISORDERS • STROKE

Paralysis

Paralysis means the loss of normal function of the muscles in some part of the body. Paralysis of a leg muscle, for example, will make walking almost impossible. Paralysis of the muscles that control a person's speech may make a person produce slurred words that are difficult to understand. A particular muscle may be completely paralyzed or only partly affected. Furthermore, paralysis may last for a short time only or it can be permanent, depending on the cause of the paralysis.

Special terms are used to describe different degrees of paralysis. Paraplegia is the condition in which both legs are paralyzed. In quadriplegia, all four limbs are affected. In hemiplegia, the paralysis affects one side of the body only. Just which areas are paralyzed depends on the site of the damage to the controlling nerves or muscles.

Causes

Paralysis can be caused by various factors, including diseases or injuries that damage the muscles themselves, damage to the nerves that control the muscles, damage to the connections between muscles and nerves, or damage to the parts of the brain that are concerned with movement. Diseases include muscular dystrophy and myositis (inflammation of the muscle cells); myasthenia gravis (which affects the nerve-muscle connections); and poliomyelitis (which affects the central nervous system).

A broken backbone can damage the nerve fibers carrying the brain's instructions down both sides of the body, so that no muscles connected to nerves below the damaged area are able to work. When a person has a stroke or receives head injuries, a particular part of the brain may be damaged so that the nerves that control speech or movement cannot work properly.

Some diseases that cause paralysis eventually resolve if the patient is well cared for. People who are partly paralyzed after a stroke often recover almost completely with careful nursing and physical therapy. However, some injuries result in permanent paralysis. Sensitive machines have been developed to make the best possible use of any movement a paralyzed person has. For example, sucking on or blowing through a straw can activate a machine to carry out a variety of tasks. Many partially paralyzed people using wheelchairs are able to lead active lives.

Q & A

My cousin's legs have been paralyzed for some time. Is there any hope of recovery for him?

It depends on the cause. If his paralysis followed an injury, there is less hope than if he was suffering from a disease that caused paralysis. However, even if the motor nerves have been badly damaged, there is often some degree of recovery, which may even allow him to walk again and lead an almost normal life.

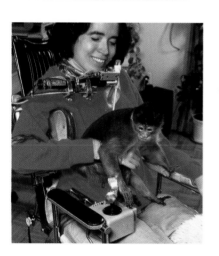

Paralyzed in all four limbs, this woman is helped by a capuchin monkey. The animal is trained to do simple tasks, such as turning on switches, putting on music, and setting up food and drink.

SEE ALSO

MUSCLE • MUSCLE DISEASES AND DISORDERS • MUSCULAR DYSTROPHY • NERVOUS SYSTEM • POLIOMYELITIS • STROKE

Parkinson's Disease

Parkinson's disease is fairly common among middle-aged and elderly people. It causes shaking limbs (particularly hands), stiff limbs, and difficulty in carrying out certain movements. It can cause problems with circulation and perspiration. There is no known cure, but drugs can help control the symptoms.

Causes

Parkinson's disease is usually caused by the degeneration of brain cells that normally control various smooth muscle movements. People make these movements without thinking—the way the arms swing when walking, for example, and facial expressions. The disease can be caused by various poisons, drug side effects, designer drugs, repeated head injuries sustained from boxing, and brain tumors, but in most cases the cause of the brain degeneration is unknown.

Symptoms and treatments

The first noticeable symptom is often trembling hands, which are most obvious when the person is at rest. The trembling often stops when a deliberate movement is made. The muscles become unusually stiff, often causing aching shoulders first thing in the morning. The person's face muscles move less than usual. Walking becomes difficult. Someone with Parkinson's leans forward and moves quickly with small, shuffling steps.

As the disease gets worse, the person's head may shake. He or she may find it difficult to speak clearly, and writing may become difficult. The patient's blood pressure may become so low that he or she frequently faints. The brain is not affected at first, but after some years, patients may become less able to think clearly and quickly, and three in 10 people may develop dementia.

Someone with Parkinson's disease should be able to lead a normal life for some years, helped by a careful diet and regular exercise. Various drugs, notably levadopa, can be given, but doctors are careful about prescribing them, because the drugs can have unpleasant side effects. Normally, the cells that control muscle movements produce a neurotransmitter (a chemical that transmits nerve impulses) called dopamine, which together with another transmitter called acetylcholine fine-tunes muscle control. In Parkinson's disease, the level of dopamine is low, and this condition affects muscle control.

Q & A

I've heard that Parkinson's disease can be caused by alcoholism. Is that true?

No. Although alcoholism does cause damage to other parts of the brain, it does not seem to attack the cells that are affected by Parkinson's disease.

Is it true that although Parkinson's disease does not affect the intellect, some psychiatric illnesses have similar symptoms?

It is true that the mind is not affected until the disease becomes very advanced, when slight mental deterioration is not uncommon. However, no mental illness has symptoms like those of Parkinson's disease.

My grandfather was disabled by Parkinson's disease. Is it possible that when I get older, I will be disabled by the disease?

The fact that your grandfather had the condition does not put you more at risk. In the unlikely event that you do develop the disease, therapies should ensure that you will not be as disabled as he was.

> **SEE ALSO**
>
> BRAIN • BRAIN DAMAGE AND DISORDERS • MUSCLE • NERVOUS SYSTEM • NERVOUS SYSTEM DISORDERS

Pelvic Inflammatory Disease

Q & A

Do sexually transmitted diseases cause pelvic inflammatory disease (PID)? What are the symptoms?

Yes. Chlamydia causes half of all cases of PID, but up to 75 percent of women and 50 percent of men have no symptoms, and chlamydia can remain dormant for many years. Symptoms include a discharge from the vagina or penis, and men have pain during urination. Gonorrhea is similar to, but less common than, chlamydia.

Is it true that other conditions have symptoms similar to PID and can be mistaken for the disease? What are some of those diseases and their symptoms?

Ectopic pregnancy and appendicitis cause pelvic pain and require immediate hospitalization. Other causes are cysts and fibroids, pelvic congestion, endometriosis, and irritable bowel syndrome. A type of intestinal inflammation called Crohn's disease leads to pain and fever. Thrush makes it easier for infections to affect the pelvic organs. Cystitis causes pain during urination.

Pelvic inflammatory disease (PID) is a common syndrome that mainly affects sexually active women under the age of 35. It is an infectious condition that causes inflammation of the fallopian tubes and the ovaries. Sometimes the infection is even more widespread, involving the lining and muscle of the uterus (womb) and the peritoneum, an area of the membrane that lines the whole abdominal cavity.

The infection is most commonly acquired via the vagina, and it ascends through the canal of the cervix and the interior of the uterus. It then passes along both fallopian tubes and may extend from the outer open ends of the tubes to involve the ovaries and other structures of the pelvis. The infection is nearly always confined to the pelvis.

Causes, symptoms, and treatments

Various microorganisms may cause PID. In most cases, they are acquired from men who have, in turn, been infected by other women. PID is thus commonly, but not always, one of the sexually transmitted diseases. Other ways in which PID can be acquired include infection spreading directly from the intestinal tract, especially following appendicitis, and direct spread from the bloodstream.

The germs that cause sexually acquired PID include *Chlamydia trachomatis* and *Neisseria gonorrhoeae* (which causes gonorrhea). Infection from the intestine is usually by *Escherichia coli* or *Streptococcus fecalis*. Blood-spread infection, although now rare, is usually by the tubercle bacillus *Mycobacterium tuberculosis*.

PID is one of the most common causes of lower abdominal pain in women. The pain may occur at any time of the month but tends to be worst during menstrual periods. Also, PID causes pain during sexual intercourse, increased vaginal discharge, irregular vaginal bleeding, nausea and vomiting, and fever. The principal complication is blocked fallopian tubes, with resulting infertility.

Treatment is by antibiotics to control the infection. If the diagnosis is made early and treatment is given, the outlook is excellent and fallopian tube damage can usually be avoided. However, delay in treatment is dangerous, because it may lead to destructive abscess formation in the tubes and in the pelvis.

SEE ALSO

APPENDICITIS • BACTERIA • GONORRHEA • NONSPECIFIC URETHRITIS • SEXUALLY TRANSMITTED DISEASES

Phenylketonuria

Phenylketonuria (PKU) is a rare genetic disease in which babies are born lacking the ability to process the amino acid phenylalanine. Amino acids are the building blocks of proteins. In most people, a body chemical called phenylalanine hydroxylase changes phenylalanine into another amino acid called tyrosine. A baby born with PKU lacks phenylalanine hydroxylase. As soon as the baby starts to take in phenylalanine from his or her food, the amino acid builds up in the blood. This buildup of phenylalanine starts to damage the baby's developing brain. Babies with PKU also lack tyrosine. Tyrosine makes the body pigment melanin. As a result, babies with the disease usually have blue eyes, fair hair, and fair skin. Other symptoms of PKU include eczema, seizures, and a musty smell to the hair, sweat, and urine.

Treatment and outlook

A newborn baby with PKU must remain on a special diet until he or she is three months old. Phenylalanine is present in both breast milk and cow's milk. As a newborn, the baby is therefore given a formula made from beef extract. After weaning, some babies can start to eat normally. However, high-protein foods, such as meat, fish, nuts, and dairy products, must be avoided. The artificial sweetener aspartame must also be avoided, because it contains a lot of phenylalanine. Starchy foods such as bread, pasta, and potatoes can be eaten, but only in moderation. In the past, doctors used to allow the diet of children with PKU to return to normal between the ages of six and 12. They now recommend that the special diet should be followed throughout life.

Genetic disease

PKU is a genetic disease. Both parents pass it on to their child as a faulty gene. If a couple has one child with PKU, there is a 25 percent risk that further children will be affected. People with a family history of PKU should consult a doctor if they wish to start a family.

Q & A

Is phenylketonuria a common problem?

Phenylketonuria is a rare disease, affecting about one in every 16,000 babies born in the United States.

Is the impairment caused by phenylketonuria a permanent impairment?

The way to prevent the effects of this disease is by screening and a special diet. Tests are carried out on newborn babies in many countries. If the condition develops untreated, intellectual impairment is 97 percent likely, and most sufferers are affected severely. A diet low in the amino acid phenylalanine can improve matters but will not restore a child who is badly affected.

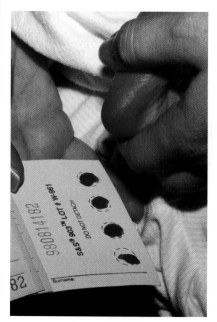

A doctor takes a blood sample from the heel of a newborn baby for a Guthrie test. This test screens for a rare genetic disease, phenylketonuria (PKU), which affects about one in 16,000 people.

SEE ALSO

BLOOD • ECZEMA • GENETIC DISEASES AND DISORDERS

Plague

Plague is one of the most dangerous infectious diseases known. In the past, epidemics of plague caused millions of deaths. For example, in the 1300s it killed one in every four people in Europe. It can now be completely cured with antibiotics.

Plague is caused by a bacterium, *Yersinia pestis*. It is present in rats and other wild rodents that live in all parts of the world except Australia. Fleas carry the bacteria from one rodent to another, and sometimes to rats that come in contact with people. When the rats die of plague, the fleas on them may move to humans. They bite humans to feed on their blood and, in so doing, infect them with plague.

The bacteria cause a sudden high fever, with a headache and vomiting. The lymph glands in the groin may swell and fill with pus. These swellings are known as buboes. They give the disease its name: bubonic plague. Its other name, the black death, comes from large, dark bruises that appear all over the body. These bruises are caused by internal bleeding. The infection can cause severe pneumonia (pneumonic plague). The patient coughs and sneezes violently, thus spreading the disease to other people. Unless it is treated quickly, plague causes death.

Because plague is still found in wild rodents, it is unlikely to disappear from humans completely. However, as living conditions and standards of hygiene improve, the number of cases is falling. People with the disease are isolated and treated with antibiotics, and those in contact with them are vaccinated. Measures are also taken to destroy all disease-carrying rats and fleas.

Q & A

My family has recently started to discuss the possibility of going to Asia for our vacation this summer. Should I be vaccinated against plague if we go to Asia?

Unless you spend your vacation in the most squalid conditions imaginable, you are unlikely to come into contact with the disease. The vaccine against plague provides protection for about six months and is intended only for people who, perhaps because of their occupation, have a high risk of exposure to the disease.

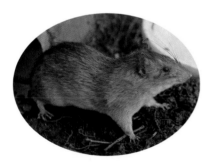

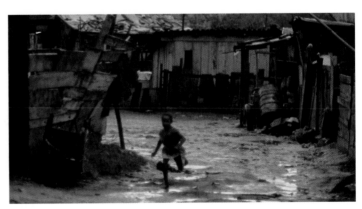

Squalid conditions in underdeveloped countries (right) are an ideal breeding ground for plague. Plague bacteria are transmitted to humans by fleas that have sucked the blood of infected rats (above). Plague used to cause terrible epidemics in which many people died, but it is now easily treated with antibiotics.

SEE ALSO

BACTERIA • BACTERIAL DISEASES • COMMUNICABLE DISEASES • EPIDEMIC • INFECTIOUS DISEASES • PNEUMONIA

Pneumonia

Q & A

Why is double pneumonia worse than ordinary pneumonia?

In double pneumonia, both lungs are infected; this is a much more serious condition than if only one lung is involved. Pneumonias involving both lungs have a higher mortality than those that are confined to a single lung.

Why are elderly people more prone to pneumonia?

Anyone who is weak, either through age or through illness, is prone to pneumonia. For this reason, pneumonia often finally leads to the death of people who are already ill with some other disease. The body's resistance to infection is reduced, and once pneumonia has become established, an elderly patient may be too weak to cough up all the infected secretions, so the infection becomes worse.

In lobar pneumonia, the alveoli (air sacs) become filled with mucus. This causes shortness of breath and pain on breathing. In this type of pneumonia, which is common in some developing countries, only one lobe of the lung tends to be affected, while the rest of the lung functions normally.

Pneumonia, inflammation of lung tissue, is often caused by infection due to bacteria, viruses, or other pathogens. The disease once caused many deaths, but antibiotics now resolve many serious cases and complications of pneumonia.

Pneumonia affects the alveoli (tiny air sacs) and the bronchioles (fine tubes) leading to them. When infected, these structures fill with mucus instead of air, leaving the patient very short of breath. On an X-ray, the infected area shows as a white patch against the normal, dark areas of the lung. Lobar pneumonia, which is usually caused by pneumococcus bacteria, affects a whole lobe of one or both of the lungs. Bronchopneumonia causes small areas of white patches scattered all over the lungs.

The symptoms of pneumonia are like those of influenza and almost always include a cough, a fever, breathlessness, and perhaps chest pains. The illness may be mild or extremely severe. Viral pneumonia cannot be treated by antibiotics, but bed rest usually clears it up in about a week. Pneumonia that has been caused by bacteria usually responds quickly to antibiotics.

The elderly, children under two, people with a serious illness (such as chronic bronchitis or heart disease), and those whose resistance is low are most likely to get pneumonia. The disease is particularly dangerous to anyone taking drugs to suppress the body's immune (defense) system.

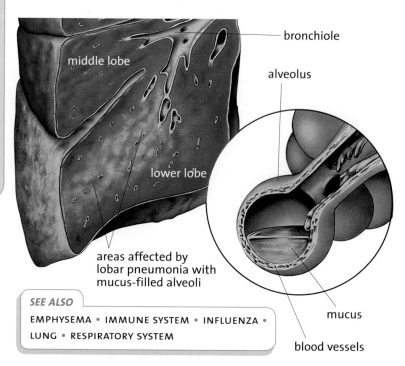

middle lobe

bronchiole

alveolus

lower lobe

areas affected by lobar pneumonia with mucus-filled alveoli

mucus

blood vessels

SEE ALSO

EMPHYSEMA • IMMUNE SYSTEM • INFLUENZA • LUNG • RESPIRATORY SYSTEM

Poison and Poisoning

People are surrounded by poisonous substances that are potential killers. Most cases of poisoning are caused by careless accidents that could be avoided. Children between the ages of two and five years are particularly at risk. They put all sorts of objects and substances into their mouths, so if there are small children in the family, anything that could be poisonous should be locked away.

What is a poison?

A poison is any substance that damages the body and interferes with its working. Many household cleansers and bleaches are poisonous if they are taken by mouth. Substances such as medicines, which are harmless in their prescribed doses, can act as poison if too much is taken. Many people poison themselves by drinking too much alcohol. Poisons can enter the body

Q & A

Do all poisons cause deep unconsciousness in the victim?

No. Tranquilizers and sleeping pills lead to coma when taken in an overdose, but others such as acetaminophen and aspirin can leave the patient wide awake for as long as 48 hours or more after being taken. The state of consciousness is not a good guide to the severity of poisoning.

Can poisoning occur in people in the form of epidemics?

Yes. An epidemic of poisoning is said to occur when a single agent is responsible for poisoning a large number of people. It can occur through contaminated food or water supplies. Therefore, the relevant authorities take great care to prevent this. However, in 1981 in Spain, a large epidemic of poisoning was caused by contaminated cooking oil.

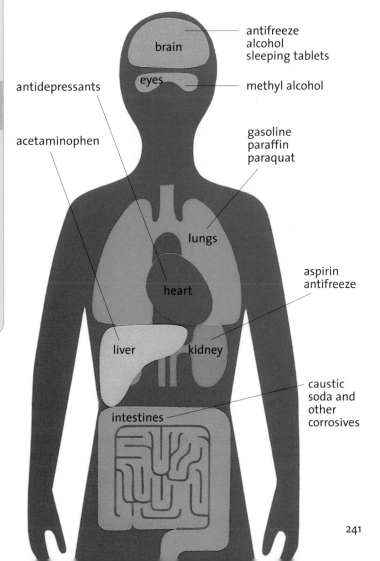

Different poisons affect different organs of the body. When taken in large quantities, the painkillers aspirin and acetaminophen can be extremely harmful. Aspirin can cause kidney failure, and an overdose of acetaminophen can cause fatal liver failure.

PREVENTING ACCIDENTS

All harmful substances must be clearly labeled and locked away from small children. Danger areas are kitchens, bathrooms, garages, and toolsheds, where bottles of cleaning fluids, bleach, weed killers, and pest killers are sometimes left on the floor or stored in unlocked cupboards where a child could easily reach them. Harmful liquids should never be poured into an empty soft drink container, because a child might think it holds something harmless to drink. All medicines should be kept in a locked cupboard. Medicine should not be taken in front of small children, because they may copy the action and poison themselves.

through the mouth or through the skin via insect bites or snakebites. Certain chemicals can make their way through the skin's surface or can be breathed in as poisonous fumes.

How poisons act

Poisons damage the body in a number of ways. Some poisons, such as sleeping tablets, tranquilizers, or excess alcohol, stop the brain from working properly so that it can no longer control the person's breathing. Because oxygen is not getting into the system, the victim dies.

Other poisons affect various organs in the body: for example, antidepressants can damage the heart, too much acetaminophen damages the liver, and petroleum compounds that are swallowed can make their way to the lungs and cause a type of pneumonia. Corrosive substances, such as acids, can burn the tissues of the mouth and throat. Some snake venoms and poisons, such as strychnine, affect the nervous system.

Many common substances, including vinegar, alcohol, shampoo, perfume, cosmetics, and detergents, are poisonous if taken in large enough quantities. For this reason, they should always be kept out of the reach of small children.

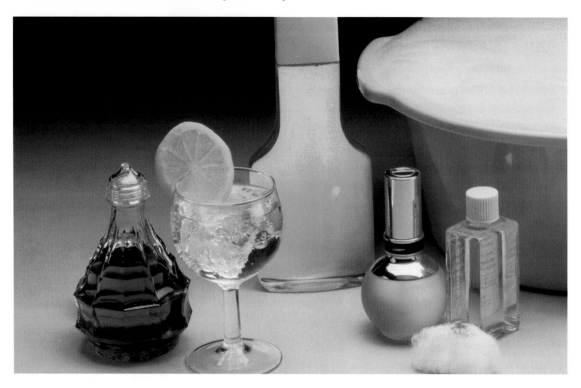

FIRST AID FOR POISONING

- If someone has swallowed poison and is unconscious, the Poison Control Center (PCC) should be called. The person's breathing and pulse should be checked; resuscitation may be necessary.
- If the person is conscious, whoever is giving first aid should try to find out what the poison was, how much was taken, and when. If there are signs of shock or breathing problems, an ambulance should be called.
- If there is a container, the person giving first aid should take the container to the telephone when calling the ambulance and the PCC.
- The PCC may advise making the victim vomit by giving him or her syrup of ipecac. Only if the PCC advises doing so should vomiting be induced or the person be given any food or drink.
- If the PCC advises the use of ipecac but a child refuses to take it, he or she should be taken to the hospital as fast as possible.
- Activated charcoal should be kept in the house. It may counteract poison that remains after vomiting. The PCC will advise when to give it.

One of the most deadly poisons is cyanide, which kills by blocking an essential enzyme called cytochrome oxidase that is necessary for the transport of oxygen to the cells.

A common symptom of poisoning is vomiting. This may occur because the poison irritates or burns the stomach, but sometimes it occurs because the poison has affected the part of the brain controlling vomiting. Other symptoms include convulsions, drowsiness, coma, and pain, depending on what the poison is.

Medical help and first aid

Anyone who has been poisoned needs medical help as soon as possible. The Poison Control Center (PCC) in the area should be called for advice. The victim must be taken to the hospital, but if it is necessary to wait for an ambulance, the first aid advice in the box (left) should be followed.

It is vitally important to find out what poison has been taken. If the victim has vomited, some of the vomit should be collected for analysis. Knowing which poison has been taken may determine the type of treatment required. If the patient is conscious, he or she may be able to say what has happened. Those giving first aid should try to find the poison container and take it with the patient to the hospital—even if it is empty—and take samples of any food and drink that could have caused the poisoning.

Treatment

Treatment includes removing as much poison from the victim's system as possible, by making the patient vomit or by washing out the stomach to prevent poison from being absorbed. Special techniques are used to flush through the kidneys and to remove poisons from the bloodstream.

Antidotes can be given to counteract the effects of some poisons. Recovery depends on the type of poison, how much was taken, and how soon treatment was started. Some people recover completely, but others may suffer permanent brain damage or even die.

> **SEE ALSO**
>
> BLOOD • BODY SYSTEMS • BRAIN • HEART • KIDNEY • LUNG • MOUTH • NERVOUS SYSTEM

Poliomyelitis

Poliomyelitis is an extremely infectious disease caused by a virus. The condition affects the nervous system, and it can kill its victims or leave them handicapped. Most children in developed countries are now immunized against polio, but in some poorer parts of the world polio is still very common.

How polio is contracted and treated

The polio virus is spread in the feces of an infected person or by ingesting food or drink contaminated with feces. At first, the virus grows and reproduces itself in the throat and stomach. There may be no symptoms at all or it may cause what seems like a mild attack of gastric influenza. In many people, the infection does not develop further. In others, the virus invades the motor cells of the spinal cord and parts of the brain. These nerves work the muscles of the limbs and those that control breathing and swallowing. Early symptoms are muscle pain and aches. Some people develop neck stiffness and sensitivity to bright light. Then, the muscles of one limb may become weaker and weaker. In severe cases, all the limbs and the muscles that control swallowing and breathing are involved, and the patient can breathe only with the help of mechanical ventilation.

There are no drugs to kill the polio virus; treatment consists of skilled nursing and physical therapy. After a time, which varies

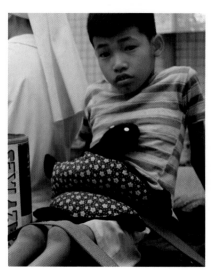

from one patient to another, the inflammation dies down. Undamaged nerve cells may be able to take over some of the work of those that have been destroyed, but once muscle fibers have wasted away, they cannot be brought back. Most polio victims make a good recovery, although some muscles may be wasted. Even people whose breathing was paralyzed are usually able to breathe unaided.

Q & A

Because polio is so rare, is it still necessary to be vaccinated against it?

Yes, it is. The disease is close to eradication only because mass immunization against polio has been successful. The poliomyelitis virus does still exist, so it is important—both for personal safety and in the interests of eradication—for immunization to continue until the threat is past.

I've heard that it's possible for someone to get polio more than once. How can that be? Shouldn't you be immune to it after you've had it?

There are three different viruses that cause polio, so it is theoretically possible to be infected three times; infection with one type does not make you immune to the others. However, the chance that this will happen is extremely low. The polio vaccine gives lifelong immunity to all three types.

Polio is still common in less developed countries. This young boy is being given treatment in a Vietnamese refugee camp.

SEE ALSO

BRAIN • INFECTIOUS DISEASES • LUNG • MUSCLE • NERVOUS SYSTEM DISORDERS • PARALYSIS • VIRUSES

Premenstrual Syndrome

Many women find that during the week before their monthly period, they put on weight and become tense, nervous, and irritable. This premenstrual syndrome, or PMS, is caused by changing hormone levels in the body during the monthly cycle, and some mild symptoms are perfectly normal.

Symptoms

For some women, PMS causes severe problems; these women will need a doctor's help. Many of the physical problems of PMS are caused by water retention. Instead of passing out of the body as urine, water builds up in body cells and tissues. Some women notice that their breasts feel tender and swollen. Swollen ankles are also common, and some women have overall swelling. Body weight may increase by 6 pounds (2.7 kg) or more just before menstruation.

Many women become emotionally upset, edgy, and easily annoyed, and they find it difficult to concentrate. Some women feel depressed and suffer fatigue.

Other physical symptoms associated with PMS are skin problems, such as pimples or blotchiness; an increase in the likelihood of cystitis; and a general feeling of being under the weather. Women who have conditions such as epilepsy, asthma, migraine, and conjunctivitis may find that their conditions worsen at this time. Some women even find that their contact lenses become uncomfortable to wear.

Treatments

Many women's symptoms are helped or eliminated by taking supplements of vitamin B complex, vitamin B_6, vitamin E, minerals, evening primrose oil, the contraceptive pill or another hormone treatment, and some complementary remedies. Various types of medication can help relieve PMS, but currently there is no one solution that is helpful to all women.

Women should try to adjust their routine in the days before a period so that they do not put themselves under physical stress. This applies particularly to dieting, which may increase the likelihood of faintness or dizziness. Women should avoid strict dieting during the premenstrual phase and ensure that they eat regularly, little but often, when premenstrual problems arise.

Q & A

Can changing diets prevent premenstrual syndrome and eliminate weight gain?

Any weight gain during the premenstrual time is almost certainly due to water retention and will disappear once the period has begun. However, a woman should eat sensibly throughout her premenstrual time. She should reduce the amount of salt in her diet, because salt increases water retention. She should not go without food for hours at a time, because this may result in her feeling faint and dizzy. Experts say that women should eat little but often during the days before a period.

Can a woman still suffer from premenstrual syndrome after reaching menopause?

At menopause, a woman no longer goes through the menstrual cycle. Therefore, she will no longer get premenstrual syndrome. Any depression, anxiety, or mood swings may be due to other hormonal cycles and should be discussed with her doctor.

SEE ALSO

ASTHMA • BODY SYSTEMS • EPILEPSY • HORMONES AND HORMONAL DISORDERS • MENSTRUAL DISORDERS • MIGRAINE

Rabies

Rabies is a fatal disease caused by a virus. It is passed to humans in the saliva of infected animals or in moisture droplets in the air. The only chance of surviving the virus is to have a series of antirabies shots before the disease develops. Rabies is present in most parts of the world except in the British Isles, where controls on importing animals are extremely strict.

Q & A

My friend says that you can get rabies months after being bitten. Is that really possible?

Yes, it is possible. The incubation period for rabies varies from days to years, although the disease usually appears within 20 to 90 days of being bitten. The incubation period is shortest in children who have been bitten on the face and longer if the site of the bite is far from the brain.

Is it possible to survive rabies?

Without early vaccination against rabies, the disease is almost invariably fatal. However, there are several known cases of survival. One of these was a young boy in the United States who was bitten by a rabid bat. He was given both serum and vaccine right away and survived even though he developed signs of the disease. In another case, a laboratory worker inhaled droplets of the virus and he, too, was given the vaccine.

These are some of the animals most likely to carry rabies in different parts of the world. In the United States, the wild skunk, fox, coyote, raccoon, and bat sometimes carry the virus.

Animals that carry rabies

There are only a few cases of rabies each year in the United States, but the disease is present in the country. Humans rarely catch the disease, because it is present in wild animals that have little contact with humans. Such animals include foxes, skunks, coyotes, raccoons, bobcats, mongooses, vampire bats, jackals, and wild dogs. They may pass on the disease to pet dogs and cats and so, in turn, to humans. An infected animal becomes irritable and snappy and develops fever, restlessness, and muscular aches, with pain at the site of the bite. Once the rabies is well developed, the animal may be very thirsty but it becomes terrified of water, and even the sight of water may bring on spasms. The term used for this condition is *hydrophobia*. The animal froths at the mouth and attacks other animals, including people, biting them and passing on the virus. The rabies virus can also be passed on in the saliva of an infected animal through a cut or a scratch.

Symptoms of rabies in humans

Once the virus has entered the body, the incubation period is usually between 20 and 90 days. During this time, the virus works its way along the victim's nerves until it reaches the brain. The symptoms include a sore throat, aching muscles, fever, restlessness, and insomnia. Then hydrophobia develops. The patient may have convulsions and back-arching spasms (any one

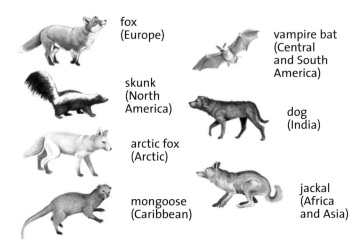

fox
(Europe)

vampire bat
(Central
and South
America)

skunk
(North
America)

dog
(India)

arctic fox
(Arctic)

mongoose
(Caribbean)

jackal
(Africa
and Asia)

FIRST AID

If someone is bitten or scratched by an animal, he or she should wash the wound with soap and water, cover it with clean dressing, and see a doctor as soon as possible. If the animal can be caught without danger to anyone, the health authority can test it for rabies. If a person is camping or hiking and is bitten by an animal that is acting strangely, he or she should keep well away from it and seek help at once. Only mammals, including bats, carry rabies. Snakes and other reptiles may be dangerous but not rabid.

of which can end in death), with periods of wild and confused excitement. The patient may sweat and salivate heavily. Some people become paralyzed. Eventually, the patient goes into a coma and dies.

Once rabies has developed, there is no cure for it. Treatment consists of keeping the patient alive while drugs are tried; but so far, only three patients have ever recovered, and they had been vaccinated soon after they were infected.

Anyone who is bitten or scratched by an animal should see a doctor immediately. In most parts of the United States, dog owners must have their animals immunized, so it is unlikely that a pet dog will be rabid. The disease is rarely caught, so there is no need for people to be frightened of contact with animals, but it is essential to act quickly if they are bitten.

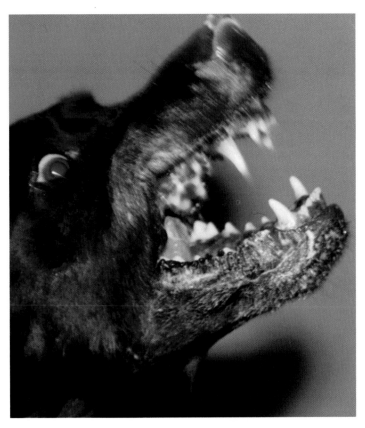

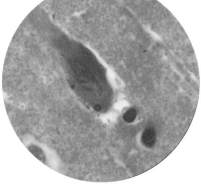

This dog (right) has rabies. The disease is transmitted by a virus (above). Once rabies affects both human and animal brains, it causes hydrophobia—terror and spasms at the sight of water.

SEE ALSO

INFECTIOUS DISEASES • NERVOUS SYSTEM • VIRUSES

Raynaud's Disease

Raynaud's disease is a sudden, intermittent narrowing of the small arteries in the hands and sometimes, more rarely, in the feet. An attack can be triggered by smoking, which constricts the arteries; exposure to cold; exposure to cold water; or handling frozen items. Stressful emotions can also trigger attacks. The fingers and toes react to the low temperature by contracting and reducing the blood flow. They become white and numb and sometimes feel painful. As they warm up, and the blood begins to flow again, they turn first blue and then deep red before returning to normal. The disease is more common in females, although the reason is unknown, and it sometimes runs in families. People in colder climates are also more likely than people in warmer areas to develop Raynaud's disease.

Raynaud's phenomenon

About half of the people who have Raynaud's disease have an underlying health problem, such as an autoimmune disorder like rheumatoid arthritis. In these cases, it is known as Raynaud's phenomenon. Other people have attacks because they work with equipment that vibrates strongly, such as pneumatic drills. Typing, playing the piano, or any other repetitive action carried out for long periods of time is often linked to Raynaud's phenomenon.

Diagnosis and treatments

Diagnosis of Raynaud's disease is usually based on a patient's history of experiencing color changes in the extremities in response to exposure to cold or emotional stress. A cold simulation test may be used to provoke symptoms for the doctor to see. A physical examination and diagnostic tests to rule out other conditions that might act like Raynaud's may be done.

Doctors may also conduct tests to find out if there is an underlying disorder. If it is an autoimmune problem, immunosuppressant drugs may be prescribed. Drugs can be taken to dilate the blood vessels during an attack. People with Raynaud's disease should keep their hands and feet warm and dry and wear thermal gloves and socks to prevent an attack. They should also stop smoking at once. If the condition is extremely severe, surgery may be required, to cut the nerves that control the constriction of the arteries. In severe cases, prolonged or repeated episodes can cause sores or tissue death (gangrene).

Q & A

When my mother puts her hands in cold water, they turn white and become painful. Her doctor says that it's due to poor circulation. Is she in danger of developing gangrene?

No, but her doctor is right. This type of bad circulation, called Raynaud's disease, is common and usually affects women. Cold water or cold air seems to cause the arteries to the fingers to close down. Your mother should try to keep her hands as warm as possible.

My grandmother gets numbness in her hands and feet every winter, at temperatures that don't affect other people. Why does this happen?

When the body is exposed to severe cold, the arteries contract automatically to cut heat loss. If your grandmother's arteries are already narrow, this additional narrowing will cause insufficient blood to get to her hands and feet. If the numbness follows changes of color from red to white to blue, the problem is probably Raynaud's disease.

SEE ALSO

ARTERY • ARTERY DISEASES AND DISORDERS • ARTHRITIS • CIRCULATORY SYSTEM • GANGRENE • IMMUNE SYSTEM

Repetitive Strain Injury

Q & A

My father is always complaining about headaches and pains in his neck. Could this be related to his job as a computer operator?

Yes. Doing repetitive work while sitting in a fixed position can cause neck problems and headaches. His posture and the design of his workstation could be at fault. A physical therapist can advise him on the posture that best suits his working environment and the correct positions for his keyboard and screen. He should not overuse the muscles that can lead to repetitive strain injury (RSI).

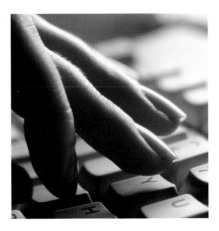

When performed regularly, repetitive actions, such as typing on a keyboard, can cause repetitive strain injury.

Repetitive strain injury (RSI) describes a range of orthopedic conditions that are caused by a prolonged and particular movement or action.

RSI is likely to occur in occupations when the work makes it necessary for the person concerned to perform a particular action repeatedly for very long periods, especially if this involves an uncomfortable or awkward position of the body. RSI commonly affects musicians, keyboard operators, production line workers, cleaners, packers, and machine operators, who all have to perform repetitive movements many, many times each day.

With the increased use of personal computers, the condition has become much more common. The widespread introduction and use of flat, light-touch keyboards that permit high-speed typing have resulted in a dramatic rise in injuries to the hands, arms, and shoulders caused by repetitive movements.

Common RSI conditions include injuries known as carpal tunnel syndrome and tendinitis. One of the most common conditions is tenosynovitis (known by many workers as teno). This is an inflammation of the narrow sheaths through which the long thin tendons of muscles, especially those of the forearm, run. The condition is usually caused by injury to a particular tendon or, more rarely, infection. Other conditions linked to RSI include bursitis, DeQuervain's syndrome, thoracic outlet syndrome, trigger finger or thumb, tennis elbow, and golfer's elbow.

RSI usually causes acute pain, cramplike stiffness, tissue swelling, and an inability to continue carrying out the repetitive movements that have caused the problem. Often, the symptoms disappear once the repetitive movements have stopped and the affected area has been rested sufficiently. However, the condition is much more difficult to treat if it has become chronic.

X-rays and blood tests are taken to eliminate conditions such as rheumatoid arthritis. Often, the condition responds to nonsteroidal anti-inflammatory drug therapy, which helps relieve pain and reduce any swelling. However, established RSI can be extremely difficult to treat. If it is work-related, a change of occupation may be necessary, because once the activity is resumed, the condition will reappear.

In some cases, those who suffer from RSI are found to dislike their work, and psychological stress is a factor.

SEE ALSO

CARPAL TUNNEL SYNDROME • MUSCLE • SPRAINS AND STRAINS • TENNIS ELBOW

Respiratory System

Q & A

My brother has been diagnosed as having small lungs. Is this serious?

Each lung has a capacity of around 0.09 cubic foot (2.5 l), but the amount of air passing in and out is often only a tenth of this, so your brother should be all right. Many people manage with only one lung.

Why are singers taught to breathe from the diaphragm?

The diaphragm controls breathing rate and depth. A voice teacher helps students develop their abdominal muscles to control their diaphragm so that they can hold long notes and create vibrato.

I broke my ribs playing basketball. Why was I not bandaged or given any treatment?

Although broken or cracked ribs can be uncomfortable or painful, the main danger is that the chest movement will be reduced, producing less airflow into and out of the underlying lung. This can cause pneumonia, so it is unusual to bandage broken ribs.

All body cells need a constant supply of oxygen to survive and to dispose of a waste product, carbon dioxide. Both requirements are fulfilled by the respiratory system and the circulatory system. The two systems deliver oxygen from the lungs to the cells and remove carbon dioxide from the cells for return to the lungs, where it is exhaled. This exchange of oxygen and carbon dioxide between the air, blood, and tissues of the body is known as respiration.

When air is breathed in, it is taken to the lungs. There, the oxygen it contains is exchanged for carbon dioxide, which, with water vapor, is expelled when people breathe out. This process is controlled by nerves that automatically send impulses to the muscles, so that people breathe in and out in an involuntary way.

Air is drawn into the body through the nose and mouth and travels down the throat (the pharynx and larynx) and the windpipe (trachea). The windpipe divides into two branches called bronchi, each leading to a lung.

How the respiratory system works

The lungs are like a pair of bellows in the chest. Around them are the rib cage and the rib muscles. Below them is a sheet of muscle called the diaphragm. The rib cage, muscles, and diaphragm form the chest cavity. When the diaphragm contracts and the chest wall rises, the space in the chest increases and air rushes into the lungs. When the muscles relax, the lungs, which are naturally elastic, collapse and air rushes out.

From the nostrils to the lungs, the air is warmed, moistened, and filtered. Tiny hairs covered with mucus line the passages and trap as much dust and germs as possible when they enter the system. However, these hairs cannot cope with cigarette smoke or very polluted air. If a large particle enters the system, it is coughed out or sneezed out. Food is prevented from entering the respiratory system by the epiglottis, a flap of tissue that closes off the windpipe as the food passes into the gullet.

The air travels into the bronchi and then into even smaller branches called bronchioles. At the ends of these narrow tubes are minute air sacs called alveoli. The alveoli are covered with a network of tiny blood vessels called capillaries. The exchange of gases—oxygen for carbon dioxide—takes place through the walls of the alveoli, which are fused with the capillary walls.

The red blood cells contain hemoglobin, a compound that picks up the oxygen from the lungs. The hemoglobin carries the oxygen to every cell in the body and releases it. At the same time, carbon dioxide passes into the blood and is carried back to the lungs, where it is breathed out.

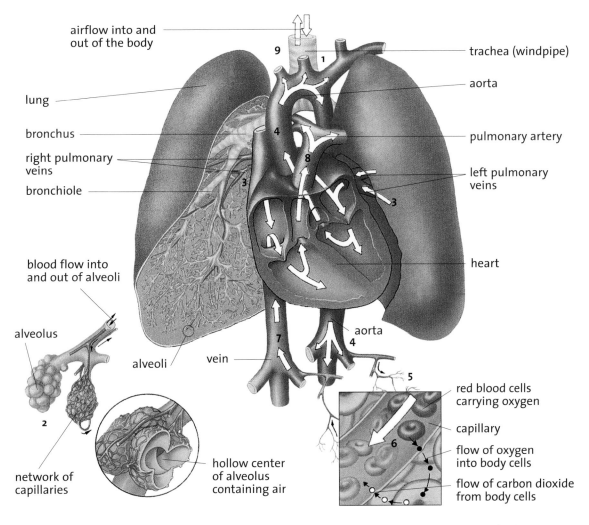

airflow into and out of the body

9

trachea (windpipe)

1

aorta

lung

bronchus

4

pulmonary artery

right pulmonary veins

8

bronchiole

3

left pulmonary veins

3

blood flow into and out of alveoli

heart

alveolus

7

aorta

4

alveoli

vein

5

red blood cells carrying oxygen

capillary

6

flow of oxygen into body cells

2

network of capillaries

hollow center of alveolus containing air

flow of carbon dioxide from body cells

Air (1) inhaled via the trachea (windpipe), bronchi, and bronchioles reaches the alveoli, where oxygen from the air is transferred to the capillaries surrounding each alveolus (2). The oxygenated blood is carried by the pulmonary veins (3) to the left side of the heart and pushed into the aorta (4), which is the body's main artery. Blood then travels around the body through the arteries to the capillaries (5). The oxygen carried by the red blood cells is given to the body cells, which transfer their waste product, carbon dioxide, to the fluid of the blood (6). This blood is carried back through the veins (7) into the right side of the heart. Finally, the blood flows through the pulmonary artery (8) into the lungs. At the site of the alveoli (2), the circulating blood gives up its carbon dioxide, which is exhaled (9), and then takes in oxygen again (1). The cycle then repeats itself.

SEE ALSO

BLOOD • CIRCULATORY SYSTEM • CIRCULATORY SYSTEM DISEASES AND DISORDERS • LUNG • LUNG DISEASES AND DISORDERS • RESPIRATORY SYSTEM DISEASES AND DISORDERS

Respiratory System Diseases and Disorders

Q & A

Can people's lungs be damaged permanently by pneumonia?

Yes. Some of the bacteria that cause pneumonia, such as staphylococcus, can lead to the formation of abscesses that remain as a scar even after treatment. However, most cases of pneumonia can be treated with antibiotics, and recovery of the lungs is complete.

I tend to get bronchitis. Will it help to leave the bedroom windows open at night?

Bronchitis often begins as an infection in the nose and throat, followed by a chest infection. The bronchi are more liable to infection if they are irritated by tobacco smoke, noxious fumes, and cold air. If there are smokers in the house, opening a window may remove some of the smoke. However, cold air and pollution coming in through the window, especially in cities, are just as bad. It is better to leave windows closed at night, because a warm atmosphere is best for all bronchial conditions.

The air people breathe contains a number of irritating substances and disease-carrying microorganisms. It is not surprising that the respiratory system is subject to a large number of infections and diseases. Many of these infections are mild, but some are very serious, and if people cannot breathe, they will die.

Oxygen enters the body through the lungs. Each lung has a great deal of spare capacity, and people with only one lung can still breathe in as much oxygen as they need, provided that the single lung is working properly. However, when the lungs stop working efficiently or when the airways to the lungs are blocked, the body cannot get enough oxygen. Inefficient lungs are also unable to get rid of the waste product, carbon dioxide, which is breathed out. People whose respiratory system is not working properly have a bluish tinge to their skin, because their blood contains too little oxygen and too much carbon dioxide. They may have to strain to breathe in enough oxygen. This effort may also strain the muscles of the heart and can eventually lead to heart failure.

It is important to remember that a person's health can be damaged by smoking, whatever his or her age, and that just one occasional cigarette does matter. It is very easy to get hooked on cigarettes and to develop the diseases associated with smoking.

Causes of respiratory diseases

Air pollution from chemical particles and mineral dust is a major cause of respiratory problems in people who live in industrial areas. People such as miners and quarry workers who work in

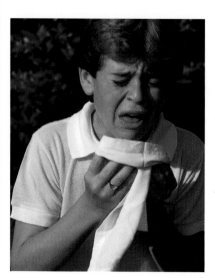

dusty conditions over a long period of time are also at risk of lung damage. Over a number of years, the irritation caused by these particles leads to patches of scar tissue on the lungs, which

The most common respiratory disease, and one for which there is no cure, is the common cold. Catching a sneeze in a handkerchief and then washing one's hands will help prevent cold germs from spreading.

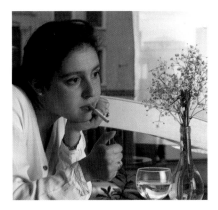

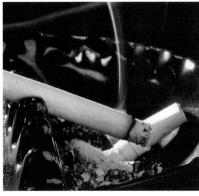

keep them from working well. This condition is called pneumoconiosis. The major symptoms are shortness of breath and coughing.

Antipollution laws and safety regulations help cut down such occupational diseases in developed countries.

Above all, smoking damages the respiratory system. It causes cancer in the lungs and throat and is a major cause of chronic (long-lasting) bronchitis. Even breathing in the smoke from other people's cigarettes can be damaging.

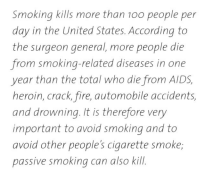

Smoking kills more than 100 people per day in the United States. According to the surgeon general, more people die from smoking-related diseases in one year than the total who die from AIDS, heroin, crack, fire, automobile accidents, and drowning. It is therefore very important to avoid smoking and to avoid other people's cigarette smoke; passive smoking can also kill.

The common cold

Everyone has a cold occasionally. It is the most common respiratory infection. Colds are caused by any one of about 200 viruses that are breathed in. Cold viruses infect the nose and throat, causing the familiar symptoms of sneezing, runny nose and eyes, and sore throat. Sometimes, the viral infection is also complicated by a bacterial infection, which may spread to the sinuses, to the larynx, and down to the lungs. Other infections of the lung include different kinds of pneumonia, which are caused by bacteria or viruses.

Disorders caused by allergies

The respiratory system is also affected by allergies. One of them, hay fever, causes the membranes lining the nose to swell, the nose to run, and the eyes to water. Asthma causes the airways of the lungs to contract. Attacks may be caused by allergic reactions to many different substances, such as house dust and food additives, or by emotional stress. Farmer's lung is a disease similar to pneumoconiosis and is caused by an allergy to a fungus growing on moldy grain or hay.

SEE ALSO

ALLERGIES • ASTHMA • BACTERIA • BRONCHITIS • CANCER • COLD • EMPHYSEMA • HEART DISEASES AND DISORDERS • INFECTIOUS DISEASES • LUNG DISEASES AND DISORDERS • PNEUMONIA • RESPIRATORY SYSTEM • VIRUSES

Retina and Retinal Disorders

Q & A

My grandmother has age-related macular degeneration and is unable to read, watch television, or even tell the time from her watch. I'm really worried about her. Will she soon be totally blind?

No. Although your grandmother is badly disabled by her loss of central vision, the disease never affects any part of the retina other than the central macular region. Therefore, her peripheral vision will be preserved.

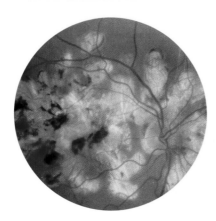

This image of a retina was taken with an ophthalmoscope. It reveals diabetic retinopathy, in which severe damage to the retina has been caused by diabetes. This condition may lead to blindness.

The human eye is much like a camera, capturing images and storing them for future viewing. Light enters the eye through a small hole called the pupil and is focused on the retina, which acts like the camera's film. The most complex part of the eye, the retina is a delicate membrane that covers the rear inner surface of the eyeball. It converts the images it captures into electrical nerve impulses that are then passed along the optic nerves and optic tracts to the rear part of the brain.

The retina is normally deep red owing to its rich blood supply. An ophthalmologist can use an ophthalmoscope to see through the pupil and lens to the retina. Any changes in the color or appearance of the retina may indicate a disease, and many such diseases can be very serious.

Diseases of the retina

Retinopathy refers to diseases of the retina. There are several types of retinopathy, all of which involve disease of the small retinal blood vessels. The most common form of these is diabetic retinopathy. The condition takes two forms: nonproliferative retinopathy (which barely affects vision and may not require any form of treatment) and proliferative retinopathy (characterized by the production of new, fragile blood vessels and bleeding into the vitreous gel of the eye). Proliferative diabetic retinopathy, caught in time, can be treated effectively with laser surgery.

A retinal detachment occurs when the retina is pulled away from its normal position; this detachment prevents the retina from working correctly and blurs the eye's vision. Some of the possible symptoms of a retinal detachment are flashing lights, a shadow in the outer edges of the eye, and a gray curtain moving across the field of vision.

Macular degeneration is an age-related disorder that involves only the central part of the retina and may progressively destroy this area, causing visual distortion that progresses slowly or quickly to total loss of central vision. In some cases, the progression can be stopped by laser treatment.

Retinitis pigmentosa is a genetic disease that causes night blindness and a progressive loss of peripheral vision so that a form of tunnel vision gradually worsens. There is no effective treatment, although the use of sunglasses to protect the retina from ultraviolet light may help preserve the patient's vision.

SEE ALSO

BLINDNESS • DIABETES • EYE AND SIGHT • EYE DISEASES AND DISORDERS • GLAUCOMA

Reye's Syndrome

Q & A

My brother insists that Reye's syndrome is a new disease that started in the 1980s. However, my cousin says that it has been around for a lot longer than that. Which one is right?

Your cousin is right. Reye's syndrome was first described in 1963, and even then it was not a new disease. The difficulty is that Reye's syndrome so closely mimics other serious conditions that, in the past, people suffering from it were wrongly diagnosed as having meningitis, encephalitis, hepatitis, diabetic hypoglycemia, a drug overdose, or accidental poisoning.

I've heard that Reye's syndrome is more likely to occur at certain times of the year. Is that true? If it is, then at what time of the year is it more likely to occur?

Yes, it is true. The highest incidence of Reye's syndrome is in late fall and winter. It is no coincidence that these are the periods in which influenza is also the most common.

Reye's syndrome is a serious and sometimes fatal illness that is most common in children between the ages of 5 and 10. In the United States, most cases occur in late fall and winter among children already affected by a viral infection such as a cold, influenza, or chicken pox.

In 1963 the Australian pathologist Ralph Douglas Reye (1922–1977) published a report of a devastating disorder that could affect young children during the week following an influenza-like viral infection. Reye's syndrome is rare, but unless it is recognized quickly at onset, the outcome is often fatal.

Doctors are uncertain about what causes the disease, but aspirin (which is usually given to alleviate the symptoms of the original infection) is known to be a factor. About 96 percent of the children who develop the disease have, in the previous week, had aspirin in the first three days of a viral infection.

Reye's syndrome has two main features: a dangerous swelling of the brain and a serious disorder of the liver. The first stage is the virus infection, which may be a minor illness. This is followed by persistent vomiting, lethargy, aggressive behavior (on about the sixth day of the illness), and rapidly progressive mental confusion (which, within hours or days, may proceed to a coma from which the patient cannot be aroused). In the late stages there may be seizures, loss of reflexes, and an inability to breathe, indicating a serious brain disorder known as encephalopathy.

Diagnosis and treatment

Successful treatment depends on early diagnosis, so that skilled intensive care may be given at once. The essential element is the maintenance of a good circulation of well-oxygenated blood to the brain. The body temperature is also monitored and carefully maintained. An intravenous drip will be set up, and hypoglycemia will be corrected by infusions of dextrose. Pressure within the skull from brain swelling is treated with intravenous steroids. If necessary, a small opening will be made in the skull to relieve pressure. If Reye's syndrome is not diagnosed early enough, the patient can go into a coma and suffer serious brain damage or even death. Because of the risk of Reye's syndrome, aspirin should never be given to children under the age of 12.

SEE ALSO

BRAIN • BRAIN DAMAGE AND DISORDERS • CHICKEN POX • COLD • HYPOGLYCEMIA • INFECTIOUS MONONUCLEOSIS • INFLUENZA • LIVER DISEASES AND DISORDERS • MEASLES • MUMPS • POLIOMYELITIS • RUBELLA • VIRUSES

Rheumatic Fever

Rheumatic fever is a serious illness in children and adolescents. An immune system reaction to streptococcus bacteria, it used to be common but has now become rare in developed countries. However, isolated outbreaks in the United States, England, and Scandinavia have alerted people to the possibility that streptococcus may become a problem again.

Symptoms and treatments

Rheumatic fever usually follows a strep throat or scarlet fever. In a few people, this type of throat infection causes something to go wrong with the body's defense system, and it reacts against normal tissues. The throat infection clears up, but from one to six weeks later, the patient begins to feel generally tired and ill, with fever, loss of appetite, and loss of weight.

The other symptoms of rheumatic fever vary from one patient to another, because it can attack several of the body's systems. Sometimes, the fever causes rheumatism, a term used to describe aches and pains of varying origin in joints, muscles, tendons, or ligaments. Rheumatic fever mainly affects the hips and knees. First one joint and then another becomes swollen and very painful. It may also affect the skin, producing a rash with pale-centered red rings. Nodules can be felt under the skin over bones in the wrists, knees, elbows, and ankles.

Most seriously, rheumatic fever inflames the lining of the heart and the heart muscle, and this condition can lead to abnormal heart valves and to heart failure. The disease can also affect the nervous system, causing chorea or Saint Vitus' dance, which results in writhing movements and facial grimacing. The movements are made worse by excitement and disappear when the child is asleep. Saint Vitus' dance seldom lasts for more than a few weeks but may recur.

Patients with rheumatic fever are kept in bed and are given large doses of aspirin. Sometimes, steroid drugs are given to reduce the possibility of inflammation of the heart. It takes about six weeks to recover. The main danger is that repeated attacks may damage the heart valves. People who have had one such episode may be given antibiotics, such as penicillin, regularly for up to five years to prevent any more attacks.

Q & A

Do you always get heart trouble after having rheumatic fever?

No. It is possible to have the disease without developing any heart trouble. Generally, severe long-term heart trouble occurs only after repeated or very prolonged attacks of rheumatic fever; it is much less likely to result from a single attack.

Is it possible to get rheumatic fever when you are an adult?

Rheumatic fever is a disease of childhood and adolescence. It rarely occurs after the age of 18.

My mother says that rheumatic fever used to be more common. Is it really more rare now?

It is still prevalent in some less developed countries, but it is less common in the United States and other developed countries owing to the more widespread use of antibiotics to treat streptococcal infections. It was almost eradicated in the United States in the early 1980s, but it resurged in 1985, and incidents have continued to occur.

SEE ALSO

BACTERIA • BACTERIAL DISEASES • HEART DISEASES AND DISORDERS • IMMUNE SYSTEM • JOINT DISORDERS • MUSCLE • NERVOUS SYSTEM • SKIN • SKIN DISEASES AND DISORDERS • STREPTOCOCCAL INFECTIONS

Rickets

Rickets is a bone condition present in children whose bodies lack sufficient amounts of vitamin D. It can cause lasting and often serious damage to their health. A similar condition in adults is known as osteomalacia.

Saltwater fish such as herring, salmon, and sardines and fish liver oils are good sources of vitamin D; lower amounts are present in butter, eggs, and milk, unless they have been fortified. Vitamin D is also made by the skin in response to sunlight. Thus, rickets is more likely to occur in children eating a poor diet and living in northern countries, where there is less sunshine. Vitamin D allows the body to absorb calcium from food and makes sure that the calcium is passed from the blood into the bone when the bone is being formed. If the level of vitamin D falls, the blood calcium level will fall, too. This could result in muscle spasms, so the body releases calcium from the bones back into the bloodstream. As a result, the bones become weak through lack of calcium, and new bones are soft, because they do not have enough calcium in them.

A substance called osteoid is laid down in large amounts at points where the bones are growing, particularly in the wrists, knees, and ankles, making these joints larger than normal. The long bones of the legs become bent by the weight of the body. The bones of the skull may become soft, and the backbone and pelvis may be deformed.

Rickets is now very unusual in the United States, where vitamin D is added to milk. Vitamin D can also be taken as tablets or drops.

However, too much vitamin D is bad for the body, so any supplements should be taken only under a doctor's supervision.

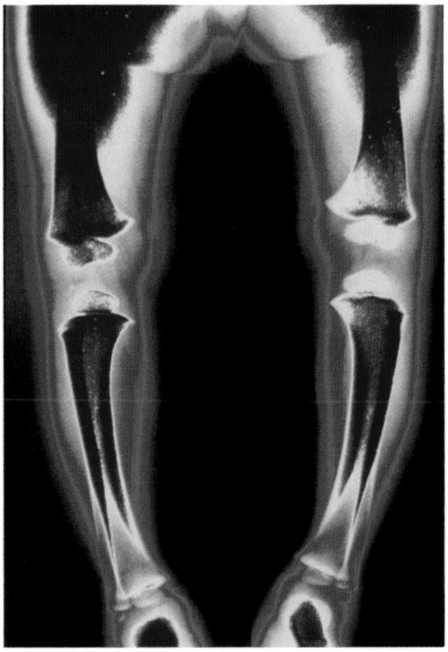

This colored X-ray shows the bones in the bowed legs of a child recovering from rickets. These bones are severely curved as a result of vitamin D deficiency.

Q & A

My great-grandmother says that if a child is given cod liver oil every day, it will prevent rickets. Is she right?

Large quantities of cod liver oil and other fish oils used to be given for this reason, but it is now known not to be such a good idea. Fish liver oils are a good source of vitamin D, and they will prevent rickets. However, high levels of vitamin D can be very dangerous, because they lead to increased calcium in the blood. Cod liver oil must not be taken indiscriminately, especially because rickets is relatively rare. Vitamin supplements are safe, if you do not take more than the stated amount; remember that too much is as dangerous as too little.

Why do the legs become bent in rickets?

The bones simply go soft as a result of the disease and are unable to support the weight of the body.

SEE ALSO

BLOOD • BONE • BONE DISEASES AND DISORDERS • MUSCLE • NUTRITIONAL DISEASES • SKELETAL SYSTEM

Rickettsial Diseases

Q & A

How did the organisms that are responsible for Rocky Mountain spotted fever and epidemic typhus get their names?

In 1916, the microorganism responsible for Rocky Mountain spotted fever was named *Rickettsia rickettsii* after the scientist Howard Ricketts, who isolated it. *Rickettsia prowazekii*, responsible for epidemic typhus, was named for a colleague, Stanislaus von Prowazek. Both men died from rickettsial infections while carrying out research on the organisms.

Is it true that Rocky Mountain spotted fever is now uncommon in the Rocky Mountains?

Yes. The name of the disease is a bit misleading because, now, fewer than 2 percent of cases occur in the Rocky Mountains area. However, the disease was first discovered there, and the name has stuck.

Can typhus cause gangrene?

Yes. In severe cases of the disease there may be gangrene of the extremities, such as the fingers, toes, ears, and genitals.

Rickettsia are microorganisms, smaller than bacteria but larger than viruses. They cause some serious illnesses, such as typhus and Rocky Mountain spotted fever. All the illnesses are carried from one human to another, or from one animal to another, by insects and arachnids: typhus by lice, and other diseases by fleas, ticks, and bloodsucking mites. Each infection can be cured by antibiotics, but treatment must be started as early as possible.

All the rickettsial infections cause fevers and a rash, so it is not easy to distinguish them from other infections. The clue lies in bites by lice or ticks. The infections have an incubation period of one to three weeks, and they all last about three or four weeks. Vaccines against these diseases have been developed, but they are not widely used. The spread of the diseases can be checked by the use of insecticides and high standards of hygiene.

Rocky Mountain spotted fever

Rocky Mountain spotted fever is a serious illness caused by a rickettsial microorganism. It is found throughout the American continent and spread from wild animals to humans and from one human to another by the bites of ticks. If left untreated, the disease can be fatal, but it can usually be cured by antibiotics.

The first symptoms of the fever appear a few days after the infecting bite. They include a headache, a high fever, and a rash on the wrists, ankles, palms of the hands, and soles of the feet that then spreads rapidly to the face, neck, and trunk. Other symptoms include pains in the joints and muscles, nausea, and chills. If the fever is not treated, the heart, liver, lungs, and kidneys may be damaged. The blood may flow around the body so slowly that gangrene develops in the fingers and toes.

In areas where there are known to be ticks, people should wear protective clothes and inspect themselves and their pets frequently for ticks. There are two methods of removing a tick from a person or a pet: putting a drop of alcohol onto the tick and covering the tick with petroleum jelly. Both of these techniques loosen the tick's hold on the skin. It can then be removed very carefully with a pair of tweezers. It is essential to avoid crushing the tick, because a crushed tick may release infected fluids or tissue into the wound it has made. Anyone who is bitten by a tick and then gets feverish symptoms should see a doctor for immediate treatment with antibiotics.

> **SEE ALSO**
> BACTERIA • GANGRENE • INFECTIOUS DISEASES • VIRUSES

Ringworm

Ringworm is a fungal infection that attacks the skin, mostly on the scalp, feet, nails, and groin. It is very easily passed from one person to another, but it is not difficult to treat. In spite of its name, ringworm is not caused by a worm and does not always appear in the shape of a ring.

Ringworm fungi feed on the dead tissues of the epidermis (the outermost layer of the skin) and then make their way into the tissues beneath, including the dermis. The fungi may produce a raised, red ring or they may make the skin gray and scaly. The symptoms vary according to which part of the body is infected, but all types of ringworm itch very badly.

Ringworm of the scalp is quite common in children and spreads rapidly through schools. The fungus usually grows outward in a ring. As the inner area begins to heal, the red, itchy area around it spreads in an even larger circle. The hairs in the center snap off but start to grow again as the skin heals. The infection can be treated with antifungal creams and with the antibiotic griseofulvin. The hair should be washed regularly, and all brushes, combs, and towels should be sterilized.

Q & A

My grandfather says that, in the past, children who got ringworm had to be kept in isolation for months and had to have their heads shaved. Why doesn't that happen now?

These measures, which were once commonplace, are not necessary any more, because antibiotics taken by mouth are effective in curing stubborn ringworm of the scalp that resists local treatment with creams. However, while a child has ringworm, he or she should be kept away from school to avoid spreading the infection.

I have recurring athlete's foot, and now I've noticed that one of my toenails has become very gnarled and odd-looking. Is there any connection?

The ringworm fungus that causes athlete's foot can also lodge itself and grow underneath the toenail, eventually leading to the condition you describe. You should seek prompt medical attention for this problem before the fungus spreads farther, or you may lose the nail altogether.

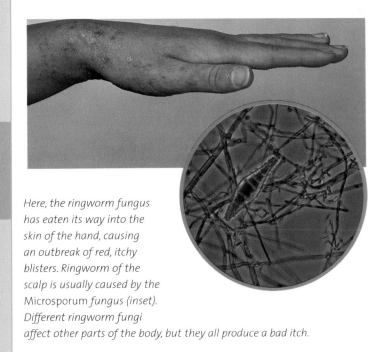

Here, the ringworm fungus has eaten its way into the skin of the hand, causing an outbreak of red, itchy blisters. Ringworm of the scalp is usually caused by the Microsporum *fungus (inset). Different ringworm fungi affect other parts of the body, but they all produce a bad itch.*

SEE ALSO

ATHLETE'S FOOT • FUNGAL INFECTIONS • INFECTIOUS DISEASES • SKIN DISEASES AND DISORDERS

Rubella

Rubella, or German measles, is an infectious disease caused by a virus. It is not serious in itself, but if a pregnant woman catches rubella in the first months of her pregnancy, her developing baby may be seriously deformed. For this reason, all girls should be immunized against rubella by the age of 13; one injection gives them protection for life.

Symptoms

Rubella is caught by breathing in droplets that have been coughed, sneezed, or breathed out by an infected person. It has an incubation period of about three weeks, during which there are no symptoms. Then, a rash of fine pink dots under the skin appears on the face and neck, spreading to the trunk, arms, and legs. Some of the lymph nodes become swollen and tender. Some patients have a low fever and sore throat. The symptoms are so mild that some people do not realize that they are ill. The rash and swollen nodes disappear after a few days. Unless the patient feels ill, there is no need to stay in bed.

People who get rubella will be infectious for about a week before the rash appears and for a few days afterward. They should tell anyone they have been in contact with during this time about the risk of infection, and they should be careful to warn and to keep away from pregnant women.

Risks to the unborn child

The virus can cause the unborn child to develop defects in its heart, nervous system, sight, hearing, bones, spleen, and liver. The developing baby may not grow properly and may have mental

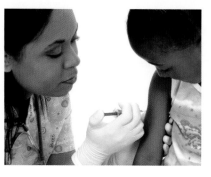

retardation. The risks are greatest before the fetus is 17 weeks old. Anyone who has had rubella becomes immune to catching it again. Any woman who is not sure if she has had rubella can have a blood test that will show whether or not she is immune.

Q & A

My aunt is six months pregnant, and she just found out that she has rubella. Is the baby at risk? What should she do?

By six months, your aunt's baby will have developed all the essential organs and systems, so the baby is unlikely to be affected. However, your aunt should see her doctor as soon as possible for reassurance.

My grandmother says that when she was young, people used to hold rubella parties so all the children could catch the illness and become immune. This sounds like a fun way to handle rubella. Why not do this now?

Years ago, if a child had rubella, all the neighborhood children would be invited over to catch it. However, this measure did not protect all children. Now, there is a vaccine that gives 100 percent protection. The vaccine may be less fun, but it is a lot safer.

A vaccination is now available that gives long-lasting protection against rubella. A single shot is needed and is given to girls between the ages of 1 and 13 years.

SEE ALSO

BONE • INFECTIOUS DISEASES • MEASLES • NERVOUS SYSTEM • SKIN • THROAT DISEASES AND DISORDERS • VIRUSES

Salmonella

Salmonellosis is a common form of food poisoning, caused by bacteria of the genus *Salmonella*. These organisms contaminate foods from domestic animals, especially eggs, poultry, meats, and dairy products, as well as fish and shellfish. Salmonella is considered one of the nation's most important communicable diseases, affecting approximately two million people each year.

Q & A

I read somewhere that the acid in a person's stomach destroys salmonella. If this is true, then how do people manage to get infected with salmonella?

It is certainly true that stomach acid provides an important barrier to infection. Food tends to stay in the stomach longer than liquids, so an infected drink may be a greater hazard than infected food. It also appears that people with no stomach acid (as a result of either illness or an operation) are more at risk of being infected by salmonella.

Bacteria killed by heat

Salmonella bacteria are killed by heat. Freshly cooked food that has been heated through quite thoroughly should be safe. However, unless the cook is hygienic, the food may be contaminated again by coming into contact with raw meat, kitchen utensils, or hands. Cooked and raw food should always be kept separate. Freezing does not kill salmonella; it simply stops bacterial growth, which will begin again as the food thaws. Frozen poultry is easily contaminated as it is prepared for freezing; it must always be thawed out completely before cooking, and then cooked thoroughly all the way through. Undercooked eggs, or foods such as mayonnaise that are made with raw eggs, may also carry the infection. These types of foods should not be given to those who are in at-risk groups, such as pregnant women, babies, young children, people with immune deficiency diseases, and seniors.

Some household pets, such as chicks, frogs, and aquarium snails, can pass on salmonella bacteria. Infection can be avoided by careful hygiene. The hands should always be washed after handling aquarium pets, and pet birds should be kept out of the kitchen or other rooms where food is usually prepared or eaten.

Symptoms and treatments

Symptoms of salmonella poisoning include severe headache, vomiting, diarrhea, stomach cramps, and sometimes fever. Treatment is usually bed rest with a diet of bland food and plenty of fluids. Patients at risk are often prescribed antibiotics.

Epidemics of salmonella poisoning can be particularly dangerous in nursing homes, where the elderly patients are vulnerable to it. Public health regulations aim to prevent outbreaks by overseeing standards of hygiene in food preparation factories, hospitals, restaurants, and hotels.

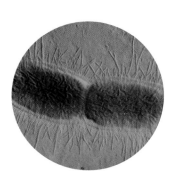

Cooked meat can be contaminated with bacilli from raw meat. The salmonella bacterium seems to thrive in poultry and eggs and in processed cooked meats prepared in unhygienic conditions.

SEE ALSO

BACTERIA • BACTERIAL DISEASES • BOTULISM • DIARRHEA • INFECTIOUS DISEASES

SARS

Severe acute respiratory syndrome (SARS) is a respiratory illness caused by a virus. First recognized as a potential worldwide threat in March 2003, the disease led the World Health Organization to issue its first global health alert warning in more than 10 years. In November 2002, cases of a new and highly infectious form of pneumonia began to appear in Guangdong province in southern China. Medical officials estimated that 792 people were infected or thought to be infected and 31 had died. This initial report of incidence and mortality was soon shown to be a serious underestimate.

By the end of April 2003, more than 1,000 cases had been reported in Guangdong, and the disease had spread to almost every province in mainland China, with a total of more than 3,000 cases. By mid-May, more than 7,600 cases had been reported worldwide from 29 countries, with 587 deaths. In the United States, 345 cases of SARS had been identified from 38 states, but there had been no deaths.

SARS is caused by a new strain of coronavirus, the same class of viruses that causes the common cold and other respiratory infections. Until the SARS outbreak, these viruses have never been particularly virulent in humans, although they can cause severe diseases in animals. For that reason, scientists originally thought that the SARS virus might have crossed from animals to humans. It now seems likely, however, that the SARS virus evolved from one or more animal viruses into a completely new strain.

Like most respiratory illnesses, SARS is most likely spread through droplets that enter the air when someone with the disease coughs, sneezes, or talks. People with SARS must be isolated and approached only by a limited number of medical personnel who are wearing masks, gowns, gloves, and eye protection. Many patients require supplementary oxygen, and in severe cases mechanical ventilation is necessary.

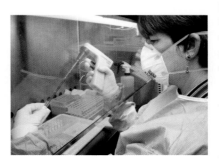

A scientist at the Special Pathogens Branch of the Centers for Disease Control processes SARS specimens.

SEE ALSO

COLD • INFECTIOUS DISEASES • PNEUMONIA • RESPIRATORY SYSTEM DISEASES AND DISORDERS • VIRUSES

Q & A

How can people minimize the risk of SARS infection when traveling in a region where the disease is a problem?

The SARS virus is spread on droplets through coughing and through contact with surfaces that have been contaminated by infected people. Viruses can easily pass through porous face masks, but these masks offer some protection against inhalation of infected droplets. As with the common cold viruses, hand-to-eye transmission is possible. Care should be taken never to rub the eyes after possible contamination of the hands. Frequent hand-washing and the use of alcohol-based disinfectants are effective against the viruses. Research in Hong Kong has shown that these measures, intelligently applied, can prevent infection.

The death rate from SARS ranges from 10 percent to more than 50 percent. Why?

The rate differs according to age groups. The overall death rate is 15 percent. For those over 60, however, the average death rate from SARS is 50 percent.

Sciatica

Sciatica, or sciatic neuritis, is pain along the large sciatic nerve that runs from the lower back down through the buttocks and along the back of each leg. It is a relatively common form of back pain. The pain is caused by pressure on the sciatic nerve as it leaves the spinal column.

Sciatica can have a variety of causes, including a herniated (slipped) disk in the spinal column, arthritis, or a fall. In most people who have sciatica, the disks in the backbone have become weakened, either with age or as a result of excessive strain. The disks are pads of tissue that separate the vertebrae. The disks and vertebrae provide the necessary flexibility for people to stretch and bend. Each disk consists of a soft center, which acts as a shock absorber, and a tough fibrous outer layer. Sometimes, this outer layer weakens in parts, and the soft center bulges out. The resulting bulge puts pressure on the nerve to the leg and causes the pain of sciatica.

Any pressure on the sciatic nerve causes sharp, stabbing pains in the buttock and down the leg. It may happen suddenly when someone is bending or stretching or it may come on gradually. Even a slight movement, such as coughing or sneezing, can bring on the pain or make it worse. For anyone suffering from sciatica, walking and sitting can be painful and difficult. The most comfortable position is lying on the back with the knees bent.

Treatments

Sciatica as a result of a slipped disk, which can be extremely unpleasant on some occasions and often disabling, usually improves on its own if the proper measures are taken. Treatment for sciatica starts with relieving the pain by resting in a firm bed and taking painkillers when necessary. Manual treatments, such as physical therapy and osteopathic or chiropractic treatments, may help relieve the pressure. Painkillers such as nonsteroidal anti-inflammatory drugs (NSAIDs), oral steroids, or epidural steroid injections can help relieve the inflammation. Muscle relaxants may be used to help relieve spasms.

It is very important to stay in bed and to resist the temptation to be up and about when the disk is only half-healed; otherwise, the patient will be back to where he or she started. Surgical treatment, a last resort, is usually reserved for those who have had repeated episodes that have not improved with bed rest.

SEE ALSO

NERVOUS SYSTEM • NERVOUS SYSTEM DISORDERS • SLIPPED DISK • SPINAL COLUMN

Q & A

I'm very confused. What is the difference between a backache and sciatica?

Sciatica is the name given to the type of back pain that radiates down the back of the leg. However, herniated (slipped) disks may start with pain limited to the back before the disk starts exerting pressure on the nerves to the leg, which causes sciatica. Most people with a bad back do not have slipped disks; they have strained ligaments and muscles.

I've heard of some people who had surgery to cure their sciatica, but that sounds extreme to me. Is surgery always necessary, or are there other ways to cure sciatica?

For a person's first attack of sciatica, the doctor will probably not recommend surgery so long as he or she is fairly confident that a slipped disk is the cause (as it usually is). Most people with sciatica find that the pain improves if they can rest their back properly and then resume exercise.

Scoliosis

Any sideways curvature seen or felt in the spine (spinal column) is called scoliosis. However, the spine is very flexible, especially in childhood, and it is easily bent to one side. A normal spine should appear straight when viewed from the back. There are other forms of spinal curvature, including kyphosis (a rounded back) and hunched shoulders in people who have poor posture.

There are two types of scoliosis, postural and structural. Postural scoliosis happens when something other than the spine causes it to bend to one side: for example, having one leg shorter than the other. When a child is sitting, however, the spine is straight. This test distinguishes postural scoliosis from the structural form. Many children have slight postural scoliosis without being aware of it. Older people with a slipped disk may have tight muscles on one side of the spine, which can also cause temporary postural scoliosis.

In structural scoliosis, there is a permanent defect in the bones of the spine or in their relationship to each other. In addition, because there is a fixed abnormal curve, there will always be a secondary curve to compensate so that the shoulders remain straight. The most common type of structural scoliosis is adolescent idiopathic scoliosis, which occurs while the spine is growing. The cause is unknown. It is usually first noticed between the ages of 10 and 15 and may affect any part of the spine. If the scoliosis is in the chest region of the spine, the ribs will protrude on the side of the curve and cause a hump. In girls, the breasts may also appear unbalanced.

Other types of structural scoliosis may be due to bone disease, bone abnormalities present from birth, or unbalanced muscle disorders that cause a sideways pull on the spine.

Treatments

First, the type of scoliosis must be diagnosed. X-rays are taken of the spine to measure the angle between the upper surface of vertebrae above and below the scoliosis. Regular checks are needed to monitor the condition. Exercises may be helpful for maintaining the flexibility of the spine, but they cannot cure scoliosis. If the curvature gets worse and the angle exceeds 20 degrees, a spinal support is required until the bones have stopped growing. When the curvature is more than 40 degrees, surgery is required to straighten the spine and fuse the bones.

> **SEE ALSO**
>
> ARTHRITIS • BONE • OSTEOPOROSIS • SKELETAL SYSTEM • SLIPPED DISK • SPINAL COLUMN

Q & A

My 10-year-old-brother has scoliosis. The doctor says that my brother may need an operation when he is older but must wear a brace until then. Why?

Scoliosis tends to worsen during growth, so your brother probably needs a brace to prevent his curve from getting any worse. Operations for scoliosis stop the spine from growing, so surgeons prefer to put off the operation until the child's growth is nearly complete.

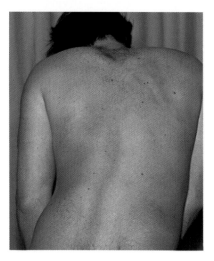

The effects of scoliosis—a twisted spine—can be clearly seen in this woman.

Scurvy

Scurvy is a disease caused by severe vitamin C deficiency. This vitamin is present mainly in fresh fruits and vegetables. In developed countries, scurvy is uncommon, but elderly people, alcoholics, and anyone who does not eat properly may develop it.

Vitamin C is needed to produce collagen, which is the basic protein that makes up all fibrous tissues in the body. Vitamin C is essential for the formation of blood vessels, bones, teeth, and ligaments. If there is insufficient vitamin C in the diet, blood vessels weaken and may bleed and other collagen problems may arise. Vitamin C is also an important antioxidant, a substance that helps reduce the risk of tissue damage from powerful chemical groups called free radicals. Free radicals are implicated in many disease processes and other health hazards, such as smoking, and are thought to be involved in the deposition of cholesterol in the arteries.

Children who do not have enough vitamin C lose weight and become irritable, their gums bleed, and their limbs may swell and become painful. Adults with scurvy also lose weight and become depressed. Their gums bleed and then draw back from the teeth, which may fall out. Large bruises appear, usually on the thighs, and sometimes there are little red bleeding marks around the roots of body hairs. As the disease gets worse, there is bleeding in the muscles or in the intestines. Wounds may not heal, because vitamin C is essential if the skin is to heal properly. The bones may become softened due to the deficiency.

Treatment for scurvy is simple—vitamin C tablets bring immediate improvement; then the patient must keep to a diet that contains enough vitamin C.

Q & A

Is scurvy an extremely painful condition?

If the teeth are still present in the mouth, it can be very painful. The pain of scurvy is most striking in babies. The disease causes bleeding into the periosteum, the fibrous covering of the bones, and this condition is so painful that the baby may adopt the characteristic froglike posture associated with scurvy.

I understand that scurvy causes the teeth to fall out, but what happens if a person has already lost all of his or her teeth?

One of the main effects of scurvy is on the teeth and gums, which bleed and become infected. If the person has already lost his or her teeth, the gums will not be affected.

Is there vitamin C in potatoes?

Yes, but the amount varies according to how long they have been stored. New potatoes contain more vitamin C than older potatoes. Also, prolonged cooking destroys the vitamin.

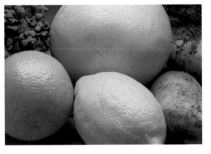

Scurvy was once a common disease among sailors who went on long ocean voyages. However, once it was recognized that eating fresh fruits and vegetables could prevent scurvy, such supplies were carried on board whenever possible.

SEE ALSO

ARTERY DISEASES AND DISORDERS • BLOOD • BONE • GUM DISEASES • MALNUTRITION • MUSCLE • NUTRITIONAL DISEASES • SKIN DISEASES AND DISORDERS

Sexually Transmitted Diseases

Q & A

Is it possible to have a sexually transmitted disease without knowing it?

Yes. People can carry the germs that cause these diseases and be unaware that they are infected. For example, about 80 percent of women who have gonorrhea have no idea that anything at all is wrong with them.

I've heard that you can catch an STD from a dirty toilet seat. Is that true?

That situation virtually never occurs, except in the case of trichomoniasis, a common cause of inflammation of the vagina. Sexually transmitted diseases are caught by having sexual intercourse with somebody who already has the disease, even if he or she is not aware of it.

Is it possible to get vaccinated against an STD?

Not at present, although a vaccine for genital herpes has been developed in a British research unit and vaccination against gonorrhea may become possible.

Sexually transmitted diseases (STDs) are passed from one person to another through sexual contact. Left untreated, some of these diseases can cause infertility; damage to joints, the brain, and other organs; and in some cases, death. STDs can also be passed to the children of infected people, either before or during birth.

HIV, a virus that can be transmitted sexually, causes AIDS. Other infections spread by sexual contact include syphilis, gonorrhea, chlamydia (which causes urethritis in men and pelvic inflammatory disease in women), and genital herpes. Other sexually transmitted diseases include trichomoniasis, candida, pubic lice, and genital warts (which has been linked to a higher chance of developing cervical cancer in women). Women who have had genital warts should have an annual cervical smear.

The symptoms of STDs include unusual discharges from the penis or vagina, sores in the genital region, and pain when urinating. Other symptoms, such as fever, pain in the abdomen, and a rash, are less easy to recognize, because they could belong to many different infections.

Despite the known risks of STDs, sexual promiscuity among young people remains very common. This has led to a noticeable increase in STDs, especially gonorrhea. Since there are usually no signs at first that someone has an infection, he or she may pass it on to a number of partners, who in turn may infect anyone with whom they have sexual contact.

As yet, there is no way of immunizing against STDs. A medical test shows if a person has an infection. People can go to their own physicians for tests and treatment or to special clinics where they can remain anonymous. Efforts are made to find and test all the sexual contacts of people with serious STDs so these contacts can be cured before they pass on the disease to more people.

People who have sex with more than one partner are more likely to pick up an infection. The easiest way to avoid becoming infected is abstinence. It is best for people not to have sex until they are old enough to cope with the consequences if it goes wrong. It is essential to practice safe sex using a latex condom and to avoid having sex with multiple partners.

SEE ALSO

AIDS AND HIV • BACTERIA • BACTERIAL DISEASES • BLOOD • COMMUNICABLE DISEASES • FUNGAL INFECTIONS • GONORRHEA • HERPES • HPV • IMMUNE SYSTEM • IMMUNODEFICIENCY • NONSPECIFIC URETHRITIS • PELVIC INFLAMMATORY DISEASE • TRICHOMONIASIS • VIRUSES

Shingles

Shingles is a very painful disease caused by herpes zoster, the same virus that causes chicken pox. Chicken pox usually affects children, but most people with shingles are over the age of 40. Although it is unproved, it seems probable that anyone who gets shingles had chicken pox at some time in the past; the virus then became dormant in the body. Doctors do not know just what triggers an attack of shingles; it cannot be caught from someone with chicken pox, although a person with shingles can pass chicken pox on to someone else. Shingles usually does no long-lasting damage, but a complete recovery can take some time.

The first sign of shingles is a pain on the surface of the skin, which then starts to redden. The patient may have a fever. A rash with little vesicles (clear spots filled with fluid) breaks out. This rash often spreads around one side of the body to form a band. As the virus spreads down a particular sensory nerve from the spinal cord or from the brain, it appears on the area of skin that this nerve supplies. The area most often affected is the chest and upper abdomen, but sometimes the limbs, neck, and face may also be involved.

The shingles rash persists for several days. At this time, the pain may lessen, but the vesicles may itch and form a crust. A lotion may sooth the itching, and the doctor may prescribe painkillers and tablets of acyclovir (Zovirax). If given early in the disease, this treatment can reduce the severity. Eventually, the rash clears up. There should be no lasting scarring, but sometimes there is depigmentation. The pain may disappear with the rash, but it can last for a while after the rash has gone. This is more likely if the trigeminal nerve—the main sensory nerve of the face—has been involved. Shingles in this area can cause damage to the eye, and the face may be paralyzed for a while.

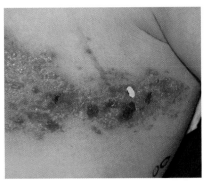

Shingles consists of a rash made up of vesicles (fluid-filled clear spots), which spread to form a band around the body.

Q & A

My grandmother had shingles, and the painful rash seemed to encircle half her body like a belt. Is this a usual reaction with shingles?

Yes. The main characteristic of this viral disease is that it is an infection that nearly always spreads out from the spinal cord through the nerves of sensation. Each nerve supplies an area of skin called a dermatome. These areas are arranged down the surface of the body like a series of belts or horizontal stripes. Normally, shingles affects one nerve's dermatome on only one side of the body, although more than one nerve can be affected in an extreme infection.

My father had shingles, and it was so painful that he could not move for a week. Is this a normal reaction?

It is normal for the condition to be painful in the early stages, but the pain often diminishes as soon as the rash has broken out. Usually, the surface tenderness is not too bad after the rash has settled down.

SEE ALSO

BRAIN • CHICKEN POX • HERPES • NERVOUS SYSTEM DISORDERS • SKIN • VIRUSES

Sickle-Cell Anemia

Q & A

Are blood transfusions needed if someone has sickle-cell disease?

Possibly. One of the problems is that the red blood cells are very unstable and break down easily, causing anemia. It may be necessary to treat this condition with blood transfusions. However, exchange transfusions are given more often. A proportion of the patient's blood is removed and replaced with normal blood. This kind of treatment is used for sickle-cell crises, in which blood vessels have been blocked off by abnormal blood cells.

Is it true that there are really many different kinds of sickle-cell diseases?

There is only one true kind of sickle-cell disease, in which the red blood cells carry the abnormal hemoglobin S, but there are some other abnormal hemoglobins, such as hemoglobin C, that can cause problems. It is possible to inherit the genes for two different types of abnormal hemoglobin from your parents, leading to diseases in which both abnormalities are present.

Red blood cells contain a substance called hemoglobin that combines with oxygen in the lungs. These cells then carry oxygen around the body. Without enough oxygen, the body cannot work efficiently. Affected people feel tired and weak, become breathless and faint, and may look pale. This condition is known as anemia. Some people are anemic because they are born with faulty hemoglobin, known as hemoglobin S, in their red blood cells. That makes the red blood cells break up unusually early, causing anemia. If the level of oxygen in the blood falls too low, the abnormal red blood cells may twist into the shape of a sickle, so the condition is known as sickle-cell anemia. This problem is most likely to happen in the hands, feet, arms, and legs. The abnormal cells tend to block small blood vessels, making the blood clot and cutting off oxygen from an area of tissue.

These crises are very painful and cause the affected tissues to die. Most organs and bones may be affected. Blood clotting may cause a stroke or heart failure. People with sickle-cell anemia have little resistance to infections.

An inherited disease

Sickle-cell anemia is an inherited disease. Only people who inherit the sickle-cell gene from both parents will have sickle-cell anemia. Some people inherit the faulty gene from only one parent and have sickle-cell trait; they have some abnormal blood cells but do not experience any serious problems unless the oxygen level in their blood falls very low. Anyone who has a sickle-cell trait or knows that it is in his or her family should have blood tests and talk to a genetic counselor before deciding to have children. If both parents carry the gene for sickle cells, their risk of having a baby with the disease is one in four.

Sickle-cell anemia seems to give some people protection against malaria. Sickle-cell anemia is often present in parts of the world where malaria is, or has been, common, such as Africa, parts of the Mediterranean, western Asia, and India. Sickle-cell anemia is also present in people whose ancestors came from these regions, including black Americans and West Indians.

Sickle-cell anemia cannot be cured, but painful crises are treated with painkillers. Transfusions of normal blood can help. In poor countries, many children die of sickle-cell anemia.

SEE ALSO

BIRTH DEFECTS • BLOOD • BLOOD DISEASES AND DISORDERS • CELLS AND CHROMOSOMES • GENES • GENETIC DISEASES AND DISORDERS • STROKE

Skeletal System

The human skeleton is strong enough to keep the body upright and protect vital organs, yet it is flexible enough to allow great freedom of movement. The skeletal system consists of the skeleton itself, which is made of bones, and the related cartilage, ligaments, and muscles.

An adult's skeleton has 206 bones. As a child grows, many bones—for example, those in the skull—fuse together. Male and female skeletons have the same number of bones, but in general the female skeleton is smaller and lighter. A woman's pelvis is broader and more boat-shaped, giving the hips their characteristic shape and allowing room for the passage of a baby's head during childbirth. A woman's shoulders are relatively narrow. In a man, the general proportions are reversed: broad shoulders and slim hips.

Each part of the skeleton has a different function. The skull protects the brain, the middle ear, the inner ear, and the eyes. The spinal column (backbone) protects the spinal cord and is made up of a chain of small bones, rather like spools, called vertebrae. Its structure gives the spinal column enormous strength, but at the same time it is very flexible. The rib cage, made up of the backbone, sternum (breastbone), and ribs, protects the heart and lungs. The pelvis shields the reproductive organs and the bladder and serves as an anchor point for the legs.

Cartilage

Cartilage is a smooth, tough, flexible tissue that forms part of the skeletal system. It is composed of cells surrounded by fibers of collagen and elastic. Cartilage gives the body strength and elasticity. There are no blood vessels or nerves in cartilage. Instead, food and oxygen are diffused from the surrounding tissue fluid.

The structure of cartilage varies according to its function. Yellow, or elastic, cartilage is extremely flexible and occurs in the earlobes, tip of the nose, and voice-producing part of the larynx. Fibrous cartilage forms the shock absorbers in the knees and the disks between the vertebrae in the spine. Hyaline cartilage lines the movable joints of the body.

Ossification

Nearly all bones begin as rods of cartilage that are gradually hardened by deposits of calcium and other minerals. This process of hardening is called ossification. It begins in the third or fourth month of an embryo's life and continues until about the age of 21. With age and wear and tear, cartilage can cause problems, particularly in the spine and knees.

Q & A

How much force is needed to break a bone?

That varies according to the position, shape, and health of the bone. The long thin bones of the arms and legs are more prone to snapping fractures than are the plate bones of the shoulder and pelvis (which are more prone to heavy blows or crushing injuries). People who are undernourished, and older people whose bones have lost part of their protein framework, have brittle bones that break easily. This is particularly the case with menopausal women who have osteoporisis.

What is a greenstick fracture?

Instead of the bone breaking into two or more separate fragments, only one side of it breaks. The other side is more bent than broken. The appearance and effect are similar to what happens if you try to break a stick of wood that is still green, hence the name. These fractures usually occur only in children whose bones have not yet fully ossified and are thus more supple.

Skeletal development

A newborn baby has more bones in its body than an adult. At birth, a baby has about 350 bones; over the years, some of these bones fuse into larger units. A baby's skull is a good example of this. During birth, the skull is squeezed through a narrow canal. If the skull were as inflexible as an adult's, it would be impossible for the baby to pass through the mother's pelvic outlet. The fontanelles, or gaps between the sections of the skull, allow the skull to be molded sufficiently to fit the birth canal. After birth, the baby's fontanelles gradually close.

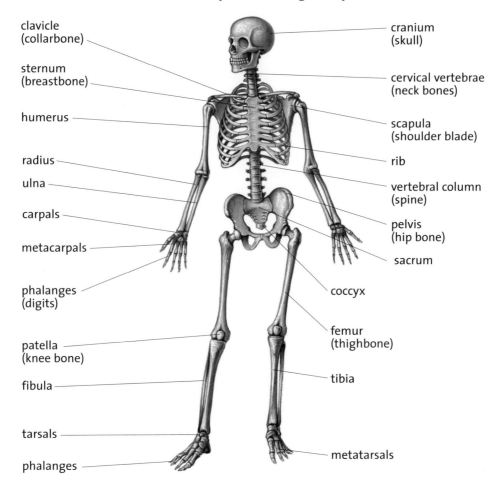

clavicle (collarbone)

sternum (breastbone)

humerus

radius

ulna

carpals

metacarpals

phalanges (digits)

patella (knee bone)

fibula

tarsals

phalanges

cranium (skull)

cervical vertebrae (neck bones)

scapula (shoulder blade)

rib

vertebral column (spine)

pelvis (hip bone)

sacrum

coccyx

femur (thighbone)

tibia

metatarsals

The human skeleton, made up of more than 200 rigid but living bones, supports the body and its vital organs and provides its shape. Here, the major bones of the skeleton are identified.

SEE ALSO

BODY SYSTEMS • BONE • BONE DISEASES AND DISORDERS • FRACTURES AND DISLOCATIONS • MUSCLE • SPINAL COLUMN

Skin

The skin is an organ—the largest the body has. It not only protects the body from injury and infection but also keeps the body's temperature and moisture content stable. Through its network of sensory nerve endings, the skin picks up information about external stimuli for transmission to the brain. The skin enables people to feel things and to experience painful and pleasant sensations through touch.

The skin is also a good indicator of the body's general health, because it is affected from within by the food eaten, by stress levels, by hormonal balance, and by physical illness. A clear, glowing complexion is regarded as a sign of good health, whereas a pallid skin could suggest anemia and a yellow tone could indicate jaundice.

Structure of the skin

The skin consists of two parts: the epidermis and the dermis. The epidermis is the upper (outer) part of the skin. It has several layers of cells, which are formed in the lower part, the dermis. Skin cells are constantly moving up to the surface, where they die and are formed into a material called keratin, which is finally shed as tiny, barely visible scales. The dermis contains the sweat glands, sebaceous glands, apocrine glands, hair follicles, and nerves. The hairs and ducts from the glands pass through the epidermis to the surface. The apocrine glands are present in the armpits and other places and produce an odor.

Skin is categorized as oily, dry, or normal, but some people have combination skin, with both oily and dry patches, usually on the face. Oily skin is more prone to problems such as acne during adolescence and early adulthood, but it ages better than dry skin, which wrinkles easily.

Skin color is due to the pigment melanin, which is produced in the lowest layer of the epidermis. The pigment-producing cells are larger in dark-skinned people than in fair-skinned people, but the number of these cells is the same. However, the amount of melanin produced varies, with dark-skinned people producing more melanin than fair-skinned people. The pigment-producing cells are also responsible for freckles.

Moles

Moles are dark spots made of collections of pigmented cells. They are very common and can be found anywhere on the body. Moles may be large or small, raised or flat, smooth or scaly, hairy or hairless. Most moles are present at birth or develop slowly during childhood. They may grow larger or darker in late adolescence or when a woman is pregnant.

Q & A

What factors affect how fast skin ages?

Inheritance is probably the most important factor in skin aging. Other influences involved are the environment, such as the amount of sun damage, and hormonal changes throughout life. The loss of elasticity that causes wrinkles in old age is due to changes in the fibers of the supporting layer of skin. Skin also becomes drier and hair becomes thinner with age.

SHAVING

During puberty, which starts at any time from age 13 to age 15, boys begin to develop facial hair. The amount of hair that grows depends on coloring and hormones. Blond men often have only a slight growth of hair, whereas those with darker hair often have a thick, dense growth. Most men prefer to remove facial hair by daily shaving.

Women often shave the hair under their arms, and those who have noticeable hair on their legs may shave them as well. To remove unwanted hair on other parts of the body, other methods of hair removal are often more suitable.

Most moles are harmless, but if a mole changes at all after adolescence, particularly if it bleeds or itches, it must be shown to a doctor. New moles that appear on adults should also be examined by a doctor. Sometimes, they may develop into a kind of skin cancer—malignant melanoma—and must be removed by surgery as soon as possible to prevent them from spreading.

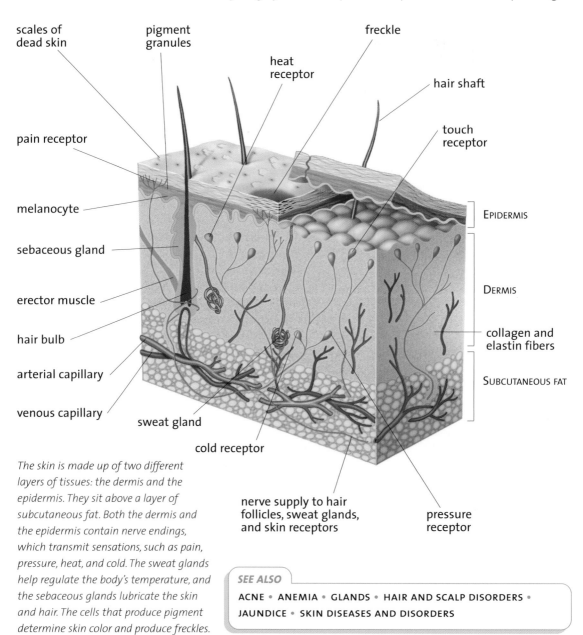

scales of dead skin

pigment granules

freckle

heat receptor

hair shaft

pain receptor

touch receptor

melanocyte

EPIDERMIS

sebaceous gland

DERMIS

erector muscle

collagen and elastin fibers

hair bulb

SUBCUTANEOUS FAT

arterial capillary

venous capillary

sweat gland

cold receptor

nerve supply to hair follicles, sweat glands, and skin receptors

pressure receptor

The skin is made up of two different layers of tissues: the dermis and the epidermis. They sit above a layer of subcutaneous fat. Both the dermis and the epidermis contain nerve endings, which transmit sensations, such as pain, pressure, heat, and cold. The sweat glands help regulate the body's temperature, and the sebaceous glands lubricate the skin and hair. The cells that produce pigment determine skin color and produce freckles.

SEE ALSO

ACNE • ANEMIA • GLANDS • HAIR AND SCALP DISORDERS • JAUNDICE • SKIN DISEASES AND DISORDERS

Skin Diseases and Disorders

The skin is an extremely important organ that fulfills many functions. Skin maintains the body at a constant temperature, ensures that it retains moisture, and protects it against heat and rain. Despite these protective qualities, skin is vulnerable to injury and infection. Sharp objects can pierce or cut skin, and it is easily scraped by anything rough or easily burned by hot appliances, hot water, or corrosive chemicals.

Potential skin problems

Skin constantly comes into contact with dirt and organisms that can cause diseases. Skin cells are continually dying off and being replaced with new ones. It is not surprising that all sorts of problems trouble the skin, but although some conditions are irritating and embarrassing, they are rarely serious and hardly ever fatal.

Childhood diseases

Babies and children have their own particular skin complaints. Cradle cap (a collection of scales and grease that sticks to the scalp) affects newborn babies, for example. It can be removed by first softening it with baby oil overnight and then gently shampooing it away. Diaper rash is an irritation of the skin caused by contact with wet or dirty diapers. Some babies also have a condition called infantile eczema, which begins with a rash. If the baby scratches it, large oozing areas develop and can become infected. This type of eczema is caused by an allergy to something, and most children grow out of it by puberty.

Q & A

Why are skin conditions so often inflamed by emotional upsets?

Most ill health is made worse by emotional upsets, and the skin is no exception. Emotion can also alter the state of the skin's irritability and sweating mechanisms. Conditions in which these factors are important, such as eczema, are aggravated by anxiety, discontent, and depression.

I developed an allergy to nickel when I wore some cheap jewelry when I was younger. Will I always have this allergy?

Allergy to nickel is fairly common in those who either wear or handle it. There is always an interval between first contact with nickel and the development of the allergy. Traces of nickel are absorbed through the skin, and the body reacts by forming antibodies so that any further contact results in an itchy, irritating skin rash. If no further contact occurs, the allergy will gradually lessen. However, it usually remains to some degree throughout life.

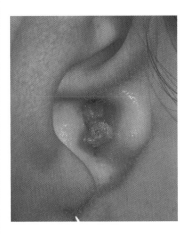

Warts are common infections that can be treated at home with salicylic acid gel.

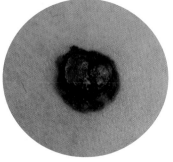

This is a malignant mole. It is characterized by itching, bleeding, or changes in color or size. Malignancy usually develops in adulthood, but if diagnosed early, it can be cured.

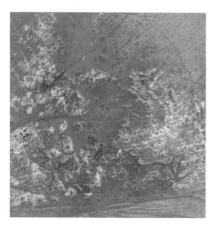

Industrial dermatitis is common among people who work with irritant substances, dust, liquids, or vapors. Rubber dermatitis, for example, may develop in someone who is in constant contact with rubber at work.

Children often get skin infections, because their bodies have not yet built up defenses against bacterial, viral, and fungal infections. Impetigo is a bacterial infection of the skin that forms crusted blisters. Ringworm and athlete's foot are fungal infections, easily spread from one child to another by towels that are contaminated. Warts are the most common viral infection of the skin; they usually appear on the hands, knees, and soles of the feet, because the virus enters wherever the skin is likely to be broken.

Skin problems in adolescence

The oil-producing glands in the skin are often affected by hormonal changes that occur at puberty. Almost all teenagers develop a few pimples at some stage, but some will develop serious acne. This is caused by the overproduction of sebum, which blocks the hair follicles. The follicles then become infected with bacteria, so that blackheads, pimples, and pustules form.

Mild acne can be helped by using lotions to control greasy skin. Moderate or severe cases of acne usually need antibiotic treatment as well as local treatment. Acne normally disappears with time.

Boils, like acne, are caused by bacterial infections of hair follicles that become filled with pus. Boils are particularly likely to occur in someone who is not in good health and whose resistance to infection is low.

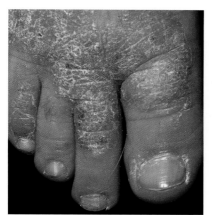

Psoriasis is a common skin disease. It is characterized by scaly red patches on the skin that cause irritation. It can occur on any part of the body, and there is no known cure.

Skin problems in adulthood

As people grow older, the skin becomes drier. Tiny cracks appear, through which irritating substances can enter. They cause inflammation of the skin, called dermatitis or eczema. An area of skin becomes red and itchy; it may flake off, and sometimes weeping blisters develop. Certain plants, such as poison ivy and sumac, can cause dermatitis. Some people may get contact dermatitis from jewelry containing a substance, such as nickel, to which they are allergic. People doing household chores often find that dermatitis is caused by cleansing products. The best way to deal with this problem is to wear rubber gloves to protect the hands from household products that cause dermatitis. Also, people should avoid any substances that are known causative agents, such as chemicals, detergents, and plants. However, some people have dermatitis for no obvious reason. It may be brought on by stress, and it tends to run in families.

In the skin rash hives, or urticaria, white welts appear, surrounded by itchy, reddened skin. It may last for weeks and is often caused by eating food to which the person is allergic.

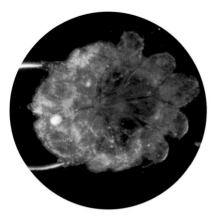

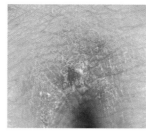

Shellfish and some fruits, food additives, and drugs can cause hives. Like many skin conditions, it is worsened by stress.

The skin replaces worn-out cells, but in psoriasis, cell reproduction in some areas is so fast that patches of skin become thickened and flaky. This condition often runs in families.

Sometimes, new skin forming a scar does not stop growing and develops into a larger scar called a keloid. It may eventually stop growing on its own or it may need medical treatment.

A different kind of thickening happens when people develop corns and calluses. They are caused by constant pressure on an area, often on the feet or hands. The area beneath the thickened skin becomes painful when it is pressed.

Lichen is another type of skin inflammation. The most common type is lichen planus, which produces red-brown itching pimples, usually on the insides of the wrists and on the cheeks. Lichen simplex causes itchy oval patches of thickened and scaly skin.

In old age, the skin becomes even drier and loses its elasticity. Many elderly people develop dry, itchy patches of skin, particularly on their legs. In addition, their skin does not easily heal itself. Some people develop keratoses (grayish patches of skin caused by the sun) and seborrheic warts (brownish-black warty patches), which are easily frozen or scraped off.

Scabies (seen greatly enlarged in the circle above) is a tiny mite that burrows under the skin. It causes intense itching and blistering of the skin, often on the hands (above right).

Skin cancers

Skin, like other parts of the body, may develop cancers. Any unusual ulcers or sores should be shown to a doctor just in case they are malignant. The sooner treatment begins, the greater the chances of its success.

It seems likely that spending a lot of time in strong sunlight may cause some kinds of skin cancer. The most serious type of skin cancer is malignant melanoma, which often develops from an existing mole.

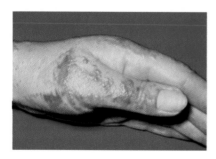

Household detergents can irritate hands and cause dermatitis. The answer is to avoid contact by wearing rubber gloves.

SEE ALSO

ACNE • ALLERGIES • ATHLETE'S FOOT • BACTERIA • BACTERIAL DISEASES • CANCER • DERMATITIS • ECZEMA • FUNGAL INFECTIONS • GLANDS • INFECTIOUS DISEASES • RINGWORM • SKIN • ULCERS • VIRUSES

Slipped Disk

Between two vertebrae of the spinal column is a disk of jellylike material, surrounded by a tough outer layer. The disk connects the vertebrae and acts as a cushion between them. Sometimes everyday wear and tear or a sudden strain makes the tough outer layer crack open. The inner layer bulges out and may press on a nerve as it leaves the spinal cord. This condition is known as a slipped or prolapsed disk. It can cause severe backache. In some cases, any movement is very painful; even coughing or sneezing can cause a sharp pain. The muscles along the spine may go into spasm or become weak or even paralyzed. The symptoms may appear suddenly or they may build up over several weeks.

The most commonly affected disks are in the lower part of the back, where the greatest strains occur, but disks in any part of the back or neck can crack open.

Most people recover from a slipped disk simply by lying flat in bed. The soft inner disk material tends to dry and shrink once it has prolapsed, thus relieving the pressure on the nerve. Lying flat keeps the pressure within the disk to a minimum. In a standing position, this pressure is higher. It is best to put a board under a soft mattress—or even put the mattress on the floor—to prevent the back from bending. In severe cases, patients may need bed rest and pain relief for two weeks or more. Great patience is needed; getting up too soon often results in a relapse.

If the patient is free of pain, physical therapy can help. If the disk is in the neck, the patient may need to wear a collar support. Painkillers and muscle relaxants will ease the pain.

In a few cases, the damaged disk may have to be removed by surgery. Patients are usually mobile again after about two weeks.

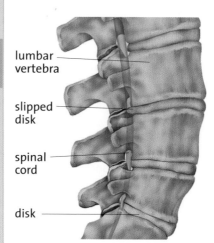

lumbar
vertebra

slipped
disk

spinal
cord

disk

A slipped disk occurs when the soft inner core of a spinal disk bulges out and presses on a nerve, causing muscle weakness and pain.

SEE ALSO

BONE • MUSCLE • SKELETAL SYSTEM • SPINAL COLUMN

Q & A

Does sleeping with a board under the mattress help prevent a slipped disk?

No, sleeping with a board under the mattress will not prevent a slipped disk. However, many people with back problems find that a firm mattress helps their back, because it is more comfortable. A soft mattress can sag in the middle, so that lying on the bed bends the back. This is an uncomfortable position. Putting a hard board under a soft mattress is an inexpensive and effective way to increase comfort.

Are women more prone to slipped disks than men?

No. Two to three times as many men as women suffer from a slipped disk. The reasons for this are not clear, and contrary to popular belief, heavy physical work is not associated with a greater risk of a slipped disk. However, a slipped disk is obviously more troublesome to someone who does heavy manual work than to someone with a more sedentary lifestyle, such as an office worker.

Smallpox

Q & A

Is it still necessary to have a smallpox vaccination?

No. The disease is now thought to have been eradicated from all parts of the world.

Did people catch smallpox even when they were vaccinated?

Yes, this might have happened. However, people were much less likely to have died from the illness if they had been vaccinated. Doctors and nurses who worked in isolation hospitals were vaccinated, and they still sometimes got a mild form of pneumonia, which was the way the disease expressed itself in an immunized person.

Did everyone with smallpox die from the disease?

There were two strains of smallpox that produced similar diseases. One of them, variola major, produced a disease that had an overall mortality of about 40 percent in people who had not been vaccinated. Variola minor, the other form, produced a similar disease that was less severe and was rarely fatal.

Smallpox is a very infectious viral disease that killed large numbers of people in many serious epidemics over the centuries. It used to be common in many parts of the world. The disease was spread from one person to another by minute droplets of saliva breathed out by infected people and had an incubation period of about 10 days.

Symptoms and treatment

During the incubation period, the disease spread from the nose and the throat of the infected person and into the lymphatic system. People with smallpox developed a fever, with aching muscles and limbs. They also developed a rash consisting of a simple outcrop of spots. In severe cases, bleeding would occur around the rash. The rash developed into raised, fluid-filled pox spots, known as vesicles. After three or four days, these vesicles became cloudy and were then called pustules. Finally, after about nine days the rash formed hard crusts that often left serious scars. Also, the virus attacked the body tissues; bleeding into internal organs could cause death.

Death could also occur in the pustular stage of the disease. Once smallpox was caught, antibiotics were given to try to prevent secondary infection of the pustules by skin bacteria. Good nursing was crucial, and great care was taken of the mouth, eyes, ears, and skin.

Prevention and eradication

In the eighteenth century, an English doctor named Edward Jenner (1749–1823) discovered that vaccination with the fluid from the spots of cowpox (a mild disease related to smallpox) could make most people immune to smallpox. Those who did get smallpox after vaccination would have only a mild case. This was the first instance of immunization. More people were vaccinated, and the disease became less common. As recently as 1967, the disease was still found in parts of the world, but an intensive program of vaccination was so successful that the World Health Organization announced in 1980 that smallpox had been completely eradicated. Carefully guarded quantities of smallpox virus are stored for research purposes.

SEE ALSO

BACTERIAL DISEASES • EPIDEMIC • IMMUNE SYSTEM • INFECTIOUS DISEASES • LYMPHATIC SYSTEM • TROPICAL DISEASES • VIRUSES

Spina Bifida

Spina bifida is a congenital condition (birth defect). Some of the bones of the baby's spine are not joined fully, so the nerves inside are not properly protected. The defect can be slight or so severe that the baby dies soon after birth or grows up handicapped.

In some cases of spina bifida there is just a dimple or a small, fatty lump over the spine. In others, the membranes covering the spinal cord may bulge out through the gap in the bones. They form a sac containing spinal fluid and sometimes nerve fibers. If the membranes are damaged, infection can enter, and the baby may develop meningitis. Babies with spina bifida often have hydrocephalus (fluid on the brain) and may be mentally retarded.

Surgeons can sometimes operate—often within 24 hours of birth—to repair the membrane. If the nerves of the spine are undamaged, the baby may grow up to be healthy. Nothing can be done to repair damaged nerves, which will cause various handicaps, depending on the region involved. Many babies with spina bifida have weak or deformed legs and will never be able to walk without help. Some are unable to control their bladder or bowels. Many can be helped by operations on their bones and tendons as they grow up. They may be able to walk, if they wear a brace for support. Pregnant women can have an amniocentesis, which shows if the baby has spina bifida.

Folic acid supplements taken daily by the mother while trying to conceive and for the first 12 weeks of pregnancy reduce the risk of spina bifida almost to zero.

Q & A

Do cases of spina bifida tend to run in families?

There is some evidence that spina bifida occurs more in some families than in others, and adults with spina bifida do have a slightly increased risk of having a baby with spina bifida. However, supplementary folic acid, taken from the start of a woman's pregnancy (or preferably before), can significantly reduce the risk of giving birth to a child with spina bifida.

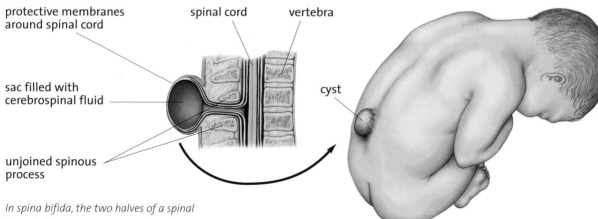

protective membranes around spinal cord

spinal cord

vertebra

sac filled with cerebrospinal fluid

cyst

unjoined spinous process

In spina bifida, the two halves of a spinal bone fail to join. A baby may be born with a soft cyst over the gap in the spine, which contains spinal fluid. Early surgery is very successful in this type of spina bifida, and the baby usually grows into a healthy adult.

SEE ALSO

BIRTH DEFECTS • BONE • GENETIC DISEASES AND DISORDERS • MENINGITIS • NERVOUS SYSTEM • NERVOUS SYSTEM DISORDERS • SKELETAL SYSTEM • SPINAL COLUMN

Spinal Column

The spinal column, or backbone, is the main bony support of the body. At the top, the spinal column supports the head. At the lower end, it is linked to the pelvis.

The spine consists of 33 small bones called vertebrae, which are stacked on top of each other to form the spinal column. The vertebrae are separated by disks with an outer fibrous ring and an inner pulpy center. These pulpy centers act as cushions and allow the spine to bend slightly. The spinal canal is a continuous channel that holds and protects the nerves that form the spinal cord. The spinal cord is further protected by membranes and is surrounded by a liquid called cerebrospinal fluid, which acts as a shock absorber.

Of the 33 bones, 24 are movable. Seven bones form the neck and are known as the cervical vertebrae. Below them are 12 thoracic (chest) vertebrae and five lumbar (lower back) vertebrae. At the lower end are two groups of bones that are fused together to form two bones (the sacrum and the coccyx).

Spinal injuries

The most common spinal injuries are a slipped disk (in which the pulpy content of the cartilage cushions moves out of place) and a fracture of the spine. A slipped disk is painful, but a fracture of the spine may cause injury to the spinal cord and lead to paralysis. A patient with a suspected fracture of the spine must be moved very carefully to avoid damaging the nerves.

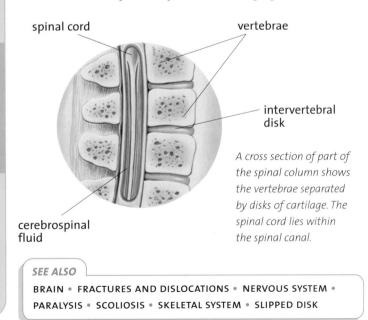

spinal cord

vertebrae

intervertebral disk

cerebrospinal fluid

A cross section of part of the spinal column shows the vertebrae separated by disks of cartilage. The spinal cord lies within the spinal canal.

SEE ALSO

BRAIN • FRACTURES AND DISLOCATIONS • NERVOUS SYSTEM • PARALYSIS • SCOLIOSIS • SKELETAL SYSTEM • SLIPPED DISK

Q & A

Is the spinal column always damaged by a broken neck?

Not always. However, spinal column damage often does occur when a person's neck is broken. The spinal cord can also be injured without there ever being a fracture of the spinal bones. This situation tends to happen when the cord is suddenly stretched or twisted in an accident. More important than the fracture is whether any bones are displaced, causing them to press onto the cord in the spinal canal that runs through the spinal bones.

My grandmother, who is 63, recently told me that she is shrinking. She says she is 2 inches (5 cm) shorter now than she was 40 years ago. I believe her, but how can she possibly be shrinking?

As the body ages, the bones in the vertebral column get smaller and the disks of cartilage between them get thinner and harder. This makes the disks shrink in size; with bone shrinkage, the person becomes shorter.

Sports Injuries

Almost every sport involves some risk of injury, from trivial cuts and bruises to more serious damage. Perhaps the most hazardous sports are those involving high speed (such as automobile racing, motorcycle racing, and skiing) and those carried out in dangerous places (such as mountaineering). Body contact sports (such as football and boxing) can also pose dangers. Some people are hurt accidentally by equipment; for example, being spiked by a fellow athlete's track shoes is a common injury.

Head injuries

Head injuries are a risk in contact sports such as boxing, where repeated blows to the head can cause long-lasting damage as the brain is knocked around inside the skull. Other sports are potentially dangerous. They include football and wrestling, as well as automobile, motorcycle, and bike racing. Horseback riding is another sport in which serious head injuries, fractures, and dislocations can occur.

Potential brain damage

All head injuries are potentially serious, because they can cause skull fractures, concussion, contusion, or internal bleeding. If a head injury is not correctly diagnosed and treated, headaches, loss of memory, and even permanent brain damage can result. However slight an injury seems, it is always best to get a doctor's

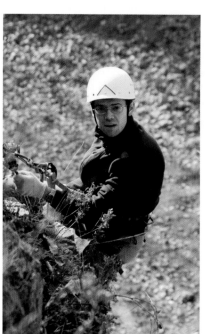

opinion. A preventive measure, such as wearing a protective helmet, provides the best safeguard.

Muscle damage and tendon injuries

Most often, a sports injury follows the overuse of some part of the body. Muscle injuries are very

This rock climber is using the proper safety equipment and wearing a protective hard hat. Young climbers should always be supervised, and only experienced climbers should tackle difficult slopes.

Q & A

I wear dental braces. Can I use a mouth protector to play football?

Anyone playing a sport that carries a risk of injury should wear a mouth protector. It will provide a barrier between your braces and your cheek or lips, limiting the risk of soft tissue injuries. Your dentist or your orthodontist will help you select the most suitable mouth protector.

I recently took up golf. Should I be aware of any potential injuries?

Although some sports such as football produce far more injuries—and more serious ones—than golf, golfers can suffer serious injury to the elbows, spine, knees, hips, or wrists. Golfer's elbow is among the most common complaints, and strengthening forearm muscles can help avoid this. The American Academy of Orthopedic Surgeons suggests some simple exercises, such as squeezing a tennis ball for five minutes at a time and doing wrist curls and reverse wrist curls with a lightweight dumbbell.

Soccer players often receive ankle injuries as a result of careless tackling.

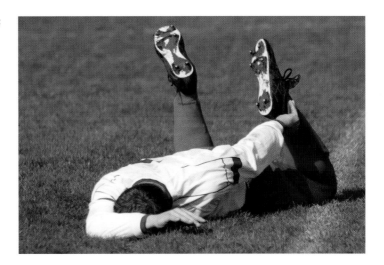

common and usually involve a rupture of some of the muscle fibers. These injuries are described in various ways: as a pull, a tear, or a strain. Soccer players frequently suffer injuries to the thigh muscles, calf muscles, and ankles; sprinters may damage the hamstrings at the back of the thigh.

The Achilles tendon above the heel is commonly injured by runners, hurdlers, and long jumpers; tendons (the fibrous cords that join muscle and bone) can also become inflamed through overuse. Rowers and racket players, for example, are at risk of inflammation of the wrist and elbow tendons. Such injuries should never be taken lightly.

Torn ligaments and tendons require just as long to heal as fractures of the bones, and inflamed tendons may need several weeks of rest from sports until the pain subsides. Even then, the return to sporting activity should be taken gradually to avoid further damage.

Knee and ankle injuries
Knee joints and ankle joints are particularly easy to injure, and once they are damaged, they are prone to weakness later on. Apart from dislocation, one of the most frequent injuries to the knee is a torn cartilage, which is very painful and makes movement of the knee difficult. Hairline fractures (shin splints) often occur in the shins of runners who overtrain on hard, jarring surfaces, such as pavements.

Avoiding injury
Most sports injuries can be avoided through a mixture of fitness training, adequate preparation for the particular sport, and

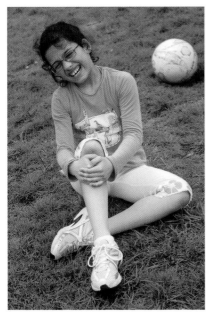

This girl fell down and hurt her knee while chasing after a ball.

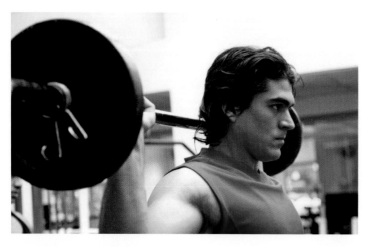

Weight lifting is an excellent activity for keeping the muscles in shape. However, it is important to receive instruction first to avoid causing unnecessary injuries.

common sense. Conditioning exercises are very important, particularly at the beginning of the sports season, when fitness levels may not be up to standard.

If people are taking part in serious or competitive sports, they should be guided by their coach, who will make sure that they have the appropriate training exercises before being allowed to play. He or she will also insist on proper stretching and warm-up routines before people undertake any strenuous sports activity. If a suitable warm-up is omitted or not properly carried out, many injuries can occur, such as strained elbows, damaged knee joints, pulled muscles, and stress fractures.

Treating sports injuries

With most sports injuries, the first thing to do is to reduce the pain and swelling in the affected areas. A coach or a doctor can advise on further treatment, which usually involves resting the injured part for a few weeks or even longer. Sometimes physical therapy may be necessary.

Apart from minor injuries, all other sports injuries should be examined by an expert. If there is any doubt, and particularly if pain is experienced, people with sports injuries should visit the emergency room.

Proceeding with caution

If people have been out of action because of illness or injury, they must regain their fitness levels before they resume play. Too many people are tempted to make up for lost time by playing too vigorously and too soon after an injury has occurred. This action can lead to permanent damage or chronic weakness in the injured part.

Mountaineering is an exhilarating but potentially dangerous sport that has claimed many lives.

SEE ALSO

BONE • BONE DISEASES AND DISORDERS • BRAIN • BRAIN DAMAGE AND DISORDERS • FRACTURES AND DISLOCATIONS • JOINT DISORDERS • MUSCLE • MUSCLE DISEASES AND DISORDERS • SKELETAL SYSTEM • SPRAINS AND STRAINS

Sprains and Strains

Sprains are common injuries that happen to almost everyone at some time. They are the result of twisting or wrenching a joint farther than it can normally move. As a result, the ligaments that hold the joint in position are stretched and some of the fibers are torn. The blood vessels in the area are usually torn, too. Strains are less serious; fibers in the muscles are stretched or torn.

People often sprain an ankle if they trip or sprain a wrist as the result of a fall. Larger joints, such as the knee or hip, may be sprained during sports. A sprained neck can occur as a result of whiplash injury in an automobile accident, although such injuries have become less common since safety belts and head restrainers were introduced.

The obvious signs of a sprain are sudden, severe pain from the stretched or torn ligaments around the joint and swelling and bruising caused by bleeding in the area around it. This pain becomes much worse if the injured person tries to move or use the joint or put weight on it.

Strained shoulder, leg, and wrist muscles and turned ankles are common sports injuries. The most frequent strains affect less active people and occur in the lower back as a result of picking up a heavy or awkward object. Learning how to lift and carry things properly can prevent back injury and pain. When lifting something heavy, it is best to keep the back straight and bend the knees, letting them take the weight.

Rest, painkillers, and heat treatment will help most strains. Any injury more serious than a minor sprain should be examined by a doctor, just in case a joint has been fractured.

Q & A

What is the best type of bandage to use for treating a sprain?

The aim is to give the joint firm support while it heals, but it should not be completely immobilized. Some form of elasticized bandage is therefore required. An ordinary cotton bandage gives too little support, but crepe, webbing, and elastic bandages are all suitable. The bandage must be tight enough to be effective but not so tight that it interferes with the circulation; impairing the circulation could cause gangrene.

My friend recommended a massage to treat my sprain. Is that a good idea?

Perhaps. Gentle massage can be started when the immediate effects of the injury have worn off, usually on the second or third day. The area will be very tender, so only light pressure should be applied.

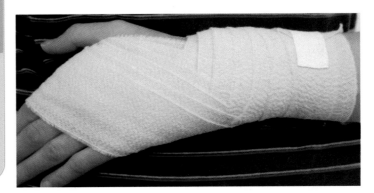

After first aid to help reduce the pain and swelling of a sprained wrist, a doctor will usually wrap the hand and wrist in an elasticized bandage to support the wrist and prevent further injury.

SEE ALSO

FRACTURES AND DISLOCATIONS • JOINT DISORDERS • MUSCLE • SPORTS INJURIES • WHIPLASH INJURY

Staphylococcal Infections

Staphylococcus bacteria are some of the most common disease-causing germs. Most infections respond well to antibiotic treatment, but a new strain called MRSA is resistant to all known antibiotics. Staphylococcus bacteria are tiny, spherical microorganisms that cluster together like grapes in the body. There are many different types of staphylococcus bacteria. The most important in medicine is *Staphylococcus aureus* (*S. aureus*), which causes diseases by producing toxins. These harmful substances break down body chemicals such as enzymes and proteins, destroy body tissue, and kill cells. *S. aureus* causes skin problems (such as abscesses, boils, and carbuncles) as well as common infections (such as food poisoning and sore throats).

MRSA

When antibiotics were first developed, they were good at treating infections caused by *S. aureus*. Over time, this bacterium became resistant to many antibiotics. Eventually only one antibiotic, methicillin, was effective. Now, a new strain of *S. aureus* has emerged that is resistant to methicillin. This methicillin-resistant *S. aureus* (MRSA) has killed many people. Most infections occur in hospitals, but more are appearing elsewhere. Doctors are now working hard to find ways to treat this dangerous new strain of *S. aureus*.

Toxic shock syndrome

Toxic shock syndrome is a very rare disease that affects women during their monthly periods. Many women use tampons to soak up the blood flow during their periods. In toxic shock syndrome,

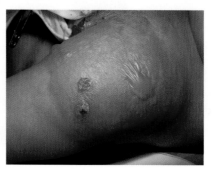

the tampon becomes infected with *S. aureus*. The bacteria then release toxins that damage blood vessels. So much blood flows out of the damaged vessels that the body goes into shock. The symptoms include fever, abdominal pains, and perhaps kidney failure.

Q & A

My brother recently had a staphylococcal infection. How did a germ get a strange-sounding name like that?

When the early bacteriologists first observed germs under a microscope, they noticed that many of them were spherical, like tiny berries. The Greek word for a berry is *kokkos*, so each one was called a coccus (plural, cocci). Some cocci formed clusters that resembled bunches of grapes. The Greek for a bunch of grapes is *staphyle*, so these cocci were called staphylococci.

My friend says that staphylococci cause food poisoning. Is that true?

Yes. A food handler with a staphylococcal skin infection, such as a boil, especially on the hands, can contaminate the food with toxins that cause an explosive attack of illness within a few hours after the food is eaten. Infected food handlers should not have access to food that will be served to the public.

A secondary staphylococcal infection has developed at the site of a smallpox vaccination on a small child.

SEE ALSO

BACTERIA • BACTERIAL DISEASES • INFECTIOUS DISEASES • SKIN DISEASES AND DISORDERS

Streptococcal Infections

Q & A

How was the streptococcus bacterium named?

A coccus is a roughly spherical germ named after the Greek word *kokkos*, meaning "berry." When streptococci germs reproduce, the daughter cells form a chain like a string of beads. The German surgeon Albert Billroth (1829–1894) named the microorganisms after the Greek word for "chain." Although he was mistaken about the meaning of the word (*strepto* means "twisted"), no one objected, and the name stuck.

Why is strep throat more serious than a regular sore throat?

Most of the germs that cause a sore throat do not usually cause additional harm. However, *Streptococcus pyogenes* causes strep throat, which may lead to a serious kidney disorder called glomerulonephritis and to a joint and heart disorder called rheumatic fever.

There are more than 85 species of streptococcus bacteria. Most are harmless, but a few cause serious and sometimes even fatal diseases. Most infections respond well to antibiotics.

Streptococcus mutans lives in the mouth. Tens of thousands of bacteria form a covering of plaque on the teeth. They break down the sugars in food and form an acid that attacks the teeth.

Streptococcus fecalis lives in the digestive system and infects the skin around the anus. It is a common cause of urinary infections, especially in women.

Streptococcus pneumoniae is the most common cause of pneumonia (an inflammation of the lungs). It also causes meningitis (an infection of the membranes covering the brain).

Streptococcus pyogenes is the most dangerous of these bacteria. It causes killer diseases such as fasciitis necroticans, in which the bacteria make chemicals that break down body tissue. *Streptococcus pyogenes* also causes infections, such as scarlet fever, strep throat, and acute tonsillitis.

Scarlet fever infection starts in the throat, where bacteria produce toxins that spread around the body. The toxins cause a fever, sore throat, and a red rash. As the rash fades, layers of skin peel away. The mouth becomes covered with a white crust, which falls away to leave the skin red and sore. Scarlet fever used to be a common childhood killer, but it is now rare as a result of the use of antibiotics.

Strep throat, another throat infection, clears up quickly with antibiotics. However, if the infection is left untreated, it may lead to kidney damage or to heart damage.

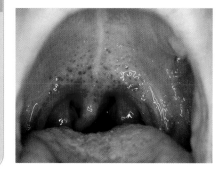

The tonsils form part of the immune system. They recognize harmful substances in food and air. Sometimes, the tonsils become infected with streptococcus bacteria, causing a painful inflammation called tonsillitis, which responds well to antibiotics.

Strep throat is caused by group A streptococcus bacteria, which are spread through direct contact with mucus from the nose or throat of infected people or contact with infected wounds or skin sores.

SEE ALSO

BACTERIAL DISEASES • DIGESTIVE SYSTEM DISEASES AND DISORDERS • KIDNEY DISEASES AND DISORDERS • MENINGITIS • PNEUMONIA • THROAT DISEASES AND DISORDERS

Stroke

When a person has a stroke, the normal blood supply to part of the brain is interrupted. A clot may form in one of the brain's arteries and block it (cerebral thrombosis). A clot or piece of artery wall from somewhere else in the body may be carried in the bloodstream to the brain and cause a blockage there (cerebral embolism). The most serious types of strokes are caused by an artery that bleeds into the brain (cerebral hemorrhage).

When the blood supply to part of the brain is cut off, that area of the brain suddenly stops working. The patient's symptoms will depend on what functions this area controlled. A stroke may cause weakness or paralysis down one side of the body, loss of sight on one side, or loss of speech or understanding. If a very large area of the brain is affected, the patient may die.

However, there are many cross-connections between neighboring areas of the brain, so the area of damage is not usually very great. The brain has spare areas that, in time, may be able to take over some of the work done by the damaged area. Thus, stroke patients may recover almost completely after a while, with physical therapy and speech therapy when necessary.

Strokes are caused by disease of the arteries and high blood pressure (which can weaken the artery walls). Smokers and people with diabetes or a high level of cholesterol in the blood are at greater risk.

Q & A

My grandfather has just had a stroke and can't speak. Will his speech return?

Yes, it is very likely that his ability to speak will come back, at least to some extent. Sometimes, people are unable to speak at all in the first few days after a stroke, but they later recover almost completely.

My uncle had a bad heart attack and then a few weeks later had a stroke that paralyzed his left side. Was this connected with his heart attack?

After a heart attack, blood clots may form on the inside wall of the chamber of the heart. Occasionally, part of a clot can dislodge and block off one of the brain's blood vessels, thus producing a stroke. Patients who have had very serious heart attacks can be given anticoagulant drugs to help prevent this.

This stroke patient has aphasia. She has difficulty in understanding words as well as speaking them. Here she attempts to name familiar objects. In time, and with good therapy, she should recover her use of language skills.

> **SEE ALSO**
> ARTERY • ARTERY DISEASES AND DISORDERS • BRAIN • BRAIN DAMAGE AND DISORDERS • CIRCULATORY SYSTEM • DIABETES • HEART ATTACK • HYPERTENSION • PARALYSIS

Sty

A sty is a painful swelling on the rim of the eyelid caused by a staphylococcal infection. The sty develops when these harmful microorganisms get into one of the tiny sebaceous glands that open into the space surrounding the shaft of an eyelash.

Dry and flaky skin, dermatitis, and dandruff all make sties more likely. Sties tend to be more common in children and adolescents, especially when these young people are run down, although adults can also get them.

For a day or two before the sty appears, the eyelid may feel itchy, and the eye may feel as if there is dirt in it. Then the sty develops into a painful red pustule. The pain in the eyelid and the feeling of grittiness increase. Bright light makes these symptoms worse, and the eye runs continuously. After a few days, the sty bursts and discharges pus; once this has happened, the eyelid soon returns to normal.

If a sty is recognized in its early stages, antibiotic ointment or drops can prevent it from forming. If the pustule has already formed, the antibiotics will not help, but they may prevent further sties from developing. A sterile pad of gauze or cotton soaked in hot sterilized water and held on the closed eye can help relieve the pain and encourage the pus to discharge.

Sties are infectious, so if a person has one, he or she should always wash the hands after touching it and use a separate washcloth and towel to avoid passing the infection on to others. During the time when people have a sty, they should avoid wearing contact lenses or eye makeup, because those items will make the eye very painful and could aggravate the infection even further.

If the sty does not go away within a week, a doctor should be consulted for oral antibiotic treatment. With this treatment, the sty should clear up within two to three days.

Q & A

Is it safe for me to pull out the eyelash in a sty?

Yes. Pulling out the eyelash allows the pus to then drain out. First, soften the eyelid with a hot compress to reduce the pain. The eyelash can be pulled out with a pair of tweezers, and the sty should discharge spontaneously. If the relevant eyelash is not obvious, the eyelids should be left alone. Either the sty is not yet ripe or it may be an internal cyst, in which case there is no eyelash to remove.

I have a small, painless nodule under my eyelid. Is this a sty?

It may be a meibomian cyst. Although sometimes called an internal sty, it is not a sty or an infection but an accumulation of trapped gland secretion. It is felt as a hard lump, like a small hailstone. There is no need to do anything, but it can be removed surgically for cosmetic reasons.

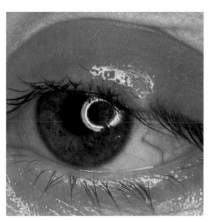

Children and adolescents often suffer from sties. A sty on the outside of the eyelid is caused by an infection in one of the sebaceous glands in the eyelid. Sometimes an eyelash is visible in the sty.

SEE ALSO

DERMATITIS • EYE DISEASES AND DISORDERS • GLANDS • STAPHYLOCOCCAL INFECTIONS

Sunburn

Sunburn is now less common than it used to be. People are gradually taking notice of doctors' warnings that too much sun is a health risk. Sunburn is very uncomfortable, painful, and dangerous. Repeated sunburn can damage the skin permanently, and skin cancer is most likely to occur in fair-skinned people who have spent a long time in strong sunlight.

Sunburn is caused by ultraviolet rays from the sun, which damage the outer layer of the skin. These rays stimulate the skin to produce a pigment called melanin, which darkens the skin to provide protection and acts as a filter for the ultraviolet rays. Sunburn occurs when there is not enough pigment produced by the cells to filter the sun's rays.

Dangers of sunburn

Sunburn is not felt until a little while after it happens. The first signs are redness and a feeling of burning caused by an increase of the blood supply to the skin. Sunburned legs and arms may swell painfully, and the victim may develop a headache and fever and may vomit. Heat exhaustion may also occur. Blisters may develop, and the surface layer of skin may peel off.

Many people think that a suntan is attractive, but repeated sun exposure over time makes the skin heavily wrinkled and leathery. Patchy areas of skin pigmentation and wartlike lumps (solar keratoses) may develop.

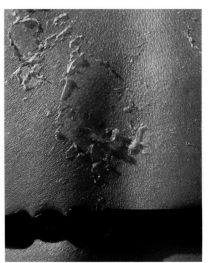

Sunburn can be treated with soothing lotions and ointments, but it is much more sensible not to get it in the first place. When out in the sun, people should use sunscreen with a high sun protection factor (SPF) to cover exposed areas of the body. Otherwise, it is best to keep out of the sun or keep the skin covered.

Q & A

I am fair-skinned and my friend is dark. Why can she spend a long time in the sun without burning while I cannot?

Being fair-skinned means that you have little pigment in your skin. Your friend has more pigment and can also make more than you when exposed to sunlight. You will burn easily, because your skin cannot produce enough protective pigment, but it is dangerous for *anyone* to spend a long time in the sun.

My family is planning a vacation to the Caribbean. What can I do to reduce the risk of sunburn?

You could have a course of ultraviolet ray therapy beforehand, to increase your pigmentation. You could also use a sunscreen preparation that filters out the sun's stronger rays, allowing a slow tan to develop. The best way to protect yourself is to stay out of the sun altogether.

A suntan does not prevent sunburn. Once the pigment-producing cells have been saturated with ultraviolet light, further exposure causes burning, unattractive peeling skin, and long-term skin damage.

SEE ALSO

BURNS • CANCER • HEAT SICKNESS • SKIN • SKIN DISEASES AND DISORDERS

Tennis Elbow

Tennis elbow is inflammation of the tendon where it attaches to the bone at the outer side of the elbow. The tendon links the muscle in the upper arm to the bone in the forearm and can become damaged owing to repeated use of the forearm, such as playing backhand shots in tennis. Other types of activities, such as excessive use of a screwdriver (where the wrist and forearm are vigorously worked), can also cause tennis elbow. The tendon becomes pulled, and small tears may occur, leading to pain and tenderness in the area.

Symptoms and treatments

When someone suffers from tennis elbow, the elbow looks normal, and bending and straightening the arm are painless and unrestricted. However, there is fairly constant pain and tenderness experienced in the elbow region. In severe cases, the pain may be felt over a much wider area, often extending well over the back of the forearm. The pain is made worse by actions such as turning a stiff doorknob or unscrewing a jar top.

Most cases of tennis elbow settle with physical therapy, ice packs, exercises to stretch and strengthen the affected muscles, ultrasound treatment, and the avoidance of any activity that causes pain. Some people have found acupuncture and heat treatment helpful.

If these actions fail, a doctor may inject a corticosteroid with a local anesthetic into the affected area. In rare cases, surgery may be needed. If the condition is caused by playing sports, expert coaching on technique may be necessary.

Q & A

If I had tennis elbow, how would I be able to recognize it?

You would have a dull ache around the elbow area and upper side of the forearm, with a particularly tender spot on the bump that can be felt on the upper side of the elbow when the forearm is placed across the chest. Typing, using a squash or tennis racket, or even picking up heavy objects may be painful.

How soon can one resume playing tennis after tennis elbow?

That depends on how serious the injury was; you should seek your doctor's advice. The symptoms vary from person to person. In mild cases, it may take only a few days until the pain and stiffness subside, and then you can resume the sport gradually. More serious cases may take longer. If the tenderness returns whenever you play, consult your doctor as soon as possible.

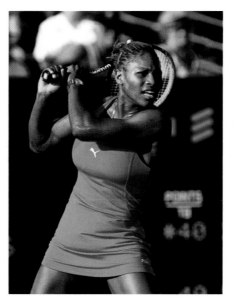

Serena Williams follows through after a backhand shot. Tennis players can suffer from tennis elbow, usually as a result of overuse of the muscles and tendons used to hit a backhand shot.

SEE ALSO

CARPAL TUNNEL SYNDROME • MUSCLE • REPETITIVE STRAIN INJURY • SPORTS INJURIES

Tetanus

Q & A

Can I be immunized against tetanus?

Yes, you can and should be. Children are given a vaccine against this serious disease with their first series of injections and are given a booster dose as they start school. Older people may not have been vaccinated and should ask their doctor for the immunization to avoid a risk of infection. If you have been vaccinated, you should have a booster dose every 10 years. People who work on farms and in stables should be especially careful to keep their immunization up to date.

Does tetanus develop only in a wound made by a rusty, rather than a clean, object?

No. Tetanus spores are very common in the environment, and it is possible to infect yourself even with an object that appears clean. However, the highest concentration of spores is found in soil and in manure. An object such as a rusty nail is perhaps more likely to have been in contact with spores; therefore, you may be more likely to get an infection from such an object.

Tetanus is a very serious and often fatal disease caused by a toxin produced by the bacterial spores of *Clostridium tetani*. If the bacteria enter a wound, the spores germinate, multiply, and produce a very strong poison that affects the muscles. Some cases of tetanus occur from wounds that are so small they are unnoticed. The spores are present in soil, dust, and animal dung.

People develop tetanus through a cut or wound that has not been properly cleaned. The toxin from the bacteria passes into the spinal cord and the brain, probably traveling along the nerves and in the bloodstream. The incubation period may be as little as a day or as long as several months, but it is usually six to 10 days. The faster the tetanus develops, the more serious it is likely to be and the less likely it is that the patient will recover.

Tetanus is very common, causing half of the deaths of newborn babies in the poorest developing countries and a quarter of newborn deaths in most other developing countries. However, immunization against tetanus is very effective.

Symptoms and treatments

The first symptoms of tetanus are headache, irritability, fever, difficulty in swallowing, and general illness. The patient's muscles become rigid. Among the worst affected are the muscles of the abdomen, which become hard; the back, which arches over; and then the jaw. The muscles of the jaw can clench shut so tightly that tetanus was often called lockjaw in the past. The patient develops extremely painful spasms—those of the throat and chest may be so severe that the patient suffocates. The toxin also interferes with the brain's control of vital functions (including the actions of the heart), and this interference can lead to death.

Tetanus patients are treated with antibiotics, antitoxin, and muscle relaxants. Sometimes the patient may be deliberately paralyzed (to prevent the painful and exhausting spasms) or put on a respirator for a while.

Once in the body, the tetanus bacterium may grow in an area that has no blood supply, making it hard for antibodies to work.

SEE ALSO

ABRASIONS AND CUTS • BACTERIA • BACTERIAL DISEASES • POISON AND POISONING • WOUNDS

Thalassemia

Thalassemia is an inherited blood disease that causes anemia. People suffering from thalassemia have abnormal formation of hemoglobin, the oxygen-carrying substance in the blood. Their red blood cells contain only a small amount of hemoglobin, and these cells live for a shorter time than normal red blood cells. The faulty red blood cells carry less oxygen than normal, so the oxygen supply to the tissues of the body is reduced. Hemoglobin for the red blood cells is normally made in the bone marrow.

Thalassemia is common in people who come from the Mediterranean regions, the Middle East, and Southeast Asia. If both parents have this condition, their children will have the illness in its most severe form. If only one parent has thalassemia, the children's condition will be mild. Thalassemia can restrict a child's development, and in its most severe form it can cause death. More than 300,000 babies severely affected with the condition are born each year.

Patients are treated with regular blood transfusions to keep the level of ordinary hemoglobin high and to provide a good supply of oxygen to their body tissues. These transfusions eventually cause a buildup of iron in the body, and drugs must be taken to help the kidneys excrete more iron. Treatment may include antibiotics to counter infection, and sometimes the spleen is removed.

If a person with severe thalassemia is to survive, he or she will need transfusions of about 25 units of blood per year. The total annual cost (about $10,000 per person) is a very heavy burden on the economy of the developing countries where most of these patients live. There is a great need for more genetic research into these conditions.

Genetic counseling

People who inherit thalassemia from only one parent develop a mild form of the disease that causes no serious problems. Inheriting faulty genes from both parents leads to a serious form of the disease. However, simple tests will show whether people have the genes causing thalassemia. Therefore, people who know of this disease in their family should have genetic counseling before having children.

Q & A

Is thalassemia found only in certain places in the world?

Thalassemia tends to occur in areas where malaria is or has been common. It is particularly prevalent on the Mediterranean coast and in the Middle East and Far East. However, because the population of the world is now so mobile, thalassemia can be found almost anywhere in the world, particularly in large cities.

Does thalassemia give a natural protection against malaria?

It is known that possessing one of the abnormal genes that give rise to thalassemia gives some protection against the effects of falciparum malaria. Some doctors believe this is because the red blood cells in the body of a thalassemic person are fragile, so when the malarial parasite gets inside a red cell, the cell breaks down and the parasite stops growing. In people who do not have thalassemia, the parasite would continue to multiply. Therefore, people with minor forms of thalassemia appear to have some protection against malaria.

> **SEE ALSO**
> ANEMIA • BLOOD • BLOOD DISEASES AND DISORDERS • GENES • GENETIC DISEASES AND DISORDERS • MALARIA

Throat Diseases and Disorders

Q & A

Why does laryngitis always tend to be more serious in children than it is in adults?

A child's trachea (airway) is much smaller than that of an adult. When it becomes inflamed, the lining swells and constricts the airway; the smaller the airway, the more potential there is for serious obstruction. In children, inflammation of the larynx (voice box) makes it more sensitive to any agents that pass down the throat. Such agents can produce bouts of coughing and spasms of the vocal cords that make it impossible to breathe.

My father has been told that he has cancer of the larynx. I am very worried. What are his chances of being cured?

Most forms of cancer of the larynx respond well to current treatments. With modern radiotherapy techniques, a cure rate of around 90 percent is common. However, the doctors will want to keep a close eye on your father for the rest of his life, to treat any recurrent problems as they arise.

The term *throat* is used to describe the area that leads from the mouth and into the respiratory and digestive tracts. The throat is composed of two main parts, the pharynx and the larynx.

The pharynx and the larynx

The pharynx is a muscular tube lined by mucous membrane. The pharynx has various openings: the mouth; the esophagus (or gullet), which leads to the stomach; the larynx, leading to the lungs; two openings leading to the nostrils; and two other openings called the eustachian tubes. These tubes connect to the middle ear and keep the air pressure on each side of the eardrum constant.

The larynx is a specialized section of the trachea (windpipe or airway), leading to the lungs. A flap valve, the epiglottis, hovers over the top of the trachea. When a person swallows, the epiglottis closes the airway so that food and liquids cannot reach the lungs. The vocal cords are in the larynx. They produce sound when air movement vibrates them.

Both the pharynx and the larynx can easily be infected by viruses and bacteria. Common and often very painful throat infections are caused by *Streptococcus* bacteria. Illnesses that involve the throat include the common cold, influenza, infectious mononucleosis, measles, and diphtheria.

Both the pharynx and the larynx can be damaged by drinking too much alcohol and by smoking (which can cause long-lasting inflammations known as chronic pharyngitis and laryngitis).

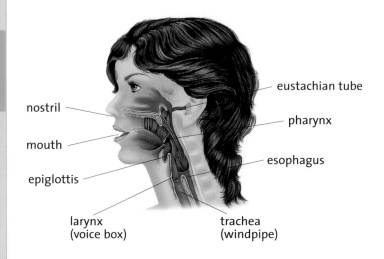

nostril

mouth

epiglottis

larynx (voice box)

eustachian tube

pharynx

esophagus

trachea (windpipe)

The throat is composed of two main parts, the pharynx (a muscular tube lined by mucous membrane) and the larynx (voice box).

HOME REMEDIES
FOR A SORE THROAT

Sore throats that occur with colds and other minor infections can be treated by gargling with a little salt dissolved in a glass of warm water. The solution should be spat out after gargling. Adults can also gargle with a solution of two soluble aspirin tablets in hot water. This solution can be swallowed after gargling, to help relieve the pain and reduce any fever. Only soft or liquid foods should be eaten, and plenty of hot liquids should be drunk. Sucking throat lozenges can soothe the throat and prevent it from becoming dry and scratchy.

Some throat infections begin with a burning feeling in the throat, which becomes increasingly uncomfortable and is made worse by speaking and swallowing. The soreness may be caused by an infection of the nasopharynx (the area just behind the nasal cavity) or an infection of the tonsils. Tonsillitis causes more severe symptoms. Repeated infections of the nasopharynx can cause the adenoids to grow larger, possibly preventing the patient from breathing properly through the nose. Enlarged adenoids may also block the drainage channel from the ear and cause infection and deafness. Badly enlarged adenoids can be removed by surgery.

Many sore throats are mild and clear up quickly. Drinking plenty of fluids and gargling with salt water can help the recovery process, and some over-the-counter remedies help ease throat pain. The throat can be rested by not talking, which also helps ease the pain. Sore throats caused by bacteria are helped by taking antibiotics prescribed by a doctor. Smokers should stop smoking immediately.

Throat growths and cancers

A virus called human papillomavirus (HPV) produces warty growths in the larynx. In time, the warts disappear of their own accord, but if they grow large enough to make breathing difficult, they can be removed by surgery. Cancers of the pharynx are unusual but may appear in middle age. They can often be successfully treated with radiotherapy or by surgery. Cancer of the larynx is more common, but it can be successfully treated if it is found early enough. Most sufferers are heavy smokers.

Foreign bodies in the throat

The pharynx can be damaged by accidentally swallowing unsuitable objects, including fishbones, bottle caps, and coins. Such objects can pierce the wall of the pharynx and cause serious infections. If the object gets stuck, it is extremely painful, and it may need to be removed under a general anesthetic. Objects inhaled into the larynx can threaten a patient's life and need immediate first-aid attention.

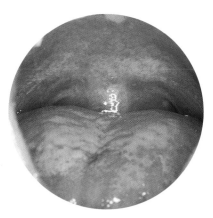

Strep throat is a common but very painful bacterial throat infection.

SEE ALSO

BACTERIAL DISEASES • CANCER • COLD • DIPHTHERIA • HPV • INFECTIOUS MONONUCLEOSIS • INFLUENZA • MEASLES • MOUTH • RESPIRATORY SYSTEM DISEASES AND DISORDERS • STREPTOCOCCAL INFECTIONS

Tourette's Syndrome

Q & A

My friend says that Tourette's syndrome is a new disease, and I say it isn't. Which of us is right?

The first full official account of Tourette's syndrome, including vocal utterances, was published by the French physician George Gilles de la Tourette (1859–1904) in 1885, but another case was described in 1825. There is every reason to suppose that the disorder existed long before the start of the nineteenth century but was simply dismissed as a form of temporary insanity. You can fairly claim to have won this argument.

My five-year-old brother has developed a very obvious tic in which he turns down the corner of his mouth and tightens a muscle in his neck. Is it likely that he's developing Tourette's syndrome?

No. Tics in young children, especially boys, are extremely common, whereas Tourette's syndrome is very rare. In the great majority of cases, childhood tics disappear spontaneously before the end of adolescence.

Tourette's syndrome is a distressing disability that takes various forms, but a key feature is a tendency to develop tics. These involuntary motions or sounds vary in severity from almost unnoticeable to quite alarming. People with Tourette's syndrome have uncontrollable attacks and may make strange faces, grind their teeth, wave their arms and legs, blink, and make noises (such as grunting and barking, clicking their tongues, and hissing). They may also shout out obscene words and remarks.

Tourette's syndrome affects about four times as many men as women and begins in childhood or adolescence.

Causes

It is unlikely that there is a single cause for Tourette's syndrome. In a high proportion of cases there is a known family history, which indicates a genetic cause. There are also likely to be environmental causes. A temporary lack of oxygen during birth has even been proposed as a possible factor.

Treatment

Although the condition remains for life, people with Tourette's syndrome can usually get a great deal of relief from the symptoms by consulting a psychiatrist and getting appropriate medication. However, many cases of Tourette's syndrome are never treated. This is partly because these cases are too mild to justify treatment, but mainly because people with the condition are embarrassed, dislike discussing the problem, and assume that the condition is beyond treatment.

Treatment is certainly difficult, but claims have been made for the effectiveness of behavior therapy, even in severe cases. Counseling may also be used. Some tranquilizing drugs are helpful, but the most frequently used medications are in the class of antipsychotic drugs known as neuroleptics. These drugs cause emotional quieting, promote indifference, and slow down bodily and mental overactivity.

The drugs may include haloperidol, clonidine, and clonazepam. For obsessive-compulsive traits that interfere significantly with daily functioning, fluoxetine (Prozac), clomipramine, sertraline, and paroxetine may be prescribed.

SEE ALSO

BRAIN DAMAGE AND DISORDERS • GENES • GENETIC DISEASES AND DISORDERS • NERVOUS SYSTEM • NERVOUS SYSTEM DISORDERS • OBSESSIVE-COMPULSIVE DISORDER

Trichomoniasis

Trichomoniasis is a sexually transmitted infection of the vagina, urethra, and bladder in women, or of the urethra and prostate gland in men. The infection is caused by a single-celled organism called *Trichomonas vaginalis*.

The condition is readily passed on, and if one sexual partner has trichomoniasis, the other partner must be assumed to be infected also. Trichomoniasis is one of the most common of the sexually transmitted diseases (STDs).

Symptoms, diagnosis, and treatment

In women, the symptoms come on suddenly: there is genital irritation, burning, itching, and a profuse, frothy, yellowish vaginal discharge. If the urethra is affected, there is burning during urination and some discharge from the urethral opening. There may be soreness and inflammation of the vulva that are severe enough to make examination by a doctor difficult and painful. The vaginal wall may be inflamed, red, and ulcerated. Men often have no symptoms, so they can pass the condition on without being aware of it. At worst, men may have a slight penile discharge and a burning sensation during urination.

The antibiotic metronidazole (Flagyl) is highly effective as a treatment for this condition. The drug selectively blocks some of the functions within the infecting organism and kills it.

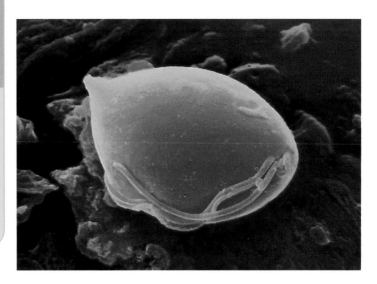

Q & A

What should a woman do if she thinks that she has a trichomonas infection?

She should see her doctor. The woman needs to take the drug that is required for the specific germ that is causing her infection. This depends on a doctor identifying the organism by examining a specimen of the discharge. It is very unwise for a woman to try to treat such an infection herself.

My friend and I have been arguing. I have said that trichomoniasis is a sexually transmitted disease, but she says you can catch it in other ways. Which one of us is right?

You are. Trichomoniasis is spread only by sexual contact. It was once thought that some cases of trichomoniasis could be acquired in a nonsexual way—for example, by using a toilet that was contaminated by an infected person a short time before—but this is not true.

The parasitic, pear-shaped organism Trichomonas vaginalis *has an undulating membrane down one side and can move around by lashing its long, hairlike tails.*

SEE ALSO

BODY SYSTEMS • SEXUALLY TRANSMITTED DISEASES

Tropical Diseases

The term *tropical diseases* is used to describe a number of illnesses present mainly in warm climates and underdeveloped areas where there is poor hygiene. Although a great deal is known about these illnesses—what causes them, how they spread, how they can be treated, and even how they can be prevented—controlling and curing them are very difficult.

The main reasons for tropical diseases are widespread poverty, lack of social development, and lack of education. The countries where they are found cannot afford large, costly health programs to provide clean water and immunization. They also have scant medical services to treat diseases. Poverty makes it hard to get rid of overcrowding and poor hygiene—conditions that make it easy for the diseases to spread. International agencies, such as the World Health Organization (WHO), have extensive programs to immunize and educate people. Despite this, tropical diseases still disable and kill many thousands of people every year.

Causes of tropical diseases

Many tropical diseases are caused by parasitic organisms. Malaria, trypanosomiasis, and leishmaniasis (a parasitic disease) are spread by insects. Yellow fever and dengue fever are viral infections that are spread through the bites of mosquitoes. Schistosomiasis (bilharzia) is caused by parasitic worms, which can be picked up by wading or swimming in the water in which the worms live. Hansen's disease (caught only by close contact over a long period), typhoid fever, cholera, and plague are caused by bacteria and are spread by direct contact with infected people or by contaminated food or water.

Doctors estimate that as many as 25 million people in tropical countries have become blind from preventable diseases. These diseases include xerophthalmia (caused by a lack of vitamin A in the diet); onchocerciasis, or river blindness (an infection of the skin by filarial larvae that may also affect the conjunctiva of the eye); and trachoma (a chronic conjunctival infection caused by the parasitic bacterium *Chlamydia trachomatis*, which is transmitted by flies or through close personal contact).

Trypanosomiasis

Trypanosomiasis is an infection by microorganisms called trypanosomes. They are transmitted from infected animals to people by the bite of an insect—in Africa by the tsetse fly (causing African sleeping sickness) and in Mexico and Central and South America by the barbeiro (causing Chagas' disease).

Once the parasites have entered the blood, they travel through the body in the bloodstream and the patient becomes feverish.

Q & A

Apart from vaccination, is there another way to prevent cholera?

A better vaccine is needed to fight cholera. At present, the vaccine provides protection in only 50 percent of cases for only a few months. Thus, the best way to avoid cholera is to avoid contaminated food and water. Cholera causes severe diarrhea, with salt and fluid loss. Prompt rehydration is vital to save life.

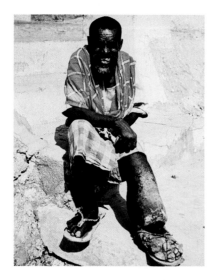

Elephantiasis, a painful swelling caused by blockage of the body's drainage system, is common in the tropics. The condition is caused by parasitic worms and their larvae.

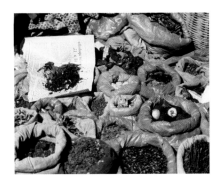

In many developing countries, herbal remedies that are prepared by tribal doctors are the only medicines available. However, few of them are effective in treating tropical diseases.

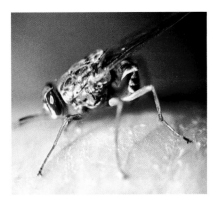

The tsetse fly spreads African sleeping sickness to both people and animals. The disease, which is difficult to treat and for which there is no vaccine, is a risk to visitors to African game parks.

IMMUNIZATION

Immunization against the following diseases may be necessary before a person visits a tropical country: diphtheria, hepatitis, malaria, meningitis, polio, rabies, tetanus, typhoid, and yellow fever.

In African sleeping sickness, the lymph nodes swell and later the brain is infected (causing twitching limbs and slurred speech). The patient becomes confused and increasingly drowsy before dying. In Chagas' disease (which usually attacks children), the eyelids, face, liver, spleen, and lymph nodes swell. The heart and brain then become affected, and this condition can cause death.

Both of these illnesses are difficult to treat. They may be fatal or quite mild. People who live in the area and have a mild attack may get better without treatment and will then be at least partly immune to further attacks. Visitors are likely to have more severe attacks. No vaccine is available to prevent African sleeping sickness, but if early medical attention is sought, the disease can be treated successfully with drugs. For people with Chagas' disease, early drug treatment is effective if given during the acute stage of infection. Once the disease has progressed to later stages, no medication has been proved to be effective.

Ebola fever

Ebola hemorrhagic fever was first reported in 1976 near the Ebola River in Democratic Republic of the Congo (formerly Zaire). This extremely contagious viral disease causes high mortality unless it is treated intensively. The symptoms include chest pain, severe abdominal pain, diarrhea, and vomiting. A non-itching skin rash that bleeds may also develop. Blood may flow from the nose, eyes, ears, gums, and rectum because the causative virus has attacked the linings of the capillaries. Eventually extensive bleeding occurs, both internally and externally. There is no known effective drug against the virus that causes Ebola fever. The main treatment is to maintain the volume of circulating blood.

Nutritional deficiency

Poor diet causes some tropical diseases, including beriberi (which comes from eating mainly white rice that lacks vitamin B_1) and kwashiorkor (which develops in children who eat a low-protein, high-carbohydrate diet). Both conditions can lead to death.

Generally, poor nutrition can make people more likely to get infections and to suffer severely. Measles, malaria, poliomyelitis, tetanus, typhoid fever, tuberculosis, diphtheria, and whooping cough kill millions of adults and children in developing countries every year. WHO has set up a program aiming to immunize all people at risk in the world against these diseases. However, the practical problems are enormous, because 80 percent of the world's population lives in remote areas and medical help cannot easily reach these people. In addition, the populations of underdeveloped countries continue to grow each year.

TRAVEL PRECAUTIONS

Disease	Protective measures	Dosage	Protection time	Effects of disease	Route of disease spread
Cholera	Immunization	2 doses, 1–4 weeks apart	6 months	Violent, severe fluid loss and dehydration	Unhygienic food handling and contaminated water
Hepatitis	Gamma-globulin injection	1 dose	2–6 months	Fever, jaundice, viral liver infection	Contact with infected people, unhygienic food handling, contaminated water
	Vaccine for hepatitis B	3 doses	Life		
Malaria	Antimalarial drugs, mosquito nets, and mosquito repellents	Start drugs before arrival; continue until 6 weeks after leaving	During period of exposure	Fever, chills, nausea, vomiting, and diarrhea	Mosquito bites
Polio	Oral polio vaccine	1 booster dose	5 years	Paralysis	Unhygienic food handling and contaminated water
Smallpox	Vaccination is no longer required or advised; the disease has been eradicated.				
Tetanus	Immunization and careful cleansing of cuts and wounds	2 doses; first booster 1 year later; then a booster every 5 years	5–10 years	Severe muscle spasms and rigidity	Contamination of a wound or wounds
Tuberculosis	BCG immunization (following skin test)	1 dose	Probably lifelong	Chronic lung disease; may damage organs	Direct contact with infected people and unpasteurized milk
Typhoid	Immunization and good hygiene	2 doses, 4 weeks apart	3 years	Fever, jaundice, and bleeding	Unhygienic food handling and contaminated water
Yellow fever	Immunization	1 dose	10 years	Fever, jaundice, and bleeding	Mosquito bites

SEE ALSO

BACTERIA • BLINDNESS • CHOLERA • HANSEN'S DISEASE •
HEPATITIS • LYMPHATIC SYSTEM • MALARIA • MALNUTRITION •
NUTRITIONAL DISEASES • PLAGUE • POLIOMYELITIS •
SMALLPOX • TETANUS • TUBERCULOSIS • TYPHOID FEVER •
VIRUSES • YELLOW FEVER

Tuberculosis

Tuberculosis (TB) is a serious disease of the lungs. It is caused by bacteria. The condition was once very common, and many people died from it. Tuberculosis is not widespread now in developed countries, and when it does occur, it can almost always be treated successfully with antibiotics. TB is still a major cause of death in developing countries, where malnutrition and poor living conditions are common and where treatment is less readily available.

How tuberculosis develops

Tuberculosis is highly infectious. It is usually caught through contact with an infected person who coughs out tiny droplets that contain the infecting bacteria. It is also possible for tuberculosis to be caught from the milk of infected cattle. The first (primary) infection is usually in the lungs. The infected patch is destroyed by the body's defenses, or the live bacteria are walled in by fibrous tissue. There are usually no symptoms.

Very often, the disease stops at this stage, but sometimes the bacteria break through the body's defenses, possibly years later. This may happen when the person's general health is low and resistance is poor. The bacteria multiply and damage the lungs, causing cavities to form. The symptoms include fever, loss of weight, chest pains, and fatigue, with a cough that is at first dry but may later produce phlegm or blood. Eventually, so much of the lung may be destroyed that the patient dies.

Affected body parts

Pulmonary (lung) tuberculosis is the most common form of the disease, but the bacteria may attack other parts of the body, including the kidneys, bones, brain, and skin. Tuberculosis of the abdomen is a common problem in Africa and India, and it is not easy to diagnose, because the symptoms apply to many illnesses.

Q & A

Can I get tuberculosis (TB) from milk?

Two strains of the TB bacterium are important causes of the disease in humans—the human strain and the bovine strain that can be passed on in milk. However, cattle are now tested for infection so that the bovine strain is not passed on in milk.

Can I be vaccinated against tuberculosis?

Yes. There is a vaccine called BCG, which is a modified form of the TB bacterium. This vaccine can fire the immune system against the disease but does not cause serious disease. Children at risk are tested for evidence of previous contact with the disease (primary TB), and if they are negative when tested, they are given BCG. Children who react when tested are known as tuberculin-positive and are immune. People at risk of the disease are tested and revaccinated as necessary.

Pulmonary tuberculosis begins as a small inflamed area in one lung. As the disease progresses, the inflamed area turns into a cavity.

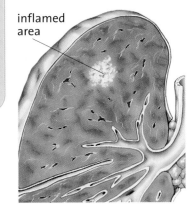
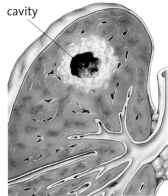

inflamed area

cavity

TB ALERT

TB was once thought to be under control, but cases of TB have been increasing all around the world. The disease spreads rapidly among populations with little resistance, owing to general poor health or immunodeficiency. Because the disease can be spread by infected people who display no symptoms themselves, it is difficult to eradicate.

In the United States, however, the number of new active TB cases has been decreasing since 1992. During 2005, about 14,000 TB cases (4.8 cases per 100,000 people) were reported in the United States.

Older children can be tested for immunity to TB and, if necessary, can be vaccinated.

However, there will probably be a cough that will not go away, coughing up of blood, a feeling of tiredness all the time, weight loss, appetite loss, and night sweats.

Treating tuberculosis

Until the 1950s, tuberculosis was often fatal. Patients were made to rest in bed to build up their strength and give their bodies a chance to fight the bacteria. Special nursing homes called sanatoriums were built in areas known for their superior air quality, particularly in mountain regions. Sometimes surgeons operated to remove the badly infected parts of the lungs.

Skin tests and X-rays now make it possible to detect and treat early cases of tuberculosis and stop its spread. Modern drugs taken in combination can stop the spread of tuberculosis within a few days, although it will take months for a complete cure (particularly for abdominal tuberculosis). Patients still need to have plenty of rest and will need regular checkups for several years after they are cured. Improved living conditions have helped to check tuberculosis in developed countries. Milk is regularly tested to make sure it is free from the bacteria. Immunization can be given to people who may be at risk.

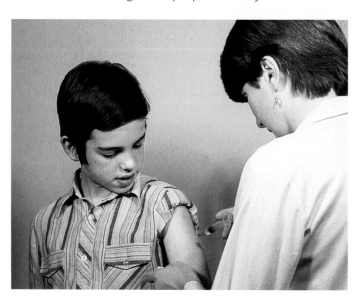

SEE ALSO

BACTERIAL DISEASES • BLOOD • BRAIN • INFECTIOUS DISEASES • LUNG DISEASES AND DISORDERS • SKIN

Typhoid Fever

Q & A

I've heard that the effect of typhoid is worse if the person has gallstones. Is this true?

No. If a person has gallstones, he or she is more likely to become a carrier of the disease. The organism seems to settle in the gallbladder, and the presence of stones in the gallbladder makes this easier.

My brother says that it is possible to catch typhoid from animals. Is he right?

No. Typhoid seems to be an exclusively human disease, with one exception—fruit-eating bats in Madagascar. If you catch the disease, therefore, you must have caught it from someone else, via contaminated food or water. It is unusual for typhoid to spread directly from person to person. On the other hand, paratyphoid seems to be less specialized, and it can attack other animals. There is at least one outbreak on record in which cattle were the source of the paratyphoid infection.

If colonies of typhoid bacteria are found in the blood, antibiotic treatment should be started immediately.

Typhoid is a very serious infectious disease caused by *Salmonella typhi* (one of the bacteria that cause salmonella food poisoning). It affects many parts of the body and may be fatal. Paratyphoid is a similar but less severe illness caused by *S. paratyphi*. Because of improved hygiene and immunization, both illnesses are now less common in developed countries, but in developing areas of the world they are still a very serious threat. Typhoid and paratyphoid are communicable diseases, so the local health authorities must be informed of any cases of infection.

Anyone traveling to an area where hygiene is poor should be vaccinated against typhoid and paratyphoid. Immunization gives protection for three years, after which booster shots are needed.

Salmonella organisms are spread by food and water that have been contaminated by the feces of an infected person. Typhoid has an incubation period of about two weeks. Some people have typhoid-causing bacteria in their bodies but have no symptoms of the illness. However, they can spread the illness to other people, especially if they handle food. Most outbreaks of typhoid that occur in developed countries are caused by such carriers.

Symptoms and treatment

The first symptoms are a headache and pains in the muscles and abdomen. The patient may have constipation and sometimes diarrhea. The temperature is raised each evening but is lower the following morning. After a week or so, it reaches about 104°F (40°C). The patient may develop chest pains and pneumonia. The abdomen swells, and pale pink patches appear on the skin.

During the second week, the untreated patient may become confused, delirious, and unconscious. Diarrhea develops, and the

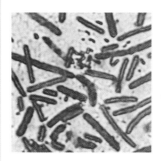

walls of the intestine may rupture, causing death. If this does not happen, the fever settles after three or four weeks, but there is always a high risk of a serious relapse.

Treatment involves antibiotics to bring the illness quickly under control. However, the salmonella organism will still be passed in the patient's feces for three months.

SEE ALSO

BACTERIAL DISEASES • DIARRHEA • INFECTIOUS DISEASES • SALMONELLA • TROPICAL DISEASES

Typhus

Typhus is a serious and sometimes fatal disease that spreads rapidly when people are crowded together in unhygienic conditions. It is one of the great drawbacks of the emergency camps that are set up to help people after natural disasters.

Causes

There are several types of typhus, all of which are caused by microorganisms called rickettsiae. These microorganisms spread from one person to another via bloodsucking insects. The most serious and widespread type is epidemic typhus, which is spread by body lice. The disease cannot be caught directly from another person, although dust from clothing contaminated with louse feces can be very infectious.

Symptoms and treatments

About 10 days after infection, the patient develops a headache, muscle pain, and a high fever. A rash of small, flat, red spots appears four days later. After another week, the spots darken to look like small bruises. The patient begins to lose consciousness for periods. The kidneys may fail, a cough develops, and the rash may turn to gangrene in the fingers and toes. Without treatment, 20 to 50 percent of patients die at this stage. Survivors recover from their fever in the third week and the brain starts working normally again, but they will not be fully well for a long time.

Typhus can be treated with antibiotics with great success, but these drugs may not be available in those areas of countries where the disease is most likely to break out.

Typhus can be prevented by good hygiene, by controlling the insects that spread the disease, and by immunization. If a person contracts typhus, he or she should see a doctor, who has to notify the local health authority of a communicable disease.

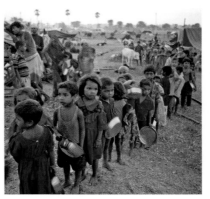

Q & A

My great-grandfather died of typhus when he liberated a concentration camp at the end of World War II. Why was typhus so common in the camps?

Typhus is found when normal social organization has broken down. The disease depends on lice for transmission from human to human, and this occurs if hygiene is poor. Also, typhus is a disease that thrives in cold conditions, such as the concentration camps in Europe.

How do lice spread typhus?

When a louse bites to eat blood, it also defecates, and louse feces contain the infection. When the bite is scratched, the infection contained in the feces is rubbed into the skin, and the disease starts. The infection survives in louse feces for a long time, so the dust from the clothes of a person who is louse-ridden can be very infective.

Children line up for food after their northern Indian village was submerged by monsoon flooding in 2007. In such emergency camps, people often live in unhygienic conditions, where body lice flourish and typhus can spread rapidly.

SEE ALSO

COMMUNICABLE DISEASES • EPIDEMIC • GANGRENE • INFECTIOUS DISEASES • RICKETTSIAL DISEASES

Ulcers

An ulcer is an open sore on the surface of the body or on an internal membrane. The base of the ulcer becomes inflamed and may eat into the tissues underneath. Some ulcers are caused by infections, others by injuries or damage to the tissues, nerves, or blood supply. Some ulcers are shallow, with only the skin lost, but others spread deep into the muscle or bone beneath.

Common sites of ulcers

Ulcers are found on the surface of the body, such as the lips and face, around the groin, on the legs, and around the hips and lower back. They are also very common inside the mouth and in the digestive tract. Tiny ulcers on the lips and face, known as cold sores, are caused by a herpes virus, which can be transmitted by someone who already has the virus in its active state. The cold sores usually clear up within a couple of weeks, but, once caught, the virus remains in the body and at different times will break out again to form another sore, particularly when the person is run down or in poor health. Another type of ulcer that occurs on the face is a rodent ulcer. It starts as a red lump, which then forms a circular ulcer. It is a form of cancer, but early treatment with radiotherapy or surgery can cure it completely.

An ulcer in the groin area may be caused by a sexually transmitted disease such as herpes or syphilis. Such a disease needs to be treated quickly if it is not to do lasting harm. Unless bedridden people are moved often, they may develop ulcers called bedsores. These ulcers are caused by constant pressure on bony areas of the body, such as the hips and base of the spine.

Leg ulcers are often caused by conditions that affect the blood vessels in the leg. If the vessels become blocked or narrowed, or the blood in them stagnates (as in varicose veins), the blood supply to the tissues is reduced. The tissues die and break down, causing an ulcer. Leg ulcers must be kept clean and free from infection. Antibiotics cure any infection, but surgery may be needed to deal with faulty blood vessels.

Mouth ulcers

Almost everyone has ulcers in the mouth from time to time. The lining of the mouth may be damaged by jagged teeth, very hot food or drink, or strong antiseptics and mouthwashes. These ulcers usually heal quickly without treatment. Other mouth ulcers are caused by infections. If mouth ulcers last for a long time or appear regularly, people should see a doctor, who will identify and treat the underlying cause. For occasional mouth ulcers, there are several effective over-the-counter preparations, such as analgesic creams and gels, that can help soothe the pain.

Q & A

Is it possible for a person to have a stomach ulcer without knowing it?

Certainly. Many people accept that a small amount of indigestion is normal. A fair proportion of these people would be found to have an active ulcer or the signs of an old ulcer if they were examined by a doctor. If the ulcer is asymptomatic (without any symptoms) and does not have any complications, then there is really no cause for great concern.

I've been told by my doctor to eat frequently, because I have a stomach ulcer. I am now worried about putting on weight. How can I avoid doing so?

The trick is to eat frequent small meals. The idea is that frequent small meals do not allow the level of acid to build up, because the acid is continually being neutralized by the food. Obviously, you do risk putting on weight, and you should aim to eat a normal amount of food, but split it into a greater number of smaller meals.

These diagrams show the development of a duodenal ulcer. Gastric juices have attacked the tissues of the duodenal wall, creating a hole and almost eating through it.

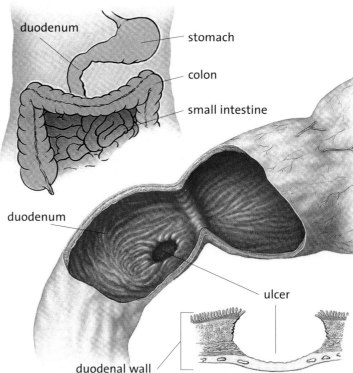

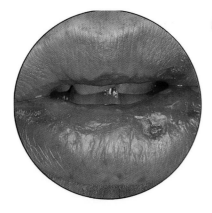

Herpes often causes clusters of small ulcers or cold sores on the lips.

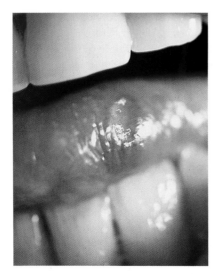

Dental hygiene can help prevent mouth ulcers, but strong antiseptics and mouthwashes should be avoided, because they can damage the lining of the mouth.

Peptic ulcers

Ulcers in the digestive tract, known as peptic ulcers, can be serious and painful. Gastric ulcers occur in the stomach. Those in the duodenum, called duodenal ulcers, can form if the body produces too much gastric acid that eats into the lining membrane. The organism *Helicobacter pylori* is associated with the development of peptic ulcers.

Peptic ulcers can be very painful and are made worse by drinking alcohol and eating spicy foods. Anyone who has frequent indigestion or stomach pains should consult a doctor.

Untreated ulcers can eat into the lining of the stomach, causing serious bleeding and eventually anemia. They may also perforate, causing life-threatening peritonitis. Treatment of peptic ulcers includes following a special diet and, if possible, leading a more relaxed lifestyle.

> **SEE ALSO**
>
> ANEMIA • CANCER • DIGESTIVE SYSTEM • DIGESTIVE SYSTEM DISEASES AND DISORDERS • MOUTH

Urinary System

The urinary system is responsible for flushing waste products out of the body. The main component of waste is urea, which is made from carbon dioxide and ammonia. Carbon dioxide is produced by metabolism (all of the chemical processes that take place in the body that are controlled by enzymes); ammonia is produced by the breakdown and buildup of proteins.

Filtering waste products

The urinary system begins with the kidneys, where waste products are filtered out of the blood. To enable the kidneys to produce sufficient urine to maintain the balance of the body's chemistry, the waste products combine with excess water to form urine, which is then excreted.

From the kidneys, the urine flows through two tubes called the ureters to the bladder, where the urine is stored. When a person feels the pressure of a full bladder, he or she urinates. The urine flows from the bladder through another tube, the urethra, and is excreted.

Urine color and composition

Disease often affects the color, chemical composition, and amount of urine. It is a valuable guide to a person's state of health, and this is why doctors often need a sample of urine to test, especially to see if it contains sugar, blood, or protein. Diabetes, for example, can be detected in a simple urine test, as can phenylketonuria, a rare inherited disease that can lead to brain damage. Doctors frequently use urine tests as part of a routine physical examination.

The color of urine is mainly due to substances produced by the metabolism of bile, which is a substance produced in the liver. A pale urine color means the urine is well diluted, and a

Q & A

Are women really more prone to urinary tract infections than men are?

Yes. Urinary system infections are more common in women than in men. This is generally thought to be because the urethra is much shorter in women than in men and its external opening is more easily contaminated than a man's.

Why does urine vary in color?

Usually urine is yellow, but it becomes darker when it is more concentrated; this occurs when the body is short of water. The color also varies from person to person and changes when certain substances are eaten or drunk. Beets and the dyes in some candies make urine redder.

My brother, who is seven, has urinary system problems. A urologist arranged for him to have an X-ray while he was urinating. Is this a real test?

Yes. It is used extensively with children and is useful in investigating abnormal bladder emptying and abnormalities in the urethra.

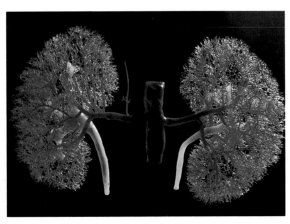

This model shows the blood vessels and ureters of healthy kidneys.

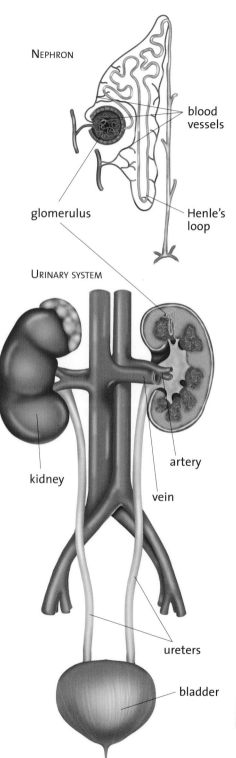

Nephron

blood vessels

glomerulus

Henle's loop

Urinary system

kidney

artery

vein

ureters

bladder

deep color means that it is concentrated. Jaundice may turn the urine dark brown. Red urine may be due to the presence of blood, but it can also be produced by eating intensely colored foods, such as beets and certain candies.

Urinary system infections

Infections of the urinary system often start in the urethral opening, especially in women. Urethritis (inflammation of the urethra) is an example. It is usually caused by a sexually transmitted disease and can be treated with antibiotics.

Cystitis, a common female complaint, is an infection of the bladder and urethra characterized by scalding pain during urination. Pus or blood in the urine can be a sign of pyelitis (inflammation of the kidneys due to infection). A doctor should always be consulted if there is blood in the urine; it could be the symptom of a tumor or of cancer of the bladder.

Lack of bladder control

Lack of bladder control, or bed-wetting, is normal in children up to the age of four but may occur in older children during a period of emotional stress, such as the birth of another child in the family. Sometimes a urinary infection is the causative factor.

Incontinence (the inability to prevent urination) is often present in adults who have had a spinal injury or brain damage or who are very elderly. Injuries in prostate operations may also cause incontinence. In women, incontinence sometimes occurs as a result of stress and physical exertion or from injuries sustained during childbirth.

This diagram shows the urinary system (bottom). Each kidney contains between one and two million filtering units called nephrons (top). The end of each nephron expands into a knot-shaped structure called a glomerulus. Minute blood vessels within each glomerulus filter the blood to extract waste products, which are then carried in the urine and taken to the bladder by the ureters before being expelled from the body during urination. The remainder of the nephron consists of a long, coiled tubule that includes Henle's loop.

SEE ALSO

BODY SYSTEMS • BRAIN DAMAGE AND DISORDERS • DIABETES • HYPERTENSION • JAUNDICE • KIDNEY • KIDNEY DISEASES AND DISORDERS • LIVER • PHENYLKETONURIA • SEXUALLY TRANSMITTED DISEASES

Vein Disorders

The blood that supplies the legs flows down the arteries to the feet and comes back to the heart through the veins. The veins contain valves, tiny folds in the linings of the veins that allow blood to flow up the limb and stop it from flowing backward.

Varicose veins

Varicose veins are twisted, knotted, and swollen veins, commonly in the lower legs. They are unsightly, can be painful, and can cause problems such as phlebitis and leg ulcers.

In people with varicose veins, the valves in the veins do not work properly. Blood can flow back down the vein, and as a result, the vein swells and twists, and its walls stretch.

Varicose veins run in families. They are also made more likely by being pregnant, being overweight, and standing for long periods. Sometimes they develop at the site of an injury. Women are more likely than men to develop varicoes veins.

Injections, followed by bandaging, can close small varicose veins permanently. Support hose prevents the veins from getting worse. Surgery for varicose veins involves removing the twisted veins and tying off the valves that are leaking. The blood then travels through some of the many other veins in the leg.

Phlebitis

Phlebitis means inflammation of a vein, generally in the veins of the legs. A thrombosis (blood clot) can form and attach itself to the wall of a vein, causing thrombophlebitis. Deep-vein phlebitis affects the large veins inside the leg muscles. Part of a clot may break off and block the main artery that supplies the lungs. A large clot can cause a blockage that leads to death. Symptoms of deep-vein phlebitis include a swollen leg and pain deep in the calf. Anticoagulant drugs can break up the clot.

Q & A

Can varicose veins be dangerous, or are they just unsightly?

Varicose veins are rarely more than an unsightly nuisance. However, varicose veins can increase the danger of a deep vein thrombosis (clot) after surgery or pregnancy. It is not uncommon for a cut or fall to cause serious bleeding from a prominent varicose vein. People who suffer from varicose veins should avoid prolonged standing and wear special support hose. In serious cases, surgery may be required to deal with the condition.

To remove varicose veins, a stripper (a long, thin tube) is introduced into an incision made in the groin. The stripper is advanced down the vein, with the surgeon's finger tracing the vein's path to ensure that the stripper's way is clear. A small incision is made on the inside of the ankle, and the stripper and the varicose vein are withdrawn through it.

SEE ALSO

CIRCULATORY SYSTEM • CIRCULATORY SYSTEM DISEASES AND DISORDERS • HEART • LUNG • ULCERS

Viruses

Viruses are infective agents that are so tiny they cannot be seen under an ordinary microscope. A virus cannot reproduce alone. Instead, it reproduces by taking over the cell of a living organism, such as a plant or animal. The cell works for the virus, making vast numbers of new, identical viruses, which spread to take over other cells. The original host cell is usually destroyed.

Common viral diseases

Viruses cause many diseases in people. Some diseases are mild and clear up within a few days, but some are serious. Rabies, for example, is always fatal unless treatment is begun immediately. Among the many diseases caused by viruses are AIDS, the common cold, influenza, some forms of pneumonia, infectious mononucleosis, mumps, measles, rubella, smallpox, chicken pox and other herpes infections, polio, yellow fever, psittacosis, rabies, hepatitis, encephalitis, some kinds of gastroenteritis, and warts.

How viruses enter the body

Many viral diseases, such as influenza, colds, and measles, are spread by droplet infection, from a cough or sneeze from an infected person. Other viruses, including the polio virus and enteroviruses, enter the body through the digestive tract when contaminated food or drink is consumed. The viruses causing yellow fever and dengue fever enter via the skin as a result of an insect bite. Hepatitis B and AIDS are caused by blood-borne viruses that enter the bloodstream. Rabies enters the body through a bite from an infected animal.

Once inside the body, viruses invade the cells near the site of entry. They may not be harmful at this point; for example, the polio virus multiplies in the digestive tract, but the symptoms of the disease arise only when the virus reaches the spinal cord.

Other viruses live in the body without causing harm. When there is a lowering of the body's resistance, viruses multiply and symptoms appear. People with the cold sore virus may develop the sores whenever they are run down; often this happens when they have a cold, which gives the sores their name.

Retroviruses

Viruses have a core of nucleic acid, which is made of either deoxyribonucleic acid (DNA) or ribonucleic acid (RNA). Viruses are thus classified as DNA viruses or RNA viruses. Because viruses can survive only by inserting DNA into that of invaded cells, viruses containing only RNA must use that RNA to make DNA.

A type of RNA virus called a retrovirus was found to cause AIDS and a type of leukemia. This was an important discovery, because

Q & A

Why can't viruses be treated with antibiotics?

Bacteria that respond to antibiotics are complicated microorganisms, although each consists of only one cell. Viruses, on the other hand, are very simple infective agents, consisting of a core of nucleic acid (genetic material) that is surrounded by a protein capsule. Antibiotics work by impeding the activity of the bacterial cell without harming human cells. However, viral metabolism and structure are quite different from those of bacteria, so antibiotics that attack bacterial structure and metabolism have no effect on viruses.

Is it likely that any new treatments will be able to affect the course of minor viral diseases, such as the common cold?

It seems unlikely that any form of direct treatment for minor viral diseases will be discovered in the near future. It has been very difficult to make a vaccine against the common cold, because the condition is caused by about 200 viruses, which are always mutating.

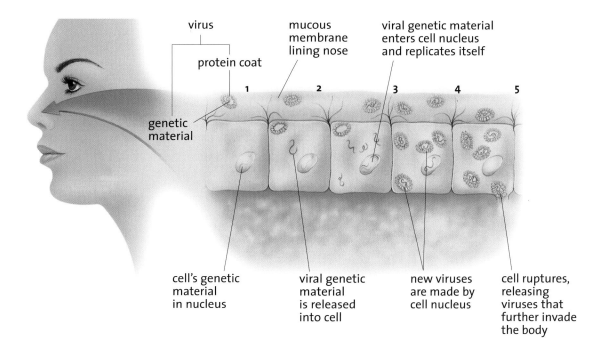

virus

protein coat

mucous
membrane
lining nose

viral genetic material
enters cell nucleus
and replicates itself

genetic
material

1   2   3   4   5

cell's genetic
material
in nucleus

viral genetic
material
is released
into cell

new viruses
are made by
cell nucleus

cell ruptures,
releasing
viruses that
further invade
the body

Viruses can multiply only in the cells of other organisms. When people have a cold, they breathe in a virus. Inside the body, the virus has the ideal conditions to multiply. First, it invades one of the nasal cells (1). Its genetic material mingles with that of the host cell (2), which then starts to produce more viral genetic material (3). Finally, the new viral particles (4) emerge from the cell (5) to invade other cells.

it led to the development of drugs that could prevent viruses from making DNA from RNA. The enzyme that is used to make DNA from RNA is called reverse transcriptase. The drugs that were developed blocked the action of this enzyme.

Difficulties of treating viral infections

Bacteria in the body are killed by antibiotics, but antibiotics have no effect on viruses. Acyclovir is an antiviral drug that kills cells infected with the herpes virus but spares normal cells. This drug may be useful against all kinds of herpes infections. Once it is known how viruses reproduce in cells and what nutrition they need, drugs can be developed to interfere with these processes. Many antivirals block the enzymes that viruses need.

Viral infections are also treated by rest and good nursing, which allows the body to concentrate its energy on fighting the infection. The immune system sends white cells and makes antibodies to destroy the virus. Drugs can be used to relieve the symptoms. Anti-inflammatory drugs bring down a fever; syrups soothe a cough; and decongestants unblock a stuffed nose.

The human immunodeficiency virus (HIV), which causes AIDS, is one of the most destructive viruses known. It destroys the white blood cells that produce antibodies to fight disease. As a result, other viral, fungal, or occasionally bacterial infections and cancers, rather than HIV itself, eventually kill the patient.

COMMON VIRAL DISEASES

DISEASE	TRANSMISSION	SYMPTOMS	TREATMENTS AND PREVENTION
AIDS	Sexual contact (via blood, semen); blood transfusion; dirty needles; mother to fetus	General illness, swollen glands, pneumonia, skin cancer, and mental changes	Treatment for secondary illnesses but no cure for AIDS viral infection
Chicken pox	Person to person by airborne droplets; from spots on skin	Fever, itchy rash, and red spots on skin	Relief of symptoms; attack produces immunity
Common cold (produced by more than 200 viruses)	Person to person by airborne droplets	Runny nose, sore throat, possible fever, coughs, and blocked nose	Relief of symptoms
Dengue fever	Certain types of tropical mosquitoes	Fever, pain in muscles and joints, headaches, and rash	Bed rest and relief of symptoms; attack produces immunity for more than 12 months
Gastroenteritis (viral and bacterial)	Person to person by airborne droplets, or by contaminated food and water	Diarrhea, vomiting, abdominal pains, and general illness	Relief of symptoms; restoring fluid balance, especially in babies and young children
Hepatitis (A, B, and C)	Type A by food or water contaminated with feces of infected person; type B by infected blood; type C by infected blood	Influenza-like symptoms, loss of appetite, nausea, vomiting, and jaundice	Relief of symptoms; prevention of type A by serum immune globulin; prevention of type B by blood screening, immune globulin, and vaccine
Herpes (simplex)	Sexual contact; cold sores by kissing	Painful sores around mouth and/or genital areas; burning sensation during urination	Relief of symptoms
Infectious mononucleosis (glandular fever)	Person to person by close contact, including kissing	Headache, chills, swollen glands, general illness, and fatigue	Rest and relief of symptoms
Influenza	Person to person by airborne droplets	Aching limbs, headache, fever, and sore throat	Relief of symptoms; prevention by vaccine moderately effective
Lassa fever	By species of rat present in West Africa; usually through contaminated food	Fever, shivering, abdominal pain, diarrhea, and vomiting	Relief of symptoms, careful nursing, and sometimes antiviral drugs; disease is often fatal
Measles	Person to person by airborne droplets	Bad cold, cough, fever, and red spots on skin	Relief of symptoms, careful nursing in severe cases; attack gives lifelong immunity; prevention by vaccine
Mumps	Person to person by airborne droplets	Influenza-like symptoms, fever, and swollen glands	Relief of symptoms; attack gives lifelong immunity; prevention by vaccine
Polio	Person to person by airborne droplets or contamination of food and water by poor hygiene habits and poor sanitation; highly contagious	Headache, sore throat, backache, listlessness, weakness and pain in muscles and limbs, and slight fever	Relief of symptoms in mild cases; paralyzed patients often need tracheotomy (surgery to allow breathing by ventilator); physical therapy; prevention by vaccine

(continued)

COMMON VIRAL DISEASES

DISEASE	TRANSMISSION	SYMPTOMS	TREATMENTS AND PREVENTION
Rabies	By bite of infected animal, such as dog or fox	Fever, sore throat, muscle pains, fear of water, spasms, and coma	No cure, established disease fatal; prevention by vaccines and by administration of serum and vaccines
Rubella	Person to person by airborne droplets	Runny nose, rash of fine pink dots under the skin, and swollen tender lymph nodes	Relief of symptoms; prevention by vaccine almost universal in developed countries for women to avoid birth defects in pregnancy
Warts	Person to person by direct skin contact or by infected towel	Small rounded growths in the skin	Childhood warts often disappear; removal by freezing or electrical-burning techniques
Yellow fever	Species of tropical mosquitoes	Fever, headache, aching limbs, jaundice, liver failure, and kidney failure	Careful nursing; attack gives lifelong immunity; prevention by control of infecting mosquitoes and by vaccines

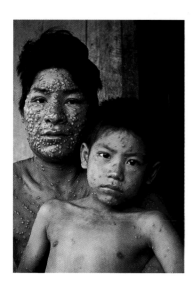

The deadly and contagious viral disease smallpox has now been completely eradicated by a worldwide immunization program. Here, two of the disease's last victims show the dreadful disfiguring symptoms that were indicative of the disease.

Prevention and immunization

Some people may develop a bacterial infection while their resistance is lowered by a virus. For example, elderly people with influenza are at risk of developing bacterial pneumonia. For this reason, antibiotics may be given as a preventive measure.

Although there is still no treatment for most viral infections, many of the serious conditions can be prevented by immunization. Smallpox (a deadly viral disease) has been wiped out by a worldwide immunization program. Someone bitten by a rabid animal can be protected from the disease if immunizing shots are given at once, before the virus multiplies. Among the many other diseases that can be prevented by vaccination are measles, rubella, yellow fever, and poliomyelitis.

> **SEE ALSO**
>
> AIDS AND HIV • CHICKEN POX • COLD • ENCEPHALITIS • GASTROENTERITIS • HEPATITIS • HERPES • HPV • IMMUNE SYSTEM • IMMUNODEFICIENCY • INFECTIOUS DISEASES • INFECTIOUS MONONUCLEOSIS • INFLUENZA • LEUKEMIA • MEASLES • MUMPS • PNEUMONIA • POLIOMYELITIS • RABIES • RUBELLA • SEXUALLY TRANSMITTED DISEASES • SMALLPOX • TROPICAL DISEASES • YELLOW FEVER

West Nile Virus

West Nile virus is a disease spread mainly by mosquitoes. The condition once infected only birds, but since the mid-1900s, increasing numbers of people have been infected. West Nile virus was first identified in a human patient in Uganda in 1937, but it was not detected as a cause of human disease in the United States until August 1999. West Nile virus is now a seasonal epidemic in North America that flares up in the summer and continues into the fall.

Illness from this virus is essentially a disease of the elderly. Although it may occur in people of all ages from five to 90, most are over the age of 50. The illness has symptoms of fever with hot flashes, night sweats, weakness, nausea, and vomiting. About one in five infected people has a measles-like rash on the skin. Common complications include encephalitis and poliomyelitis. In encephalitis, headache, stiff neck, bladder dysfunction, altered mental state, and respiratory distress occur; if the spinal cord is involved, the infection may look like poliomyelitis.

Diagnosis and treatment

The diagnosis of West Nile virus infection can be made by culture of the virus from the blood, by finding specific antibodies to the virus, and by detecting the RNA of the virus in tissue samples. These tests are done if the disease is suspected and if these signs occur in the presence of an epidemic of the disease.

There is no specific treatment for West Nile virus, but the symptoms of the disease are treated to make the patient comfortable until the virus completes its life cycle in the body. When encephalitis or meningitis develops, that disease is treated accordingly.

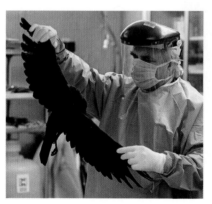

A pathologist examines a crow suspected to have died from West Nile virus.

SEE ALSO

BRAIN • ENCEPHALITIS • EPIDEMIC • INFECTIOUS DISEASES • MENINGITIS • POLIOMYELITIS • RESPIRATORY SYSTEM DISEASES AND DISORDERS • VIRUSES

Q & A

I heard that West Nile virus is an arbovirus. What is that?

The term *arbovirus* does not refer to a particular kind of virus. It refers to any of the viruses spread by blood-feeding insects, such as mosquitoes and sand flies. About 100 of these viruses can cause disease in humans. *Arbovirus* is a contraction of "arthropod-borne virus" (an arthropod is any jointed-legged animal, such as an insect, spider, tick, centipede, or millipede). Arthropods form the largest phylum (major grouping) in the whole animal kingdom. The West Nile virus is transmitted by mosquitoes.

Is it true that West Nile virus can affect the brain?

Yes. Although most people affected by West Nile virus suffer only a very mild and brief illness, a proportion develop brain inflammation (encephalitis) or meningitis (inflammation of the brain coverings). This complication occurs rarely in young people, but in the older age groups, it carries a death rate of around 9 percent.

Whiplash Injury

Whiplash injury is a type of neck sprain. It is nearly always caused by an automobile accident. Someone in a car that is hit from behind is suddenly thrown forward, but his or her head lags behind for a moment and then jolts forward. This jolt puts the muscles and ligaments at the front of the neck and throat under sudden strain. In severe cases, one or more of the small joints in the neck may be dislocated or the neck bones may be fractured.

Symptoms

People with whiplash injury may feel little pain immediately after the injury happens. The next day, however, they may have pain and stiffness in the neck, spreading to the shoulders.

People with bad cases of whiplash may experience blurred vision, headaches, dizziness, or difficulty in swallowing. Most cases recover completely within a month, but pain and stiffness may last a year or more. Some of these pains may be due to underlying arthritis in the joints of the neck, which is triggered by the injury. In other cases, there is a vicious circle of pain and stiffness giving rise to muscle spasms, which in turn cause more pain and stiffness.

The main danger of whiplash is that the symptoms will become persistent. However, serious injury to the neck is rare; fractures of the neck bones, a slipped disk, dislocations of the joints, spinal cord injuries, and nerve root injuries are more commonly caused by bending the neck forward or by direct force applied to the top of the head.

Q & A

Will wearing a seat belt in an automobile prevent a person from getting a whiplash injury?

No. The injury occurs when the head snaps back suddenly if a vehicle is struck from behind. Properly adjusted headrests can prevent most of these injuries. Seat belts may lessen the severity of the injury by preventing the wearer from bouncing forward again once the initial blow is over. Wearing a seat belt may also prevent a driver or passenger from being flung against a windshield.

Is it true that a whiplash injury can occur when a baby is physically abused?

It is possible for a whiplash injury to occur in these circumstances. It may, however, be much more difficult to diagnose than more obvious injuries caused by child abuse, because there are usually no outward signs of injury at all. Because a baby cannot complain, especially of neck pain, such an injury might never be detected.

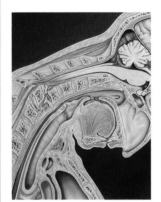

Treatment

The initial treatment is to allow the neck muscles to rest and relax by wearing a surgical collar or neck brace. Painkillers will prevent sore muscles from going into spasm. If the pain lasts for more than a week, physical therapy (including heat treatment and traction) may help. Surgery to fuse the neck bones may be needed. Constant headaches and dizziness may require medication.

In extremely severe whiplash injury, the spinal joints of the neck are dislocated.

SEE ALSO

ARTHRITIS • FRACTURES AND DISLOCATIONS • MUSCLE • SLIPPED DISK • SPRAINS AND STRAINS

Whooping Cough

Q & A

Do most doctors now advise giving children the whooping cough vaccine?

Yes, if there is no history of convulsions or brain damage. The risks of severe illness are greater from whooping cough than from the vaccine.

Why is whooping cough such a dangerous illness in babies and small children?

Whooping cough produces very thick, sticky mucus in the air passages to the lungs, which can prevent air from getting to the lungs unless the mucus is coughed away. Small children and babies can be too weak to cough up this mucus, so their lungs get blocked.

My sister had whooping cough. Since then, she has had a series of coughs and colds. Did the illness weaken her resistance to infection?

No. It is probably just bad luck. However, your parents should ask her doctor to check her over, because sometimes part of the lung collapses after whooping cough.

Whooping cough (pertussis) is a very infectious illness caused by the bacterium *Bordetella pertussis*, which inflames the lining of the lungs, trachea (windpipe), and throat. The infection causes coughing and produces a thick, sticky mucus. It is the most serious and distressing of the infectious diseases of childhood. Many babies are now immunized against whooping cough, and the illness is no longer widespread in developed countries.

Whooping cough bacteria are released into the air as droplets by an infected person and then inhaled by someone nearby. The first symptoms develop between six and 20 days after contact. They include running nose and eyes, a slight cough, and a fever. This coldlike stage lasts about two weeks. Then patients start to have bouts of coughing, consisting of five to 10 repetitive coughs, followed by an effort to breathe in, with a gasping whoop. During the coughing fit, the patient's face turns red or blue, the eyes bulge, and the eyes and nose run. At the end of the bout, the patient may vomit. These coughing spells may happen 40 times a day and are very tiring. This whooping stage lasts from two to four weeks. Then the coughing, whooping, and vomiting gradually die down, although the cough and whoop may come back if the patient catches a cold or throat infection.

Complications and treatment

Whooping cough may cause serious complications, including pneumonia and collapse of the lung. Lack of oxygen to the brain during a bad coughing spell can cause convulsions or unconsciousness, or brain damage in small children. It can even cause death, particularly in children under a year old. Treatment is with antibiotics; babies and small children may be treated in a hospital if complications develop.

Immunization

Children are vaccinated against diphtheria, tetanus, and pertussis using one vaccine called DTaP. Babies are given their first DTaP immunization at eight weeks, with booster shots at four and six months, at 15 to 18 months, and between four and six years. Immunization may not always prevent a child from getting whooping cough, but only a mild case should develop.

SEE ALSO

BACTERIA • BACTERIAL DISEASES • BRAIN DAMAGE AND DISORDERS • COLD • INFECTIOUS DISEASES • LUNG DISEASES AND DISORDERS • PNEUMONIA

Worms

Q & A

Can you avoid worms by cooking food thoroughly?

Yes, some worms can be avoided by cooking food thoroughly. Both types of common tapeworms are spread by undercooked beef and pork, for example. The larvae die at 144°F (62°C), so extremely high temperatures are not necessary to kill them. A tapeworm (*Diphyllobothrium latum*) that lives in fish occurs in Scandinavia; it is caught by eating raw fish. *Anisakis marina* is a parasite of herrings that can also be ingested with raw fish; it infects humans in Holland and Japan, where some people eat raw herring and sushi. There are also two forms of liver flukes living in Asia that can be caught only by eating raw or undercooked fish.

I had hookworms three years ago. Could I still be infected?

Left untreated, hookworms usually disappear after about two years, although they can live for up to five years. Provided you have not been reinfected and have no symptoms now, it is unlikely that the worms have survived.

Worldwide, people become ill from worms living as parasites in their bodies. Some of these infestations are serious, particularly some of those present in tropical countries.

Many of the worms that infest humans spend part of their lives as eggs, larvae, or adults in other animals. Some worms burrow into the skin. In other cases, people eat infested meat or ingest food or water that has been contaminated by animal feces containing the worms. Some worms enter people through insect bites.

Pinworms (threadworms) are very common, particularly in children. These worms are nematodes or roundworms. Worms called filariae live in tropical countries and cause filariasis. Trichina worms live in pigs and cause trichinosis. Hookworms and ascaris are common in the tropics and live in people's intestines.

Dogs and cats may be infested with toxocara roundworms, and people may become infected with their larvae if they do not wash their hands after playing with their pets. The larvae move around in the body and may harm the liver and eyes. Pets should be wormed regularly to rid them of such parasitic worms.

Another group of worms are trematodes (flatworms or flukes), which cause schistosomiasis. Cestodes (tapeworms) are caught by eating meat containing their larvae. The typical tapeworm is *Taenia saginata*, the beef tapeworm. The worm anchors itself to the wall of the upper intestine, producing a long string of egg-bearing segments (the tape). Eggs pass out in the feces. For the infestation to be passed on, the eggs must be eaten by a suitable intermediate host, such as a cow. In this host, the eggs hatch into larvae, which spread to the animal's muscles. The life cycle continues if a human eats the infested, undercooked meat. The other common tapeworm is *Taenia solium*, the pig tapeworm.

Treating worm diseases

Worm infestations are a major public health problem. Although drugs are available to kill the worms that infest humans, some of these drugs are harmful in themselves. Preventing infestation is the answer to the problem. Prevention means better sanitation and hygiene, and in particular reducing the risk of food and water being contaminated with human and animal feces.

SEE ALSO

DIGESTIVE SYSTEM • SKIN • TROPICAL DISEASES

Wounds

A wound is an injury that breaks the skin, removes part of the skin surface, or causes damage just beneath it. A wound may occur as the result of an accident or of surgery. Most wounds are not serious and heal without difficulty, but some wounds are so bad that they can cause permanent scars or disabilities. Healing depends on avoiding wound infection and on the alignment of the edges of the wound. If the wound is clean and well closed, healing should be complete in a few weeks; open wounds can take much longer and may leave more obvious scarring.

Types of wounds

Wounds are grouped into several basic categories. Abrasions (grazes) happen when the outer layer of skin is rubbed away by something rough. Small broken blood vessels bleed a little, and exposed nerve endings make abrasions very painful. Abrasions that scrape only the epidermis (outer skin layer) heal with little or no scarring; deep abrasions usually leave a scar.

Contusions (bruises) are caused by a blow from something blunt. The skin is not broken, but the tissues beneath the skin are damaged. Small blood vessels are broken, and blood leaks into the tissues, causing them to swell and turn purplish blue.

A laceration is a tear, but the term is used for any form of cut from a surface wound to a deep one. Lacerations can be caused by something sharp (such as a knife or a piece of glass) or by a blow from a blunt object that splits the skin. A deep laceration may require stitching to avoid leaving a puckered scar. A clean, well-closed laceration should not leave obvious scarring.

An incision is a deliberate cut by a clean, sharp instrument (as in a surgical operation). A puncture is a wound made by a needle or thorn that is deeper than it is wide. Although a puncture may heal quickly, there is a risk of infection.

Minor wounds heal easily if they are cleaned and kept free from infection. The wound should be dressed with a sterile, unmedicated dressing after bleeding has stopped.

After ensuring that a wound does not contain glass, grit, or other foreign bodies, major bleeding should be controlled by putting pressure on the wound with the thumb and fingers. The injured part of the body should be raised, and the wound should be bandaged firmly. Medical attention should then be sought.

Q & A

When I grazed my arm, why did my mother not cover the wound?

It is usually best to allow a graze to dry up. Over the first few hours, it will form a dry scab that serves as an effective dressing. Covering a graze makes the area moist and may cause an infection.

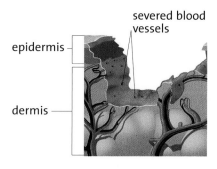

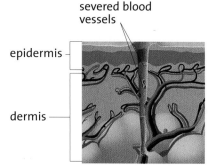

Lacerations (top) and puncture wounds (bottom) are often serious and can take a long time to heal. They should be kept covered until medical attention is available.

SEE ALSO

ABRASIONS AND CUTS • BLOOD • CIRCULATORY SYSTEM • SKIN • TETANUS

Yellow Fever

Yellow fever is a dangerous viral disease that is present in tropical countries. It attacks the liver and causes severe jaundice, in which the patient develops yellowing skin and eyes. Most people do recover completely from the disease, but about 5 percent of cases result in the death of the patient.

Symptoms and treatment

People catch the yellow fever virus from the bite of a mosquito that has previously bitten an infected monkey or person. After a few days, the patient develops a fever and a headache, as well as pain in the abdomen, back, and limbs. Internal bleeding may cause the patient to vomit blood, and the virus injures and destroys liver cells. Jaundice is common. The kidneys may start to bleed, and this results in blood in the urine.

Once the disease has developed, there is no curative treatment; the patient can only rest and drink plenty of fluids. Recovery can start at any stage. The outlook for patients is generally good if a fair standard of medical care is available.

An attack of yellow fever gives immunity for life, and relapses do not occur. The disease can pass almost unnoticed, especially in people raised in areas where yellow fever is endemic.

Prevention

Yellow fever can be prevented by vaccination and by control of mosquitoes, but because it is present in the monkeys of the tropical forests, eradicating the disease completely will probably be impossible.

Yellow fever began in West Africa, but it is now present all over tropical Africa, in South America, and in the Caribbean. It was probably carried across the Atlantic Ocean on ships. It is not present in tropical parts of Asia or in Europe, and there are strict controls on aircraft movements and rules for disinfection to prevent the accidental spread of the mosquitoes that carry it.

An effective vaccine against yellow fever is available worldwide and is recommended for anyone traveling to or through the tropics. A certificate of vaccination is required for many countries. The vaccine provides protection from 10 days after the shot and lasts for about 10 years. Babies should not be vaccinated.

Q & A

Is it possible for someone to get yellow fever twice?

No. One infection provides extremely good immunity. People who are brought up in tropical rain forest areas do not often suffer the effects of the disease, and examination of their blood shows a high level of immunity.

My friend says we can't catch yellow fever, because we live in the United States. Is she right?

Yellow fever may be brought to the United States by travelers incubating the disease, but it is unlikely to spread here. The infection has to be carried from person to person by mosquitoes, and the species of mosquito that the virus infects does not exist in the United States.

Can you be vaccinated against yellow fever?

Yes. There is an effective vaccine that is used around the world. Vaccination is sometimes a legal requirement for anyone visiting many parts of the tropics, but it is also a sensible precaution to take.

SEE ALSO

IMMUNE SYSTEM • INFECTIOUS DISEASES • JAUNDICE • KIDNEY • LIVER • LIVER DISEASES AND DISORDERS • SKIN • TROPICAL DISEASES • VIRUSES

Index

Page numbers in **bold** type refer to main entries; *italic* type refers to illustrations or captions.

A

abrasion **5**, 316
abscess 34, 35, 170, 284
acetaminophen 241
acetylcholine 28, *159*
acne **6–7**, 271, 274
acquired immunodeficiency syndrome (AIDS) **8–10**, 37, 78, 110, 158, 168, 172, 174, 266, 308, 309–310
Addison's disease 165
adenoid 199, *213*, 293
adolescence 6–7
adrenal gland 47, *48*, 135, *136*, 159–160, 165
adrenalin 135, 160
aerobic exercise 148, 232
aging 169
AIDS *see* acquired immunodeficiency syndrome
alcohol 14, 92, 180, 192, 225, 229, 241–243, 265, 292
alimentary canal 89–91
allergen 11–12, 84
allergy **11–12**, 28–29, *40*, 84, *84*, 88, 104, 178–179, 194, 253, 273, 274–275
alopecia 142, 143
alveoli 46, 57, *57*, 106, *106*, 193, 240, 250, *251*
Alzheimer's disease **13**, 55–56
amino acid 47, 90, 190, 238
amniocentesis 36, 97, 278
amylase 89
anabolic steroid 234
anaphylaxis 11, 12
anemia **14–15**, 42, 92, 208, 229, 271, 291, 304
Falconi's 134
hemolytic 15
pernicious 14–15
sickle-cell 15, 37, 67, 134, **268**
aneurysm 24, 73, 75, 205
angina 23, 73, 148, 149, 150–151
ankylosing spondylitis 26
anorexia nervosa **16–18**, 203, 208
antibiotic 33, 34, 170, 174, 284, 308, 309
antibody **19**, 33, 34, 40, 41, 45, 135, 167, 169, 199
antidiuretic hormone 160
antihistamine 12
antioxidant 76, 265
anus 47, *91*, 93, 155
aorta 21, 22, 24, 72, *72*, 73, 146, *147*, *151*, *251*
appendicitis **20**, 92, 214, 237
appendix 20, *20*, *91*
artery **21**, 44, 72–75, 146
blocked 22, 73, 74, 75, 130, 148, 150–151, *151*, 265
diseases and disorders **22–24**, 73–75, 146
arthritis **25–27**, 35, 139, 263
aspergillus 126, 127, *127*
aspirin 25, 76, 241, 255
asthma 11, **28–29**, 104, 127, 194, *195*, 196, 253

astigmatism 116, 117
atheroma 22–23, 73
atherosclerosis 22–24, 73, 74, 75, 130, 148
athlete's foot **30**, 78, 126, *127*, *172*, 259, 274
atrial fibrillation 151
autoimmune illnesses 25
autonomic system 223, *224*
avian influenza **31–32**, 110, 177

B

backache 49, 263
backbone *see* spinal column
bacteria **33**, 41, 111, 168, 170–171, 284–285, 308, 309
pathogenic 34–35
bacterial diseases **34–35**, 78, 92
bad breath *see* halitosis
balance 48, 52, 82, 100, 103
baldness 143
B cell 41, 167–169, *167*, *168*
Becker muscular dystrophy 222
beriberi 229, 297
bile *48*, 89, 128–129, 180, 190, 190, 305
bile duct 89, *128*, 190, *190*
bilharzia *see* schistosomiasis
bird flu *see* avian influenza
birth defect **36–37**, 67, 68, 83, 96–97, 102, 278
bladder 47, 305–306, *306*
blastomycosis 127
blindness **38–39**, 99, 117, 254
blood **40–41**, 72, 136
cells 190
clotting 154
diseases and disorders **42**, 154
fluid 105
glucose 40, 47, 85, 87, 135, 165–166, 191
hypoglycemia 85, **165–166**
plasma 40–41, 58
platelets 40–41, *40*, 42
pressure 74–75, 164, 185
proteins 105
red cells 14–15, 40–41, *40*, 41, 42, 66, 183, 268
white cells 33, 34, 40–41, *40*, 41, 42, 45, 49, 167–169, 171, *171*, 175, 189, 199–200
see also anemia; circulatory system; heart; hemoglobin
blood transfusion 9, 41
blood vessels *see* artery; capillary; vein
body odor 135, 271
body systems **43–48**
boil 34, 35, 101, 274, 284
bone 43, 44, **49**, 234, 269–270
diseases and disorders **50**, 257
fractures and dislocations 50, 54, **122–124**, 181, 234, 269, 281
osteoporosis 50, 122, **234**
see also joint; skeletal system
bone marrow 41, 42, 49, 189

botulism 35, **51**, 92
bovine spongiform encephalopathy (BSE) 79
bowel 48, 178–179
brain 47, *48*, **52–53**, 223, *224*, 225
Alzheimer's disease **13**
cerebral embolism 74, 286
cerebral thrombosis 74, 286
damage and disorders **54–56**
encephalitis 55, 56, 69, **107**
tumor 55, *55*
see also stroke
brain stem 52, 53, 54
brain tumor 55, *55*, 120, 225–226, 236
breast cancer 62, 63
breast-feeding 88
breathing 11, 28–29, 46, 193, 213, 223, 230, 250
bronchi 28, 46, 57, *57*, 193, *195*, 196, 250, *251*
bronchiole 46, 57, *57*, *106*, *195*, 240, 250, *251*
bronchitis 29, **57**, 76, 110, *195*, 196, 252–253
bronchopneumonia 240
bulimia **16–18**
burn **58–60**, 288
bursitis 249

C

calcium 49, 90, 135, 234, 269
cancer **61–63**, 67, 167, 169, 199, 293
bone 50
brain tumors 55, *55*
cervical 161–162, 266
colon 77
digestive system 94
leukemia 42, 62, 169, **189**
lung 62, 194, *195*, 196
lymphoma 62, 199, 200, **201**
primary tumors 61
secondary tumors 50, 62
skin 8, 9, 272, 273, 275, 288
candida (thrush) 78, 126, *127*, *172*, 213, 214, 266
capillary 21, 40, 42, 44, 72, 90, 146, 250
carbuncle 284
carcinoma 61
cardiac arrest 151
cardiomyopathy 150, 151
carpal tunnel syndrome **64**, 249
cartilage 26, *26*, 43, 44, 49, 182, *182*, 269
cataract 38, 117, 119
celiac disease **65**, 88
cell 43, 61, **66–67**, 72, 73
central nervous system (CMS) 47, *48*, 52, 215, 223
cerebellum 52, *52*, 53, 100, *224*
cerebral cortex 53
cerebral embolism 74, 286
cerebral hemorrhage 286
cerebral palsy 54, **68**, 225
cerebral thrombosis 74, 286
cerebrospinal fluid (CSF) 207, 279, *279*
cerebrum *224*

cervical cancer 161–162, 266
cervical smear 162, 266
Chagas' disease 296–297
chicken pox **69**, 78, 107, 158, 171, 173, 255, 267, 308, 310
chlamydia 78, 170, 174, 227, 237, 266
cholangitis 129
cholera 2, 35, **70**, 78, 170, 171, 296, 298
cholesterol 22, 24, 73, 75, *129*, 148, 265, 286
chorea 256
Huntington's 37, 55, 134, **163**
chorionic villus sampling 36
chromosome **66–67**, 96, 133, 134, 154
chronic fatigue syndrome **71**
chyme 89, *90*, *91*
circulatory system 40, 44, 45, **72**, 135, 146–147, 167, 250
diseases and disorders **73–75**, 130, 248
pulmonary circulation 146
smoking 24, *24*
systemic circulation 146
see also artery; capillary; heart; vein
cirrhosis 191–192, *191*
cleft palate and/or lip 36, 37, 213
clostridia 130
clubfoot 37
cochlea 82, 99–100, *100*
cognitive behavior therapy 71
cold, common 19, 29, 34, **76**, 78, 170, 173, 253, 255, 292, 308, 310
cold sore 78, 158, 213, 214, 303, *304*, 308
colitis 77, 92
pancolitis 88
ulcerative 77, 88
collagen 49, 265, *272*
colon (large intestine) 47, *47*, **77**, 88, 89, 90, *91*, 94
colostomy 77
communicable diseases **78**, 170
computed axial tomography (CAT) 79
computed tomography (CT) scan 55
congenital defect *see* birth defect
conjunctivitis 78, 117, 119, 229
constipation 92, 93, 94, 155, 178, 208
contact dermatitis 84, *84*, 274, *274*, *275*
contagious diseases 78
contusion 316
corn 275
cornea 114, *115*, 119
coronary arteries 21, 22–23, *22*, 73, 146–147, 150–151, *151*
coronary thrombosis 23, 149, *151*
coronavirus 262
corpus callosum 53
corticosteroid hormone 135
cortisol 135
cortisone 165
coughing 76, 106, 194
cradle cap 273

D

dandruff 84, 143, 287
deafness **82–83**, 101–103
dehydration 131, 132
dementia 13, 23, 56, 225–226, 229
dendrite 223
dengue fever 78, 296, 310
deoxyribonucleic acid (DNA) 43, 66, *67*, 133, 308–309
DeQuervain's syndrome 249
dermatitis 11, **84**, 229, 274, *274*, *275*, 287
dermatome 267
dermis 7, 271, *272*
diabetes 73, **85–87**, 119, 130, 153, 165, 169, 185, 209, 230, 286, 305
diabetic retinopathy 254, *254*
insipidus 160
type 1 (insulin-dependent) 85, 135
type 2 (noninsulin-dependent) 86, 165
dialysis 186–187
diaper rash 273
diaphragm 45, *46*, 250
diarrhea 88, 92, 94, 98, 132–133, 178–179, 229
spurious 92
diet 89, 92, 178–179, 230
acne 6
birth defects 36–37
breast-feeding 88
carbohydrates 165–166
cholesterol 24, 73, 75, 148
eating disorders 16–18
fat 24, 73, 89, 148
fiber 47, 92, 155, 179
intestinal cancer 62
malnutrition 169, **203**
nutritional diseases **229**
protein 203
salt 73
sugar 165–166
digestive system 44, 46–47, *47*, **89–91**, 128–129, 136, 159, 212
bacteria 33, 34
diseases and disorders 65, 80, **92–94**, 131–132
diphtheria 35, 78, **95**, 111, 171, 172, 173, 292, 297, 314
discoid lupus erythematosus (DLE) 197
dislocation 50, 54, **124**, 181
diverticular disease 94
DNA *see* deoxyribonucleic acid
double vision 116, 117, 119
Down syndrome 36, 37, 67, **96–97**, 134
drug addiction 8–9, 10
duodenum 47, 89, *91*, 92, 159–160, *159*, 304

dysentery 35, 78, **98**, 174
    amebic 78, 92, 98, 191
    bacillary 78, 98
dysmenorrhea 208
dyspepsia 92
dysuria 227

E

ear 48, 52, 82–83, **99–100**
    diseases and disorders
        101–103
earache 101
eardrum 99, *100*, 102
earwax 82, 101, 102, 136
eating disorders **16–18**
Ebola fever 297
E. coli 131
eczema 84, **104**, 273, 274
edema **105**, 151
electric shock 58
electrocardiogram (ECG) 148,
    149
elephantiasis 200, *296*
embolism 22–23, 74–75, 286
emphysema 57, **106**, 194, *195*,
    196
encephalitis 55, 56, 69, **107**,
    206, 225, 308, 312
encephalopathy 255
endemic diseases 111
endocarditis 150
endometriosis **108–109**, 237
endothelium 21
energy 45–46, *87*, 90, 190
enteritis 131
environmental disorders
    36–37
enzyme 89–90, 159
epidemic **110–111**
epidemiology 110
epidermis 7, 271, 272
epiglottis 213, *213*, 250, 292,
    292
epilepsy 56, **112–113**, 225–226
epithelial tissues 43, *43*, 44
esophagus 46, 89, 90, 94, 292,
    292
estrogen 142, 234
eustachian tube 99, *100*, 101,
    102, *213*, 292, *292*
eye 39, 48, 52, 53, **114–115**, 136,
    254
    blindness **38–39**, 254
    diseases and disorders 26,
        116–119, 137, 254, 287

F

fainting 73
fallopian tube 48, *48*, 237
Farmer's lung 253
fat 44, 230
fatty acid 90
feces 47, *48*, 90
fertilization 48, 66
fetus 49
fibroid **120**, 208, 237
fibromyalgia (fibrositis) **121**,
    220
fistulas 80
flatulence 92, 178
flea 110, 170, 239
flu *see* influenza
fluid retention 105
fluke 78, 315
folic acid 14, 278
fontanelle 270
food allergy 11–12, 88, 178–179,
    210
food poisoning 35, 78, 88, 92,
    284
    botulism 35, **51**, 92
    salmonella 92, 98, 131, *131*,
        261

fracture 50, 54, **122–124**
freckle 271, *272*
frostbite **125**, 130
fungal infections 30, 78,
    126–127, *170*, *172*, 214,
    274

G

gallbladder 48, 89, *91*,
    128–129, *190*, *190*
gallstone **128–129**, 230, 301
gangrene **130**, 145, 248, 258
gas gangrene 130
gastric juices 46, 89
gastritis 93, 131
gastroenteritis 78, 93, 98,
    131–132, 308, 310
gene 43, 66, *67*, **133**
    chromosomes **66–67**
    diseases and disorders
        36–37, 67, 96–97, 133, **134**,
        154, 163, 209, 291
    genetic mutations 65, 67, 133,
        134
genital herpes 158, 266
genital warts 161–162, 266
German measles *see* rubella
gingivitis 141, 214
glands 47, *48*, **135–136**, 223
    endocrine 47, 135, *136*, 159
    exocrine 47, 135, *136*, *136*
glandular fever *see* infectious
    mononucleosis
glaucoma 39, 117, 119, **137**
glomerulus 183, *183*, *306*
glucose 40, 47, *87*, 89,
    165–166, 190, 191
gluten 65
glycerol 90
glycogen 166, 190
goiter 229
golfer's elbow 249, 280
gonorrhea 26, 34, 35, 78, **138**,
    237, 266
gout **139**
grand mal 112
greenstick fracture 122, *123*,
    269
Guillain-Barré syndrome **140**
gum 33, **141**, 213, 214, 265
Guthrie test 238

H

hair 44, *142*, 271, *272*
    hair and scalp disorders
        142–143
halitosis 93, 214
hamstring injury **144**
Hansen's disease 35, 78, **145**,
    296
hay fever 11, 104, 253
headache 225
    see also migraine
hearing 52, 52, 82–83, **99–100**
heart 22, 40, 72, **146–147**,
    218–219
    congenital malformation
        37
    diseases and disorders
        149–151
    muscles 44
    pacemaker 73, 151
    valves 146, 149–150
heart attack 23, 74, **148**, 151,
    230
heartbeat 72, 150–151, 223
heartburn 92, 94
heart failure 150, 151
heart murmur 149
heart rate 135, 146, 150–151
heat exhaustion 152, 288
heat sickness **152**
Heberden's node 233

hemiplegia 235
hemochromatosis **153**
hemodialysis 186–187
hemoglobin 14, 40–41, 250,
    268, 291
hemophilia 9, 36, 37, 42, 134,
    154
hemorrhage 38, 229, 286
hemorrhoids 14, 93, **155**
Henle's loop 183, *183*, *306*
hepatitis 78, **156**, 169, 170, 173,
    174, 180, 191–192, 297,
    298, 308, 310
hereditary diseases 81
hernia 93, 94, **157**
herpes 69, 78, **158**, 170, 214,
    266, 267, 303, *304*, 308,
    309–310
high blood pressure *see*
    hypertension
hirsutism 142
histamine 11, 12, 28
HIV *see* human
    immunodeficiency virus
hives 11, 274–275
Hodgkin's disease 199, 200,
    201
hookworm 14, 78, 315
hormone 41, 47, **159–160**
    disorders **159–160**
hormone replacement
    therapy (HRT) 234
human immunodeficiency
    virus (HIV) **8–10**, 266,
    309–310
human papillomavirus (HPV)
    161–162, 293
Huntington's disease 37, 55,
    134, **163**
hydrocephalus 54, 278
hygiene 34, 170, 261, 296
hyperopia 116, 117, *118*, 119
hypertension 73, 75, 119, 130,
    164, 185, 230, 286
hypoglycemia 85, **165–166**
hypothalamus 53, *53*, 135
hysterectomy 108

I

immune system 1, 44–45,
    167–168, 169, 171, 199
    antibodies 19
    autoimmune illnesses 25
immunization 19, 34, 78, 107,
    110, 170, 171–172, 277, 299,
    311, 314
immunodeficiency **169**
impetigo 78, 274
impotence 160
incontinence 306
incubation 171
incus 82, 99, *100*
indigestion 92, 304
infectious diseases **170–174**
infectious mononucleosis 78,
    135, 156, 158, 169, **175**, 199,
    200, 292, 308, 310
infertility 109
influenza 31–32, 78, 107,
    110–111, 170, 173, **176–177**,
    255, 292, 308, 310, 311
insect bites 8, 11, 45, 78, 107,
    110, 170, 198, 242, 296,
    302, 312, 317
insulin 85–87, 135, 160, 165, 209
intestine
    large *see* colon
    small 20, 47, *47*, 65, 89–90,
        90, *91*
iron 14–15, 41, 90, 153, 229
irritable bowel syndrome 94,
    178–179, 237

J

jaundice 129, 156, **180**, 192, 271,
    306, 317
jejunum *47*
joint 44, *45*, 49, 139, 230
    arthritis **25–27**
    disorders **181–182**
    double-jointedness 181
    osteoarthritis **232–233**
    replacement 27, 182
    sprains and strains **283**
jugular vein 72

K

Kaposi's sarcoma 8, *9*
keratin 271
kidney failure 187
kidneys 47, *48*, **183–184**, 305,
    305, *306*
    dialysis 186–187
    diseases and disorders 105,
        185–187
kidney stone 185–186, *186*
knee 27, *45*, 181, *182*, 232, 233,
    269, 281
Koplik's spots 206
kwashiorkor 203, 297

L

labor 135
Landouzy–Dejerine dystrophy
    222
laryngitis 292
larynx 213, *213*, 250, 292–293,
    292
lassa fever 310
laxative 92
Legionnaires' disease 78, 173,
    188
leprosy *see* Hansen's disease
leptospirosis 35, 191
leukemia 42, 62, 169, **189**,
    308–309
leukocytosis 42
lice 258, 266, 302
ligament 43, 44, 49, 121, 281
limbic system 52, 53, *53*
lipase 89
lips 212
liver 47, *48*, *87*, 156, 166, 170,
    180, **190**
    diseases and disorders
        191–192, 317
lockjaw 290
Lou Gehrig's disease 211, 221,
    225
lung 21, 44, 45–46, *46*, *48*, 72,
    193, 250–253, *251*
    cancer 62, 194, *195*, 196
    diseases and disorders
        194–196, 240, 299–300,
        314
    emphysema 57, **106**
    fluid on 151
    pulmonary circulation 146
    pulmonary embolism 74,
        75
lupus erythematosus **197**
Lyme disease **198**
lymphatic system 42, 90, 135,
    136, 167, **199–200**, 201
lymphedema 200
lymph node *48*, 61–63, *62*, 136,
    199–201
lymphocyte 40, 41, 135, 136,
    167–169, *167*, 175,
    199–200
lymphoma *62*, 199, 200, **201**

M

macular degeneration 39, 117,
    254

mad cow disease 79
magnetic resonance imaging
    (MRI) 79, *79*
malabsorption 93
malaria 78, *172*, 173, 180, **202**,
    268, 296, 297, 298
malleus 82, 99, *100*
malnutrition 169, **203**
maltose 89, 165–166
mammary gland 47, 136, *136*
Marfan syndrome **205**
mastoidectomy 101
measles 78, 82, 101, 107, 111,
    114, 169, 171, 172, 173, 174,
    194, **206**, 292, 297, 308,
    310, 311
melanin 238
melanoma 272, *273*, 275
melatonin 136
memory 13, 52, 53
Ménière's disease 82, 102, 103,
    225–226
meninges 52, 207
meningitis 35, 55, 56, 78, 107,
    127, 173, **207**, 225–226,
    297, 312
menopause 160, 234, 245
menstruation 14, 108–109,
    120, **208**, 245
metabolic disorders **209**
metabolism 48, 135, 305
migraine 11, **210**, 225
milk 47, 135, 136, *159*, 160
minerals 40, 90
mitosis 67
mole 271–272, 275
mosquito 8, 45, 107, 170, 202,
    296, 312, 317
motor neuron disease **211**, 221
mouth 45, 46, *46*, 89, *91*, 141,
    212–213, 285
    diseases and disorders **214**,
        303, 304
    plaque 33, 141, *141*, 285
MRSA 284
mucus 89, 92, 212
multiple sclerosis (MS) 55, 56,
    140, **215**, 225–226
mumps 78, 111, 171, 172, 173, 214,
    216, 308, 310
Munchausen syndrome **217**
muscle 44, *45*, **218–219**, 235,
    269
    cardiac 218
    diseases and disorders
        220–221
    fibromyalgia **121**
    skeletal (voluntary) 44, 218
    smooth (involuntary) 44,
        218
    sprains and strains **283**
    tissue 43, *43*
muscular dystrophy 37, 221,
    222, 235
myasthenia gravis 235
myelin 140, 215, 223, 225
myopia 39, 116, 117, *118*
myositis 220–221, 235

N

nasopharynx 293
nausea 92, 93
nephrectomy 187
nephritis 185, *186*, 227
nephron 183, *183*, 185, *306*
nervous system 43, 44, 47–48,
    48, 66, 140, 211, **223–224**,
    271
    disorders **225–226**
neuralgia 225–226
neuritis 225–226, 263
neuron 52, 211, 223, 225
neurotransmitter 223

nonspecific urethritis (NSU) **227**
noradrenalin 135
nose 45, 46, 52, 250
nosebleed 108, **228**
nutritional diseases **229**

O

obesity 86, **230**, 233
obsessive-compulsive disorder **231**
optic nerve 38, 39, 114, 115, 254
optic neuritis 118
organelle 43
ossicle 82
ossification 269
osteoarthritis 25, 182, **232–233**
osteoid 257
osteomalacia 50, 229, 257
osteomyelitis 35, 50
osteoporosis 50, 122, **234**
ovarian cyst 108–109
ovary 48, 48, 135, 136, 159, 237
ovum 48, 66
oxygen 45, 68, 193, 250–252
    transportation 14–15, 21, 40, 42, 44, 46, 54, 55, 72, 73, 106, 146, 268

P

pacemaker 73, 151
Paget's disease 50
palpitations 14, 150, 151
pancreas 87, 89, 91, 135, 136, 136, 159–160, 159
pandemic 31, 32, 110
paralysis 225, 226, **235**, 286
    hyperkalemic 221
    hypokalemic 221
    spastic 68
paraplegia 235
parasites 78, 93, 170, 202, 258, 296–298, 302, 312
    amoebas 98
    lice 258, 266, 302
    ticks 198, 258
    Toxocara canis 39, 315
    Toxoplasma gondi 39
    worms 14, 20, 78, **315**
parathyroid gland 135, 136, 159–160
Parkinson's disease 55, 56, 225–226, **236**
parotid gland 213, 216
pathogen 170
peanut allergy 11–12
pelvic inflammatory disease (PID) 227, **237**, 266
pepsin 89
peripheral vascular disease 75, 130
peristalsis 90, 91, 178
peritonitis 20, 93, 304
perspiration 135, 152, 152, 271
pertussis *see* whooping cough
petit mal 112
phagocyte 168
pharyngitis 35, 78, 292
pharynx 213, 213, 250, 292–293, 292
phenylketonuria (PKU) 36, 37, 209, **238**, 305
phlebitis 74, 75, 307
phosphorus 49, 135, 234
photophobia 114
piles *see* hemorrhoids
pineal gland 136, 136
pituitary gland 47, 48, 135, 159–160, 159
placenta 47
plague 35, 78, 110, 171, 174, **239**

plaque 33, 141, 141, 285
plasma 40–41
pleurisy 194
pneumoconiosis 253
pneumonia 35, 78, 170, 172, 173, 194, 196, 206, **240**, 252, 253, 285, 308, 311
pneumonic plague 239
poisons and poisoning **241–243**
    see also toxins
poliomyelitis 78, 172, 225–226, 235, **244**, 297, 298, 308, 310, 311, 312
pollution 28, 194, 250, 252–253
polymyalgia rheumatica 221
pregnancy 9, 14, 37, 47, 142, 260
    amniocentesis 36, 97
    birth defects **36–37**
    ectopic 237
premenstrual syndrome (PMS) 208, **245**
progressive muscular atrophy 211
prolactin 135, 160
protein 40, 46–47, 89, 90, 105, 190, 305
protozoa 170
psittacosis 78, 308
psoriasis 26, 143, 274, 275
psychoneuroimmunology 43
pulmonary artery 21, 72, 195
pulmonary circulation 146
pulmonary embolism 74, 75
pulmonary vein 72, 195
Putti-Platt operation 181
pyelitis 306

Q

Q fever 78
quadriplegia 235
quarantine 78, 171

R

rabies 170, **246–247**, 297, 311
radioisotope scan 55
radiotherapy 61, 63, 201
rash 11, 126, 197, 206, 267, 273
Raynaud's disease **248**
Raynaud's phenomenon 248
rectum 47, 47, 91, 155
Reiter's syndrome 227
repetitive strain injury (RSI) **249**
reproductive systems 47, 48, 48, 66
respiratory system 45–46, 46, **250–251**
    diseases and disorders **252–253**
retina 39, 39, 114, 115, 254
    detached 39, 117, 119, 254
retinitis pigmentosa 118, 254
retrovirus 308–309
Reye's syndrome 76, **255**
rheumatic fever 26, 149, 150, **256**
rheumatism 153, 182, 256
rheumatoid arthritis 25–27
ribonucleic acid (RNA) 308–309
rickets 50, 229, **257**
rickettsial diseases 78, 172, 174, **258**, 302
ringworm 78, 126, 127, 173, **259**, 274
Rocky Mountain spotted fever 78, 258
rubella 36, 37, 38–39, 78, 102, 107, 113, 171, 172, 191, **260**, 308, 311

S

Saint Vitus' dance 256
saliva 46, 89, 212
salivary gland 47, 48, 89, 91, 136, 136, 212, 213, 214, 216
salmonella 35, 92, 98, 131, 131, **261**, 301
sarcoma 62
saturated fat 148
scabies 275
scalding 58
scalp disorders **142–143**
scapula 124
scar 5, 6, 275, 316
scarlet fever 34, 35, 78, 171, 173, 285
schistosomiasis 78, 296, 315
sciatica 225–226, **263**
sclerosing cholangitis 129
scoliosis 205, **264**
scurvy 229, **265**
sebaceous gland 6, 136, 142, 271, 272, 274
sebum 6, 7, 136, 274
semicircular canal 100, 100
septicemia 170
severe acute respiratory syndrome (SARS) 110, 111, **262**
sex chromosomes 66
sex hormones 135, 142, 159–160, 254
sexually transmitted diseases (STDs) 8–10, 78, 138, 158, 161–162, 170, 227, 237, **266**, 295, 303, 306
shingles 158, 225–226, **267**
shock 58, 74–75
sight 52, 52, **114–117**
sinusitis 29, 228
skeletal system 44, 45, 49, **269–270**
skeletal tissue 43
skin 43, 44, 48, 136, **271–272**
    abrasions **5**, 316
    acne **6–7**
    allergic reactions 11–12, 273
    burns **58–60**
    cancer 8, 9, 62, 272, 273, 275, 288
    dermatitis **84**
    diseases and disorders **273–275**
    eczema 84, **104**
    grafts 59–60
    wounds 5, 45, **316**
    wrinkles 271, 288
skull 49, 49, 54, 269, 270
sleeping sickness 296–297, 297
slipped disk 181, 263, **276**, 279
smallpox 78, 171, **277**, 298, 308, 311, 311
smoking 22, 24, 24, 57, 62, 63, 73, 76, 92, 106, 130, 148, 164, 193, 194, 196, 214, 248, 250, 252–253, 265, 286, 292, 293
somatic system 223, 224
sperm 48, 66
spina bifida 36, 36, 37, **278**
spinal column 49, 49, 181–182, 264, 269, 276, **279**
spinal cord 47, 48, 52, 223, 224, 225
spinal muscular atrophy 211
spondylitis 26, 225
spongiform encephalopathies 79
sporotrichosis 126
sports injuries **280–282**, 283
squint 116, 117, 118, 119
stapes 82, 99, 100

staphylococci 34, 35, 35, 92, 170, 252, **284**, 287
stem cell 134
stomach 46–47, 47, 89, 91, 92, 93, 303–304
strep throat 34, 285, 292–293
streptococci 34, 35, 191, 256, **285**, 292
stress 164, 208, 273, 275
    asthma 28, 29, 253
    dermatitis 84
    diarrhea 88, 178–179
    eating disorders 18
    eczema 104
    irritable colon 77
    migraine 210
    ulcers 92
stroke 23, 55, 56, 74, 75, 82, 225–226, 230, 235, **286**
sty 118, 119, **287**
sunburn 58, **288**
sweat gland 44, 135, 136, 136, 152, 152, 271, 272
swine flu 177
syphilis 34, 35, 37, 78, 83, 266
systemic lupus erythematosus (SLE) **197**

T

tachycardia 151
tapeworm 14, 78, 315
Tay-Sachs disease 37
T cell 41, 167–169, 167, 168, 200
teeth 93, 141, 203, 212, 214, 265
    plaque 33, 141, 141, 285
tendinitis 249
tendon 43, 44, 120, 281
tennis elbow 249, **289**
tenosynovitis (teno) 249
testes 48, 135, 159
tetanus 35, 170, 172, 172, 173, **290**, 297, 298, 314
thalamus 53, 53
thalassemia 15, 37, **291**
throat diseases and disorders 284, 285, **292–293**
thrombosis 22–23, 74–75, 149, 151, 286, 307
thrush 126, 172, 213, 214, 237
thymus gland 136, 169, 199–200
thyroid gland 47, 48, 135, 136, 150, 159–160, 229, 230
tinnitus 83, 103
tongue 52, 213, 213
tonsilitis 35, 199, 200, 285, 293
Tourette's syndrome **294**
toxic shock syndrome 35, 284
toxins 34, 51, 92, 170
    endotoxins 34
    exotoxins 34
    see also poisons and poisoning
Toxocara canis 39, 315
Toxoplasma gondi 39
trachea 28, 45–46, 46, 193, 195, 213, 213, 250, 251, 292, 292
trachoma 38, 118, 119, 296
trematode 315
trichiosis 315
trichology 142
trichomoniasis 266, **295**
trigger finger 249
tropical diseases **296–298**
trypanosomiasis 296–297
trypsin 89–90
tuberculosis (TB) 26, 34, 35, 42, 78, 173, 174, 194, 207, 297, 298, **299–300**
tularemia 35, 78
tumor 38, 61–63, 93, 159
    benign 55
    fibroids **120**

malignant 55, 61
    secondary 50
    see also brain tumor
tunnel vision 116, 118, 137
tympanic membrane *see* eardrum
typhoid fever 34, 35, 42, 78, 92, 98, 111, 172, 173, 296, 297, 298, **301**
typhus 78, 171, 258, **302**

U

ulcer 14, **303–304**, 307
    corneal 119
    gastric 25, 92, 303, 304, 304
    mouth 141, 213, 214, 304
    peptic 304, 304
ulcerative colitis 77, 88
urea 48, 305
ureter 47, 183, 183, 305, 305, 306
urethra 47, 227, 305–306
urethritis **227**, 266, 306
uric acid 139
urinary system 47, 183, **305–306**
urinary tract infection (UTI) 227, 305–306
urine 47, 160, 183, 305–306
uterus 48, 120, 135

V

vaccination *see* immunization
vagina 48
varicella-zoster virus (CMV) 158
varicose vein 74, 75, 105, 303
vein 44, 72, 74, 146
    disorders 74, 75, 105, **307**
    hemorrhoids 14, 93, **155**
venae cavae 72, 72
vertebra 49, 49, 181, 279, 279
vestibular neuronitis 226
villi 47, 65, 65, 90, 90
virus 19, 34, 78, 111, 167–168, 170–171, 176, **308–311**
vision *see* sight
vitamins 33, 40, 90, 203–204
    A 229
    B 229
    B1 229
    B12 14–15, 229
    C 76, 229, 265
    D 50, 221, 229, 257
vomiting 92, 93, 132–133

W

wart 273, 274, 308, 311
    genital 161–162, 266
    seborrheic 275
waste products 44, 45–47, 48, 72, 90, 183, 185–187, 190, 250, 252, 305–306
water, contaminated 70, 98
West Nile virus **312**
whiplash injury 283, **313**
whooping cough 78, 111, 171, 172, 297, **314**
Wilson's disease 209
windpipe *see* trachea
worms 14, 20, 78, **315**
wound 5, 34, 45, 170, 265, **316**

X

xerophthalmia 296
X-ray 61, 133, 189

Y

yeast infection 78, 126–127
yellow fever 111, 191, 296, 297, 298, 308, 311, **317**